SO-AUI-336

MANUAL OF AMBULATORY PEDIATRICS

WITHDRAWN

Withdrawn
Outdated Material

MANUAL OF AMBULATORY PEDIATRICS

FOURTH EDITION

Rose W. Boynton, RN, CPNP
Pediatric Nurse Practitioner
Clinical Consultant N-PACE
Nurse Practitioner Associates for Continuing Education
and Clinical Consultant International Journal of N-PACE
"Clinical Excellence for Nurse Practitioners"

Elizabeth S. Dunn, BSN, RNC, PNP
Pediatric Nurse Practitioner
Gleason and Greenfield Pediatrics
Marion, Massachusetts
and
Massachusetts Maritime Academy
Buzzards Bay, Massachusetts
Consultant
Wareham School System
Wareham, Massachusetts

Geraldine R. Stephens, BS, RN, MED, PNP
Volunteer Child Advocate
Massachusetts Society for the Prevention of Cruelty to Children
Boston, Massachusetts

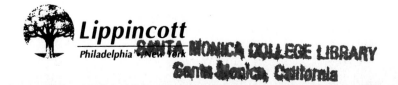

Lippincott
Philadelphia • New York

Sponsoring Editor: Jennifer E. Brogan
Coordinating Editorial Assistant: Susan V. Barta
Project Editor: Erika Kors
Senior Production Manager: Helen Ewan
Production Coordinator: Sharon McCarthy
Assistant Art Director: Kathy Kelley-Luedtke

4th Edition

9 8 7 6 5 4 3 2 1

Library of Congress Cataloging-in-Publications Data

Boynton, Rose W.
 Manual of ambulatory pediatrics/Rose W. Boynton, Elizabeth S. Dunn,
Geraldine R. Stephens.—4th ed.
    p.   cm.
 Includes bibliographical references and index.
 ISBN 0-397-55472-9 (alk. paper)
 1. Pediatrics—Handbooks, manuals, etc. 2. Ambulatory
medical care for children—Handbooks, manuals, etc. 3. Pediatric nursing—
Handbooks, manuals, etc. I. Dunn, Elizabeth S. II. Stephens,
Geraldine R. III. Title.
 [DNLM: 1. Ambulatory Care—in infancy & childhood—handbooks.
2. Nursing Care—in infancy & childhood—handbooks. 3. Pediatrics—
methods—handbooks. 4. Drug Therapy—in infancy & childhood—
handbooks. WS 39 B792m 1998]
 RJ48.B69 1998
 618.92—dc21
 DNLM/DLC
 for Library of Congress   97-35923
                                                            CIP

Care has been taken to confirm the accuracy of the information presented and to describe generally accepted practices. However, the authors, editors, and publisher are not responsible for errors or omissions or for any consequences from application of the information in this book and make no warranty, express or implied, with respect to the contents of the publication.

The authors, editors and publisher have exerted every effort to ensure that drug selection and dosage set forth in this text are in accordance with current recommendations and practice at the time of publication. However, in view of ongoing research, changes in government regulations, and the constant flow of information relating to drug therapy and drug reactions, the reader is urged to check the package insert for each drug for any change in indications and dosage and for added warnings and precautions. This is particularly important when the recommended agent is a new or infrequently employed drug.

Some drugs and medical devices presented in this publication have Food and Drug Administration (FDA) clearance for limited use in restricted research settings. It is the responsibility of the health care provider to ascertain the FDA status of each drug or device planned for use in their clinical practice.

To Glenn W., John, Cathy, Peter, Sheila and Nathan
with love—R.W.B.

Dedicated with a heart full of love and laughter to my grandchildren:
Maggie, Anna Lee, Caroline, Elizabeth, Brendan, and Christopher.
My pot of gold at the end of the rainbow.
XXXOOO   E.S.D.

Dedicated to my family for their understanding and loving support.
Special thanks to Susan L. McCarthy for helping to prepare the manuscript.
G.R.S.

PREFACE

The first edition of the Manual of Ambulatory Pediatrics was written to provide a concise reference book for health care providers in ambulatory settings. In the early 1980s when we were faculty members at the Nurse Practitioner Program at Northeastern University in Boston, we identified the need for a book of this type. Not an in-depth reference book or textbook—Nelson, Oski, and others do that very well—but a handbook that could easily be used in the practice setting. An impetus for the development of this book was the fact that Nurse Practitioners have to develop mutually approved protocols for management of common health problems in the practice setting and follow standards for well child care. This manual was originally developed to fill that need as well as to provide an educational tool for students preparing for the expanded role. To that end, it is imperative that they be reviewed by the physician and nurse practitioner or physician's assistant to define the boundaries of practice and standards of medical care for each setting.

This fourth edition has been developed to continue to fill the educational and practice needs for which the manual was originally intended—a concise, ready reference for well child care and its attendant problems; a compilation of the most common management problems seen in the average pediatric practice; and a drug reference. The revision reflects changes in pediatric well child care and management of illnesses, and the drug index has been expanded to include additional pharmaceuticals.

Again, the manual has been written with each of the authors assuming responsibility for a specific section. Part I provides comprehensive guidelines for well child visits from birth through adolescence, which enable the health provider to assist the parent in providing optimal care for the child. A number of child-rearing issues of major concern to parents and health care providers are included in this section.

Part II of the manual is composed of protocols for the management of the most commonly seen illnesses in pediatric practice. This section has been developed according to the SOAP format (Subjective data, Objective data, Assessment, and Plan), which was widely accepted in the first three editions. Each protocol has been researched in current literature from multidisciplinary sources and presents pertinent background information, such as communicability, incubation period, etiology, incidence, and the current recommended pharmacological treatment. Also, each protocol has in-depth education as well as indications for follow-up and referral.

A concise review of pharmaceuticals commonly used in pediatric practice is included in Part III. The indications and dosages of all the drugs in this book are recommended in the medical literature and conform to the practices of the medical community. This index includes dosages, side effects, drug interactions, and directions for administration and specific education for parents. Since standards for usage change, it is advisable to check package inserts for revised recommendation, particularly with regard to new drugs.

Again, as in the previous editions, the author of Part II wishes to acknowledge the contribution made by Charles S. Gleason, M.D., F.A.A.P. A friend, mentor, "boss," colleague, consultant, and advocate of nurse practitioners since the concept was introduced 30 years ago, he has spent many hours answering questions and reviewing protocols. Additionally, his pediatric practice in Wareham, MA, a model of comprehensive pediatric care, has served as a preceptor site for nurse practitioners for the 26 years that we have been in practice together.

Once again for the mechanics of Part II, special acknowledgment to Cate and Dan Arkins and to Dina and Michael Dunn. Their invaluable computer expertise and continuing support have enabled this author to prepare a manuscript efficiently and to learn new skills in the process. Also, to Brian Dunn, who has been my sounding board, who put my office together, and who frequently rescued me when I lost something in "that little box" that contained all my manuscript; and to Sue and Tom Dunn who have used the manual both as medical professionals and as parents and have given input into its development; and to Mom and Bill. Thank you for your patience and understanding when I was buried deep in revisions with little time for my family. With special thoughts also to my Dad who made bowls of popcorn while I was creating the original manuscript and, this time, "popped" down from his big white cloud and sat on my shoulder throughout the revisions.

To MaryAnn Ashe, the secretary at the Marion Board of Health, thank you for your willingness to drop everything and run to my home—not for our BOH business, but to do a little training session.

We believe that this manual will continue to serve as an educational and practice tool and fill the need for which it was originally written—for nurse practitioners, physicians assistants, and nurses involved in primary care. Use of it will help to enhance pediatric ambulatory care by providing an up-to-date, ready reference for ambulatory care providers.

CONTENTS

Part I: Well Child Care
Geraldine R. Stephens

Initial History 3
Physical Examination..9
Well Child Visits 13
Injury Prevention Guidelines..15
Child Abuse Guidelines...17
Breast-Feeding Guidelines...19
2-Week Well Child Visit 26
Anticipatory Guidance for the Period of 2–8 Weeks 32
2-Month Well Child Visit..38
Anticipatory Guidance for the Period of 2–4 Months 44
4-Month Well Child Visit..50
Anticipatory Guidance for the Period of 4–6 Months 56
6-Month Well Child Visit..62
Anticipatory Guidance for the Period of 6–8 Months 68
8-Month Well Child Visit..78
Anticipatory Guidance for the Period of 8–14 Months 83
14-Month Well Child Visit..92
Anticipatory Guidance for the Period of 14–18 Months 96
18-Month Well Child Visit..103
Anticipatory Guidance for the Period of 18–24 Months 108
24-Month Well Child Visit..116
Anticipatory Guidance for the Period of 24–36 Months 121
3-Year Well Child Visit..131
Anticipatory Guidance for the Period of 3–6 Years 138
6-Year Well Child Visit..148
Anticipatory Guidance for the Period of 6–9 Years 154
9- to 11-Year Well Child Visit 165
Anticipatory Guidance for the Period of 9–11 Years 171
12- to 17-Year Well Child Visit 178
Anticipatory Guidance for the Adolescent Years...185
Common Childrearing Concerns: Temper Tantrums..189
Common Childrearing Concerns: Toilet Training..192
Common Childrearing Concerns: Limit Setting (by Elizabeth S. Dunn).................194
Common Childrearing Concerns: Sibling Rivalry (by Rose W. Boynton)...............197
Child Abuse (by Rose W. Boynton) 201
Bibliography...205

Part II: Management of Common Pediatric Problems
Elizabeth S. Dunn

Acne 209
AIDS (Acquired Immune Deficiency Syndrome) 215
Allergic Response to Hymenoptera 223
Allergic Rhinitis and Conjunctivitis 227
Anorexia Nervosa 232
Aphthous Stomatitis 237
Asthma 240
Bulimia 249
Candidiasis (Diaper Rash) 253
Cervical Adenitis, Acute 255
Colic 258
Conjunctivitis 262
Constipation 267
Diaper Rash—Primary Irritant 271
Diarrhea, Acute 274
Dysmenorrhea, Primary 280
Enuresis 284
Environmental Control for the Atopic Child 290
Erythema Infectiosum (Fifth Disease) 293
External Otitis 296
Fever Control 300
Frostbite 304
Hand, Food, and Mouth Disease 308
Herpangina 310
Herpes Simplex Type 1 313
Herpes Simplex Type 2 316
Herpes Zoster 320
Herpetic Gingivostomatitis 323
Hordeolum (Stye) 326
Impetigo 328
Infectious Mononucleosis 331
Intertrigo 335
Iron-Deficiency Anemia 338
Lyme Disease 342
Marginal Blepharitis 347
Metatarsus Adductus 349
Miliaria Rubra 351
Molluscum Contagiosum 353
Mycoplasmal Pneumonia 356
Otitis Media, Acute 359
Pediculosis Capitis, Corporis, and Pubis 364
Pertussis 370

Pinworms 374
Pityriasis Rosea 377
Poison Ivy or Poison Oak Dermatitis 380
Roseola (Exanthem Subitum) 383
Scabies 386
Scarlet Fever 391
Seborrhea of the Scalp (Cradle Cap) 394
Serous Otitis Media 396
Sinusitis, Bacterial 400
Streptococcal Pharyngitis 403
Suicide Prevention 407
Thrush 410
Tinea Corporis 412
Tinea Cruris 414
Tinea Pedis 417
Tinea Versicolor 420
Umbilical Cord Care 422
Umbilical Granuloma 424
Urinary Tract Infection 426
Varicella (Chickenpox) 431
Viral Croup 435
Viral Gastroenteritis 442
Vomiting, Acute 446
Vulvovaginitis in the Prepubertal Child 450
Warts, Common and Plantar 454
Bibliography 458

Part III: Drug Index
Rose W. Boynton

Aclovate (Topical Cream, Ointment) 463
Actifed (Antihistamine-Decongestant) 464
Adrenalin Chloride Solution (Epinephrine Hydrochloride) 464
Amoxicillin (Synthetic Antibiotic) 465
Ampicillin (Antibiotic) 466
Anaprox (Nonsteroidal Anti-inflammatory) 467
Aristocort A (Topical Cream) 468
Aspirin (Analgesic) 469
Atarax (Antianxiety, Antihistamine) 470
Augmentin (Oral Antibiotic) 471
Auralgan Otic Solution (Topical Otic Analgesic) 471
Azmacort (Oral Inhaler) 472
Bactrim or Septra (Synthetic Antibacterial) 473
Bactroban 2% Ointment (Topical Ointment, Dermatologic Use) 474

Biaxin (Semisynthetic Macrolide Antibiotic) 475

Bromfed DM (Cough Syrup) 476

Bromfed PD (Antihistamine/Decongestant) 477

Cefaclor (Semisynthetic Cephalosporin Antibiotic) 477

Ceftin (Second-Generation Cephalosporin Antibiotic) 478

Cefzil (Second-Generation Cephalosporin Antibiotic) 479

Claritin (Antihistamine) 480

Colace (Stool Softener) 481

Domeboro Powder Packets (Topical Solution) 482

Donnagel (Antidiarrheal) 482

Donnatal (Anticholinergic/Antispasmodic, Mild Sedation) 483

Dorcol Pediatric Cough Syrup 484

Duricef (First-Generation Cephalosporin Antibiotic) 485

Erycette Topical Solution 486

Erythromycin (Antibiotic) 487

Eurax (Scabicide, Antipruritic) 488

Feosol Elixir (Nonprescription Iron Supplement) 489

Ilotycin Ophthalmic Ointment (Erythromycin) 489

Intal Inhaler (Antiasthmatic) 490

Keflex (Cephalosporin Antibiotic) 491

Kwell Lotion (Pediculocide, Scabicide) 492

Kwell Shampoo (Antiparasitic) 493

Lorabid (Second-Generation Antibiotic) 493

Lotrimin Cream 1% (Antifungal) 495

Luride (Flouride Supplement) 495

Monistat 7 Vaginal Cream (Antifungal) 496

Monistat 3 Vaginal Suppositories (Antifungal) 497

Motrin for Children (Nonsteroidal Anti-inflammatory Analgesic) 498

Motrin IB (Antirheumatic, Analgesic, Fever Reducer) 498

Mycelex-G500 mg (Antifungal Vaginal Tablet) 499

Mycostatin (Antifungal) 500

Nasacort Inhaler 501

Nix (Topical Pediculicide) 502

Novahistine DMX (Antitussive/Expectorant) 502

PediaCare 503

Pedialyte (Oral Electrolyte Solution) 505

Penicillin V Potassium (Antibiotic) 505

Phenergan Expectorant with Codeine (Cough Formula) 506

Ponstel (Anti-inflammatory, Non-narcotic Analgesic) 507

Prostaphilin (Antibiotic) 508

Proventil Syrup (Bronchodilator-Antiasthmatic) 508

Pyridium (Urinary Analgesic) 509

Rondec-DM (Antihistamine/Decongestant/Antitussive) 510

Sudafed (Adrenergic) 511

Suprax (Semisynthetic Cephalosporin Antibiotic) 512
Tavist Syrup (Antihistamine)...513
Tetracycline Capsules (Antibiotic) 514
Tinactin (Antifungal)..515
Tofranil (Antidepressant)...516
Tussi-Organidin DM (Antitussive/Expectorant) 517
Vantin (Second-Generation Cephalosporin Antibiotic) 517
Ventolin Inhaler (Aerosol Bronchodilator)..519
Vermox Chewable Tablets (Anthelmintic)..520
Zithromax (Macrolide Antibiotic) 521
References 523
Appendices...525
Index...557

I

Well Child Care

Geraldine R. Stephens

Part I of this manual develops criteria for individualizing the delivery of well child care. The emotional, intellectual, social, and physical components of development are integrated to show their inseparable interrelationship in the progress of each child toward maturity. Growth periods are divided into three cycles. The first cycle, from birth to about 3 years of age, is a period of rapid growth, laying the foundation for the future individual pattern of development. The second cycle, from 3 years through the early school years, is a period of slower physical development but rapidly expanding emotional, social, and intellectual growth. The third cycle, from preadolescence through adolescence, is again a period of rapid physical growth, with the drive for maturity affecting social, emotional, and intellectual development.

In each cycle, guidelines have been developed identifying factors to be considered in all health supervision visits. Outlines for the initial history and general physical examination are presented to establish the baseline information from which to begin individualizing the care plan. For each well child visit, specific factors are outlined for obtaining a broad-based history, and the age-specific factors to be evaluated during the physical examination are given. From these, problem lists and appropriate care plans can be established. Also included are outlines of the developmental tasks for each age period. These outlines can be used to help parents reach a positive understanding of the path their child is taking toward developing his or her capabilities in the maturation process.

This edition adds protocols for injury prevention and physical abuse, and guidelines are given for assessing these areas.

INITIAL HISTORY

The initial history is obtained at the child's initial health care visit. Because taking the history is time-consuming, allow an additional 30 minutes for that visit. When the appointment is scheduled, the secretary should advise the parent or child of the extended visit and request that he or she have immunization, birth, developmental, and illness records available.

I. **Informant's relationship to patient**
II. **Family history**
   A. Parents
       1. Age
       2. Health status
   B. Chronological listing of mother's pregnancies, including miscarriages. List name, age, sex, and health, and consanguinity of children.
   C. Familial review of systems (including parents, siblings, grandparents, aunts, uncles)
       1. Skin: Atopic dermatitis, cancer, birthmarks
       2. Head: Headaches (migraine, cluster)
       3. Eyes: Visual problems, strabismus
       4. Ears: Hearing deficiencies, ear infections, malformation
       5. Nose: Allergies, sinus problems
       6. Mouth: Cleft palate, dental status
       7. Throat: Frequent infections
       8. Respiratory: Asthma, chronic bronchitis, tuberculosis
       9. Cardiovascular: Cardiac disease, hypertension
      10. Hematologic: Anemias, hemophilia
      11. Immunologic deficiencies
      12. Gastrointestinal: Ulcers, pyloric stenosis, chronic constipation or diarrhea
      13. Genitourinary: Renal disease, enuresis
      14. Endocrine: Diabetes, thyroid problems, abnormal pattern of sexual maturation
      15. Musculoskeletal: Dislocated hips, scoliosis, arthritis, deformities
      16. Neurologic: Convulsive disorders, learning disabilities, craniosynostosis, mental retardation, mental illness
      17. General: Obesity, unusual familial pattern of growth, cystic fibrosis
III. **Social history**
   A. Occupation
       1. Mother
       2. Father
   B. Housing
       1. Ownership of home
       2. Age and condition of home

    C. Parents' marital status

        1. Duration of marriage

        2. Marital relationship

        3. Single parent, support system

    D. Parents' source of medical care

    E. Medical insurance

    F. Financial status and source of support

    G. Social outlets of parents and family

IV. Pregnancy

    A. Prenatal care

        1. Location and duration

        2. Prenatal classes

    B. Mother's health

        1. Complications: Vaginal bleeding, excessive weight gain, edema, headaches, hypertension, glycosuria

        2. Infection: Rubella, urinary tract infection

        3. Exposure to radiation, drugs (alcohol, medications, smoking)

    C. Planning of pregnancy

        1. Methods of contraception

        2. When contraception discontinued

V. Birth

    A. Location

    B. Gestational age in weeks

    C. Labor

        1. Induction

        2. Duration

        3. Medication, natural birth

        4. Father present

    D. Delivery

        1. Presentation: Vertex, breech, transverse

        2. Method: Spontaneous, forceps, cesarean section (repeat, emergency)

    E. Parents' reaction to labor and delivery, including mother's physical and mental recuperation

    F. Complications

    G. Neonatal health

        1. Birth weight

        2. Condition at birth

            a. Apgar score

            b. Resuscitation, oxygen

            c. Special nursery

            d. Congenital anomalies

        3. Hospital course

            a. Respiratory distress

      b. Cyanosis

      c. Jaundice: Physiologic, ABO, Rh, other

      d. Difficulty sucking

      e. Vomiting

      f. Other complications

         (1) Infection

         (2) Seizures

      g. Length of stay

      h. Low weight and discharge weight

VI. Nutrition

    A. Feeding

      1. Breast: Duration

      2. Formula: Amount, type

    B. Problems

      1. Scheduling

      2. Vomiting

      3. Diarrhea

      4. Colic

    C. Vitamins and fluoride

    D. Solids

      1. When introduced—cereal, vegetables, fruits, meats, eggs, juices

      2. How prepared

      3. Infant's tolerance

    E. Present diet

      1. Appetite

         a. Balanced—relate to growth pattern

      2. Food intolerances and dislikes

VII. Growth and development

    A. Physical

      1. Height and weight at birth, 6 months, 1 year, etc.

      2. Consistent growth rate

    B. Motor

      1. Gross motor

         a. Sits by 6 months.

         b. Crawls by 8 months.

         c. Stands alone by 12 months.

         d. Walks by 16 months.

         e. Undresses, dresses by 2.5 years.

         f. Pedals tricycle by 3 years.

         g. Ties shoes by 6 years.

      2. Fine motor

         a. Reaches for objects by 4 months.

         b. Pincer grasp by 1 year.

       c. Holds and drinks from cup by 1.5 years.

       d. Feeds self by 2 years.

       e. Catches ball by 3 years.

       f. Uses pencils by 4 years.

  C. Language

    1. Single words other than "mama" and "dada" by 1 year

    2. Phrases (two or three words) by 1.5 years

    3. Sentences by 3 years

  D. Toilet training

    1. When started

    2. Technique used

    3. When achieved

  E. School

    1. Grade appropriate for age

    2. Academic performance

    3. Social adjustment to school

      a. To teachers

      b. To peers

  F. Personality traits as viewed by parents

    1. Relationships with parents: Happy, self-actualizing, exhibits self-control, takes responsibility for own actions according to developmental stage

    2. Relationships with siblings: Cooperative rather than aggressive interaction

    3. Relationships with peers: By school age, can be part of a peer group

  G. Behavioral traits

    1. Pica, tantrums, thumb sucking, rocking, etc.

    2. Sleep patterns

    3. Hobbies, activities

    4. Smoking, drugs, sexual practices

    5. Ability to control behavior

    6. Ability to anticipate and take responsibility for consequence of behavior

    7. Ability to accept and return affection

VIII. Parental reaction to child's development

  A. Proud, understanding

IX. Immunizations and screening tests

  A. Types and dates of immunizations, including boosters

    1. DPT

    2. Td

    3. TOPV

    4. Measles

    5. Rubella

    6. Mumps

    7. Other (per office protocol)

  B. Reactions to immunizations

C. Screening and dates of last tests
  1. Tuberculin
  2. Sickle cell
  3. Lead
  4. Hearing
  5. Vision
  6. Urine
  7. Hemoglobin, hematocrit

X. Previous illnesses
  A. Contagious diseases
    1. Dates
    2. Severity
    3. Sequelae
  B. Infections
    1. Dates
    2. Severity
    3. Sequelae
  C. Other illnesses and complications
  D. Hospitalizations
    1. Illnesses, operations, injuries
    2. Dates
    3. Places
    4. Complications
  E. Injuries
    1. Accidents
    2. Abuse

XI. Review of systems
  A. Skin: Birthmarks, rashes, skin type
  B. HEENT (Head, Eyes, Ears, Nose, Throat)
    1. Hair and scalp: Seborrhea, hair loss, pediculosis
    2. Head: Injuries, headache
    3. Eyes: Vision test, glasses, strabismus, infections
    4. Ears: Hearing test, infections, discharge
    5. Nose: Epistaxis, allergies, frequent colds, snoring, sense of smell
    6. Mouth: Dental hygiene, visits to dentist, mouth breathing
    7. Throat: Sore throats, swollen glands, difficulty swallowing, hoarseness
  C. Respiratory: Bronchitis, pneumonia, asthma, croup, persistent cough
  D. Cardiovascular: Heart murmur, cyanosis, dyspnea, shortness of breath, edema, syncope, energy level
  E. Gastrointestinal: Appetite, diet, abdominal pain, vomiting, diarrhea, constipation, type and frequency of stools, jaundice
  F. Genitourinary: Enuresis, urinary tract infection, dysuria, urinary frequency, hematuria, vaginal discharge

G. Skeletal: Deformities, joint pains, swelling, limp, orthopedic appliances, injuries

H. Neurologic: Fainting spells, dizziness, tremors, loss of consciousness, seizures, ataxia

I. Endocrine
   1. Sexual maturation
      a. Male: Hair, beard, voice, acne
      b. Female: Breast development; menarche, duration, regularity, amount of menstrual flow, dysmenorrhea; acne; pregnancies, miscarriages, abortions
   2. Growth disturbances
      a. Consistent growth rate
      b. Excessive weight gain
   3. Excessive thirst

XII. **Assessment**
   A. Problems identified from subjective and objective data
   B. Problem list developed with parent or child

NOTES

PHYSICAL EXAMINATION

The following outline of the physical examination should be used, age-appropriately, at each well child visit. Refer to the well child examination schedule of the American Academy of Pediatrics.

I. **General appearance and behavior**
   A. Habitus
      1. Body build and constitution
      2. Size
      3. Nutrition
   B. General
      1. Alertness
      2. Cooperativeness
      3. Activity level
II. **Measurements**
   A. Temperature
   B. Pulse rate
   C. Respiratory rate
   D. Blood pressure, with use of proper cuff size; examination routine from 3 years of age
   E. Height; percentile plotted on growth chart
   F. Weight; percentile plotted on growth chart
   G. Head circumference; percentile plotted on growth chart
III. **Skin and hair**
   A. Inspection
      1. Color: Normal, cyanosis, pallor, jaundice, carotenemia, hair color and distribution
      2. Eruptions: Macules, papules, vesicles, bullae, pustules, wheals, petechiae, ecchymoses
      3. Pigmentation: Hemangiomas, nevi
   B. Palpation
      1. Skin texture: Smooth, soft, flexible, moist, rough, dry, scaly, edematous
      2. Scars
      3. Hair texture: Fine, coarse, dry, oily
IV. **Head and face**
   A. Inspection
      1. Size: Normal, microcephalic, macrocephalic
      2. Shape: Symmetry, bossing, flattening
      3. Control: Mobility, head lag
   B. Palpation
      1. Fontanelles: Size, shape, bulging, depression
      2. Suture lines: Separated, overriding, closed
      3. Craniotabes

4. Caput succedaneum, cephalhematoma
C. Percussion
   1. Sinuses
   2. Macewen's sign (cracked-pot sound)
D. Auscultation: Bruits

V. **Eyes**
A. Inspection
   1. Size and shape: Equal, symmetric
   2. Control: Ptosis, nystagmus, strabismus, blinking
   3. Pupils: Shape, equality, size, reaction to light, accommodation
   4. Conjunctivae and sclerae: Clarity, hemorrhage, color, pigmentation
   5. Eyelids: Ptosis, blepharitis, styes
A. Examination
   1. Ophthalmoscopic: Red reflex, cataract, eye grounds
   2. Dacryocystitis, dacryostenosis
   3. Visual acuity

VI. **Ears**
A. Inspection
   1. Size and shape: Lop ears, skin tags, dimples, sinus tracts, anomalies
   2. Position: Low-set
   3. Otoscopic examination
      a. External canal: Cerumen, discharge, inflammation, foreign bodies
      b. Tympanic membrane: Color, light reflex, bony landmarks, mobility, perforation, bulging, retraction, scars
   4. Auditory acuity: Whisper test, audiometry, Rinnie's test, Weber's test, tuning fork
   5. Impedance audiometry
B. Palpation
   1. Auricle: Pain on retraction
   2. Mastoid: Tenderness

VII. **Nose**
A. Inspection
   1. Size and shape
   2. Mucosa: Color, discharge, polyps
   3. Turbinates: Size, color
   4. Septum: Deviation, bleeding points
   5. Foreign bodies
B. Palpation: Tenderness, crepitus, deformity

VIII. **Mouth**
A. Lips: Symmetry, color, eruptions, fissures, edema
B. Gums: Color, cysts, infection, ulcerations, mucous membranes
C. Tongue: Symmetry, tongue-tie, color, anomalies
D. Teeth: Number, alignment, caries

IX. Throat
    A. Palate: Symmetry, shape, color, cleft, arch, eruptions
    B. Uvula: Symmetry, shape, bifid
    C. Tonsils: Symmetry, shape, size, color, exudate, ulcerations
    D. Epiglottis: Size, shape, color

X. Neck
    A. Inspection: Size, shape, webbing, fistulas, masses, neck veins, cysts
    B. Palpation
        1. Trachea: Position
        2. Thyroid: Size, masses
        3. Neck: Masses, mobility, torticollis

XI. Lymph nodes: Suboccipital, postauricular, anterior and posterior cervical, supraclavicular, axillary, epitrochlear, inguinal
    A. Inspection: Size, overlying skin color, lymphangitis
    B. Palpation: Size, consistency, tenderness, mobility

XII. Chest
    A. Inspection
        1. Shape: Funnel, pigeon, barrel, precordial bulge, protruding xiphoid, Harrison's groove
        2. Size, symmetry, mobility: Expansion, flaring, retraction
        3. Respirations: Rate, type, tachypnea, dyspnea, hyperpnea
    B. Palpation
        1. Tactile fremitus
        2. Breast: Consistency, masses
    C. Percussion: Tympany, resonance, dullness, flatness
    D. Auscultation
        1. Breath sounds: Vesicular, bronchovesicular, bronchial
        2. Adventitial sounds: Rales, rhonchi, wheezes, rubs
        3. Vocal resonance

XIII. Heart
    A. Palpation
        1. Point of maximum impact (PMI)
        2. Thrills
    B. Percussion: Heart border
    C. Auscultation
        1. Rate, rhythm, character of first and second heart sounds, third heart sound, splitting
        2. Sinus arrhythmia, gallop, premature beats, murmurs (systolic, diastolic), clicks, rubs

XIV. Abdomen
    A. Inspection
        1. Size and shape: Distention, respiratory movements, peristalsis
        2. Umbilicus: Granuloma, hernia
        3. Diastasis recti

    4. Veins
B. Auscultation: Bowel sounds
C. Palpation
    1. Tone: Rigidity, tenderness, rebound
    2. Liver, spleen, kidneys, bladder: Masses
    3. Femoral pulses
D. Percussion: Organ size, tympany, fluid

XV. Genitalia
  A. Inspection
    1. Male
      a. Penis: Size, foreskin (phimosis), circumcision, urethral meatus (hypospadias, epispadias, chordee)
      b. Scrotum: Size, testicles (size, shape), hydrocele, hernia
      c. Hair distribution
    2. Female
      a. Labia, clitoris, vagina: Foreign bodies, adhesions, discharge
      b. Urethra
      c. Hair distribution
  B. Palpation (male)
    1. Testicles: Descended, undescended, position
    2. Hernia: Direct, indirect
    3. Masses

XVI. Anus and rectum
  A. Inspection
    1. General: Position, fissures, fistulas, prolapse, hemorrhoids
    2. Sacrococcygeal area
      a. Pilonidal dimple or fistula
      b. Masses: Teratoma, meningocele
    3. Palpation: Sphincter tone, masses, tenderness

XVII. Musculoskeletal
  A. Hands: Clubbing, polydactyly, syndactyly, nails, dermatoglyphics
  B. Legs and feet: Symmetry, forefoot adduction, pes planus, clubbed feet, knock-knees, bowed legs, tibial torsion, gait, anteversion of femoral head, limp, length, paralysis
  C. Hips: Symmetry of skin folds
  D. Back: Scoliosis, kyphosis, lordosis

WELL CHILD VISITS

Although the well child visits defined here are labeled for a specific age span, they are intended to be used as a continuum in following each child's own developmental progress. Broad guidelines for well child visits are as follows:

I. **First cycle of growth**
  A. 0–8 weeks (neonatal period)
    1. Establishment of general well-being of parents and baby
    2. Development of a good working relationship between parents and baby
  B. 2–4 months: Continuing period of symbiosis of parents and baby
    1. Stabilization of physical systems
    2. Development of contentment for both parents and baby
  C. 4–6 months: Period of awareness
    1. Physical system stability and beginning of body control
    2. Beginning of the separation of the individuality of parents and baby
    3. Established reliance of the baby on the goodness or unreliability of the environment
      a. Primary caregiver
  D. 6–8 months: Becoming the student
    1. Watching intently what is going on around him or her
    2. Progressing from random to purposeful movements
    3. Building up memory store of people and objects in the environment
  E. 8–14 months: A watershed period
    1. Past physical and emotional development provides the building blocks for the next stage.
    2. Reaching out into the environment to fashion confidence in developing skills
    3. Expanding emotional responses
    4. New physical mobility
  F. 14–18 months: Exploration and self-confidence
    1. Refinement of physical skills
    2. Beginning to use language as a tool
    3. Development of self-esteem versus self-doubt, reflecting encouragement or discouragement by primary caregiver
  G. 18–24 months: Experimenting with establishing independence
    1. Using "no" as a test of power
    2. Learning that behavior has consequences
    3. Safety of primary concern
  H. 24–36 months: Definitive year to complete the development of the physical and emotional tasks of the first period of growth
    1. Maturation of physical systems
    2. Establishment of the emotional maturity needed to move away from the security of family and join peer group

II. **Second cycle of growth**
   A. 3–5 years
      1. Increase in muscle strength, but slower development of endurance
      2. Progressing from fantasy and magical thinking to a world of reality
      3. Sexual identity established
   B. 6–9 years
      1. Halcyon years of good health, intellectual curiosity, few responsibilities, and high adventures
      2. Strength and endurance increased (dependent on exercise and use, not on sex)

III. **Third cycle of growth**
   A. 9–11 years
      1. Physical changes
      2. Transitional period from childhood to adolescence
      3. Need for child and parent to understand and appreciate the individual pattern of each child's development
   B. 12–16 years
      1. Physical stability
      2. Establishing independence by making appropriate decisions
      3. Understanding the consequences of and accepting responsibility for one's actions
      4. Learning to accept and appreciate one's own uniqueness

The general outline used for the presentation of the rest of Part I is as follows:

I. **Well Child Visit**
   A. Visit overview
   B. Injury prevention protocol and child abuse
   C. Developmental process
   D. Family status
   E. Health habits
   F. Growth and development
   G. Risk factors
   H. Physical examination
   I. Assessment
   J. Plan

II. **Anticipatory Guidance**
   A. Overview
   B. Expectations for development
   C. Family status
   D. Health patterns
   E. Growth and development
   F. Risk factors
   G. Childrearing practices
   H. Stimulation

|INJURY PREVENTION GUIDELINES

The number one health threat to children is injuries. Primary care providers can significantly reduce the number of victims by reviewing the causes of age-specific injuries with the caregivers at each visit. The following is a protocol of basic safety practices. For each well child visit, specific age-appropriate injury prevention plans are included.

I. **Safety strategies**
  A. Caregivers
     1. Provide a safe environment.
     2. Be aware of safety precautions.
     3. Have first-aid training.
  B. Child
     1. As child develops ability to comprehend cause and effect of activities and to control behavior, responsibility for safety must be given to him or her.

II. **Safe environment**
  A. House
     1. Heating and electric systems
     2. Windows and doors: Locks
     3. Stairs: Repairs and lighting
     4. Water below 120°F
  B. Play areas
     1. Fence as needed
     2. Safe equipment
  C. Car
     1. Safety features, doors, tires
     2. Car seats appropriate for age of passenger
     3. Responsible driver
  D. All appropriate phone numbers posted near phone

III. **Injury prevention**
  A. Fire
     1. Smoke detectors throughout house
     2. No smoking in house
     3. Fire drills and designated meeting place outside house rehearsed
     4. Fire extinguishers in kitchen, checked monthly
  B. Burns
     1. Water heater set below 120°F, or scald valve on water taps
     2. Hot drinks kept away from child's area
     3. Hot pans and wood stoves placed so child cannot get to them
     4. Fireplaces securely screened
  C. Falls
     1. Stairwells lighted
     2. Toys, small rugs, slippery floors attended to

3. Gates on stairs as needed
4. Awareness of things to climb on, such as boxes, stools, small trees
5. No baby walkers

D. Suffocation
1. Remove window drapes, blind cords near crib.
2. Keep plastic bags and coverings out of reach.
3. Do not put baby on soft mattresses, couches, waterbeds, bean bags, fluffy pillows, or blankets.
4. Do not have baby sleep in bed with adult.

E. Water
1. Keep hot water temperature in house below 120°F, or install scald valves on water taps.
2. Baby can drown in 1″ of water (tubs or puddles).
3. Children can fall into toilet, bucket of water, open can of paint.
4. All pool areas must be fenced and supervised when in use.

F. Furniture
1. Crib
   a. If old, check for lead paint.
   b. Slats no more than 1.75″ apart
   c. Firm mattress with no gaps between mattress and frame
   d. Sides stay as placed.
2. Sharp edges of furniture, fireplace, stairs, etc. covered

G. Poisons
1. Cleaning equipment locked in cabinets, not kept where child can reach it
2. Medications kept in locked cabinet
3. Drugs and alcohol kept in locked cabinets
4. Rubbish kept out of child's area

IV. **Most accidents happen:**
A. After stressful events
B. When caregiver is tired or ill
C. When routine changes, as on holidays, vacation, visitors
D. Late in the day (emergency rooms are busiest from 4 to 8 p.m.)

V. **Special counseling needed for:**
A. Single parents with little support from family and friends
B. Fathers with feelings of isolation and abandonment
C. Caregivers using alcohol and drugs
D. Medicaid families—not that they are careless parents, but because they often cannot provide a safe environment and lack adequate health care

VI. **Not all injuries are accidents; indications of abuse must be considered.**

VII. **Reference**
American Academy of Pediatrics. *TIPP—The Injury Prevention Program: A Guide to Safety Counseling in Office Practice.* 141 Northwest Point Boulevard, Elk Grove Village, IL 60009

| CHILD ABUSE GUIDELINES

Prevention, identification, and reporting of abuse are important aspects of-child care. Physical abuse is the most obvious abuse assessed by professionals. However, adults, siblings, caregivers, and teachers who degrade and debase children are also abusers; verbal and psychological abuse must be carefully evaluated. Helping children to develop their full potential, with a strong sense of self-worth and self-esteem, is as important as protecting them from physical abuse. The developmental milestones of childhood are identified throughout this part of the book, and the progress toward these tasks must be evaluated.

I. **Characteristics of children who have been or may be abused**
   A. More boys abused than girls
   B. Difficult children to care for
      1. Frequent illnesses, physically handicapped, mental retardation, premature babies
   C. Behavior characteristics
      1. Stubborn, overly shy, fearful, passive to explosive behavior, disturbed sleep patterns, gaining attention by acting out
   D. Language
      1. Speaks grudgingly
      2. Expresses self with difficulty
      3. Uses foul language

II. **Characteristics of abusers**
   A. Parent
      1. One abuse victim in the family may mean that other members are abused as well.
      2. Delayed treatment for less-than-emergency injury
      3. History of abuse in their own childhood
      4. Ethnic values of accepted behavior may not identify this behavior as abuse.
   B. Mother
      1. Single parent four times more often an abuser
      2. Difficult pregnancy
      3. Little prenatal care
      4. Unwanted child
      5. Poorly educated about child care, but can otherwise be a well-educated person
      6. Adolescent with no support system, low self-esteem, depressed, alcohol or drug user, poor environment, poverty
   C. Father
      1. Feelings of displacement and isolation
      2. Reactive pattern of aggression
      3. Alcohol or drug user

III. **Types of abuse**
   A. Corporal punishment as a cultural pattern of behavior

    B. Failure to thrive—parent uneducated about child care, not always a poor environment

    C. Falls

        1. Children under 12 years old falling from moderate heights seldom have broken bones; history of short fall with significant injury can indicate abuse.

    D. Head injury

        1. Head injury in a child under 2 years old indicates abuse.

        2. Accidental injury seldom causes brain damage.

        3. In the absence of sufficient history, retinal hemorrhage may indicate abuse.

    E. Abdominal trauma

        1. Can be indicated when there are multiple injuries

        2. Second highest mortality rate of abused children

    F. Shaken baby syndrome

        1. Usually indicated in child under 1 year old with abuse in other family members

        2. Abnormal respiratory patterns and bulging fontanelle may be present.

    G. Sudden infant death syndrome

        1. History of abuse of all family members important to investigate

    H. Frequent illnesses

        1. Parent reports unrealistic and unconfirmed symptoms.

        2. Parent demands repeated testing and hospitalization of child.

        3. Child is unresponsive and seems overwhelmed.

    I. Burns

        1. Either too severe or in areas of body that would not normally be exposed to burns

        2. Confused history of actual occurrence

    J. Sexual abuse

        1. Question all family members if they are afraid of anyone or are being hurt by anyone.

IV. **References**

American Academy of Pediatrics. *Child Abuse: A Guide to References and Resources in Child Abuse and Neglect.* 141 Northwest Point Boulevard, Elk Grove Village, IL 60009

BREAST-FEEDING GUIDELINES

Breast-feeding is the most natural way to feed a baby. It should be something a mother does because she wants to, because she and the baby find it satisfying. If, for any reason, it does not work out, there is no cause for guilt. The method of feeding is much less important than the general quality of the relationship between mother and baby.

I. **Mother**

A. Bras

1. Should fit well and provide support without causing pressure on any part of the breast

2. Most women are more comfortable if they wear a bra around the clock during the early postpartum weeks.

B. Appetite and thirst

1. May increase during lactation; add 500 calories to the prepregnant diet.

2. Control weight by eliminating sweets and cutting back on fatty foods. Do not skimp on fruits, vegetables, meat, fish, poultry, cereals, and breads. Do not diet. Breast-feeding aids maternal weight loss.

3. Drink at least 3 quarts of liquid a day, including some milk. Other milk products include yogurt, ice cream, cheese, and custards. Coffee or tea should be decaffeinated, because caffeine is excreted in breast milk. Avoid colas with caffeine.

4. Rarely does a food that agrees with the mother cause a problem for the baby; however, onions and garlic may affect the taste of the mother's milk, causing the baby to protest. This may be a cause of the baby's fussiness.

5. Avoid beer and other alcoholic drinks; alcohol is excreted in breast milk.

C. Drugs

1. Check with doctor before taking any medication.

2. Most doctors discourage use of birth-control pills during lactation because they often decrease the milk supply and possibly its nutrient value.

3. Because many drugs pass into the milk, always consider their effect on the baby.

4. Avoid nicotine: It accumulates in breast milk and can limit the amount of milk produced.

D. Menstruation

1. Return of periods may be delayed for as long as breast-feeding is continued without supplementation with formula or solids.

2. Absence of periods does not mean that the mother cannot get pregnant; breast-feeding is not a reliable form of birth control.

3. Menstruation has no effect on the quality of milk.

E. Fatigue and discouragement

1. Mother will probably be surprised at how tired and on edge she feels during the early postpartum weeks; she will get little else done besides meeting the baby's needs.

2. Fatigue and emotional stress decrease milk supply and affect the way mother and baby get along. If the mother is upset, the baby will be too.

    3. Do not feel guilty about:

        a. Admitting fatigue and accepting (or demanding) help from others

        b. Napping when the baby sleeps (curl up together)

        c. Cutting activities down to bare essentials—ignore the dust and resort to simple meals for a while

F. Sore breasts

    1. Usual cause is blockage of one of the milk ducts due to engorgement, a tight bra, or poor or delayed emptying of that breast. There will probably be a lump or two in the tender area. Because an infection is possible, treat immediately.

    2. Nurse very frequently on the sore side to "empty" it; offer it to the baby first.

    3. Gently massage the area while taking a hot shower; make sure no crusted milk is covering part of the nipple.

    4. Try different nursing positions to change pressure areas.

    5. Remove bra if too tight, or get a bra extender.

    6. Extra fluids and rest help.

    7. If the lump does not disappear after two or three feedings, if the area becomes red and more tender, or if a fever is present with flulike aches, call the health care provider; an antibiotic may be necessary.

    8. Do not stop nursing; the milk will not harm the baby.

G. Sore nipples

    1. Some discomfort is usual during the first week or two of nursing.

    2. Soreness is temporary and should not be a reason to stop nursing or resort to nipple shields.

    3. To reduce soreness:

        a. Always:

            (1) Get the milk flow started manually before putting the baby to the breast. This prevents irritation from the initial "dry" sucking necessary to draw the milk down.

            (2) Nurse frequently for short periods (5–10 minutes on each side every 2–3 hours).

            (3) Break the suction before removing the baby.

            (4) Offer both breasts at each feeding (if 10 minutes on one side fills the baby up, nurse for 5 minutes on each side).

            (5) Make sure the baby takes the nipple and most of the areola into the mouth. The mother should be able to see the brown area pucker slightly as the baby nurses.

            (6) Wash breasts with water only.

            (7) Rotate pressure areas by experimenting with different positions for both mother and baby.

            (8) Begin on the less painful breast, and then switch to the sore side after letdown has occurred and the baby's hunger has eased a bit.

            (9) Take a hot shower to help relax and get the milk flowing before nursing.

          (10) Expose nipples to sunlight for brief periods.

   b. Never:
      (1) Skip a feeding or avoid nursing on the sore side.
      (2) Use a nipple shield. This only postpones the toughening process and often adds to the irritation, because the baby must get the milk by suction alone.
      (3) Use excessive amounts of cream on nipples. A thick layer of cream tends to trap moisture and also makes the nipples slippery, which forces the baby to clamp down repeatedly in an effort to stay on.
      (4) Use plastic-covered bra pads.
      (5) Use soap or drying agents on nipples.
   c. When soreness diminishes, increase the nursing time to meet the baby's needs.

II. Baby

A. Feeding schedule

1. Nurse 10–15 minutes on the first side, then allow the baby to nurse until satisfied on the second.
2. At times the baby may fall asleep, yet by reflex the lower jaw will move rhythmically without effective sucking. After a minute or two of this, the baby will usually remain asleep when removed from the breast.
3. Follow the baby's signals rather than the clock. Most breast-fed babies want to nurse every 2–3 hours during the early weeks. Human milk is easier to digest than formula, so a breast-fed stomach empties sooner than a formula-fed one. As the mother's milk supply increases, the number of feedings will decrease. If the baby is small and consistently sleeps 4–5 hours between feedings, the mother should attempt to nurse at least every 3 hours during her waking hours.

B. Indications that the baby is getting enough milk

1. Six to eight wet diapers over a 24-hour period (not a good indication if the baby is also getting a lot of water)
2. Contented, vigorous, frequent (every 2–3 hours) nursing periods of at least 5 minutes per side
3. An alert, responsive baby
4. Do not test for hunger by offering the baby a bottle after feeding. Often babies take an extra ounce or two just because it is there, because they like to suck, and because they are not used to a nipple that allows milk to flow so quickly and easily.
5. Adequate weight gain

C. Supplementary feeding

1. Although frequent bottles can interfere with the mother's milk supply, an occasional bottle of breast milk or formula can be given without creating a problem.
2. The most convenient kind of substitute is ready-to-feed formula that comes in a bottle and requires only attaching a sterile nipple, but powdered formula (mixed with boiling water) is more economical.
3. Mother can express milk before or after feedings to freeze for supplementary feedings.
   a. Manual expression. Baby gets milk by squeezing the areola with gums, not by direct suction. To imitate this action, grasp the edge of the

areola with a thumb and forefinger and gently squeeze the fingers together while pressing inward toward the chest. Never pull or squeeze just the nipple itself. Because there are many ducts arranged around the nipple somewhat like the spokes of a wheel, change the position of the fingers often.

    b. Hand or electric pump (bulb type). While taking a hot shower, gently massage each breast, starting at the chest wall and working toward the nipple. Immediately afterward, moisten the pump's cone with warm water, compress the bulb halfway, and apply the cone to the breast so the nipple points toward the bulb. Gently and rhythmically apply and release pressure on the bulb. It probably will take a minute or two before the milk starts flowing.

    c. Collecting milk

        (1) Cleanliness is essential.

        (2) Take apart and wash all equipment in hot, soapy water; rinse well.

        (3) Place parts in a covered pan and cover with water.

        (4) Boil for at least 5 minutes.

        (5) Turn off heat and allow pan to cool on burner.

        (6) Drain water and store parts in the covered pan until ready to use.

        (7) Wash hands before reassembling equipment; be careful not to touch parts that will come in contact with milk.

        (8) Repeat step (2) immediately after use.

    d. Storing milk

        (1) Plastic or glass bottles may be used for freezing. Disposable bottle liners may be frozen in the outer case and then sealed with a twist-tie.

        (2) Label the container with the date if it is to be frozen.

        (3) Breast milk should be used within a day after it is refrigerated. It will stay fresh up to 2 weeks in the freezer, at 0°F or below.

        (4) Milk separates into layers as it cools but will mix again when thawed.

    e. Thawing milk

        (1) Do not thaw milk slowly at room temperature.

        (2) Place bottle in a pan of cold water and bring water to a boil.

        (3) Remove pan from heat and take bottle out when milk is warm.

        (4) Refrigerate leftover milk, but discard if not used within 2–3 hours.

D. Weaning

  1. The baby's age or the appearance of teeth should not be the reason to stop breast-feeding. The decision should be based on the mother's feelings and needs as well as on the baby's cues and needs.

  2. Delay weaning if the baby is irritable from teething or sick or if some other stress is present.

  3. Weaning can be accomplished in a matter of days if necessary, but doing it so rapidly can be extra-hard on both mother and baby. The weaning process should be spaced over a period of weeks so there is time to adjust gradually.

4. Choose the feeding in which there is the least milk or in which the baby is least interested, and replace it with a cup or bottle of formula or milk, depending on the baby's age and nutritional and sucking needs. If breasts become uncomfortably full, nurse (or express) a short time to relieve the discomfort.

5. When supply and demand are again balanced, skip another feeding. Continue this pattern until the baby is completely off the breast.

NOTES

|OVERVIEW

2-WEEK WELL CHILD VISIT

I. **Parents**
   A. Adjustment to new responsibilities and appreciation of continued emotional stress and fatigue
   B. Identify any abuse of family members.

II. **Mother**
   A. Physical status
   B. Breast-feeding
      1. Attitude toward breast feeding
      2. Problem identified
   C. Fear of abuse

III. **Baby**
   A. Physical
      1. Quality of care
         a. Consistent caregiver responding to needs of baby
      2. Good color, lusty cry
      3. Sleeping and nursing appropriately
      4. Physical problems not already under care identified: Referrals
   B. Emotional
      1. Quieting easily: Contented baby
      2. Responding to parents by eye contact
   C. Intellectual
      1. Searching for eye contact with caregiver

IV. **Risk factors**
   A. Apathetic
   B. Low weight gain
   C. Cannot be comforted
   D. No consistent, caring caregiver

V. **See guidelines for specific factors to be noted in physical examination.**

|INJURY PREVENTION

I. **Review safety protocol**
   A. Safe environment
      1. Cradle or crib in safe area
      2. Baby not placed on soft mattress, couch, bean bag, fluffy blankets
      3. Baby not sleeping in bed with adult
      4. Siblings and pets supervised
      5. Appropriate car seat—facing backwards if in front seat; in back seat if there is an air bag in passenger side of front seat

II. **At-risk Caregivers**
   A. Difficult responses to birth and postpartum recovery
   B. Support system and basic needs not being met
   C. Fear of violence or abuse
III. **Not all injuries are accidents.**

CHILD ABUSE

I. **Physical identification**
   A. Failure to thrive; physical bruises, burns
   B. Any injury with delayed office visit or unreliable history
II. **At-risk baby**
   A. Cranky baby, physical abnormalities, premature birth
III. **Identify:**
   A. Siblings and adults near baby who have aggressive behavioral patterns
   B. Drug users and those with history of being physical abusers or being abused

NOTES

| **2-WEEK WELL CHILD VISIT**

This is the settling-in period for parents and baby. Adequate physical care and the development of emotional ties are the essential factors to be evaluated.

I. **Developmental process**
   A. Parents
      1. Energy level and general health adequate for demands of family and baby
      2. Expectations of having and caring for baby and expectations of baby's physical appearance fulfilled and accepted
      3. Acceptance of and coping with actual situation
      4. Report of being threatened or abused
   B. Baby
      1. Good sucking instinct, eats and sleeps well, is gaining weight
      2. Cries appropriately and quiets easily
      3. Responds to parent's voice, touch, presence

II. **Family status**
   A. Basic needs being met; referrals as needed with follow-up
   B. Family members
      1. Adjusting to change in family routine
      2. Appreciating emotional stress during this adjustment period
   C. Support system
      1. Father: Giving help and getting pleasure from new role
      2. Mother: Having time to regain energy, catch up on sleep, and have free, peaceful periods with baby
   D. Health status of all family members reviewed

III. **Health habits**
   A. Nutrition
      1. Mother
         a. Breast-feeding: See Breast-Feeding Guidelines
         b. Adequate diet, weight control, referrals as needed
      2. Baby
         a. Stomach holds about 4 oz and empties every 3–4 hours. Digestive system is still immature, so formula or breast milk is the only food appropriate at this time.
         b. Requirement: 50 cal/lb/day or 110 kcal/kg/day, so a 10-lb baby needs 10 × 50, or 500 cal, per day; a 4.54-kg baby needs 4.54 × 110, or 500 cal, per day.
         c. Standard formulas and breast milk have 20 cal/oz.
         d. $\dfrac{500 \text{ cal}}{20 \text{ cal/oz}}$ = 25 oz or 750 ml of formula per day
         e. Number of feedings and amount per 24 hours
         f. If reflux occurs, identify whether too many ounces are being given. Advise caregiver to prop baby up after feedings.
         g. Projectile vomiting: Refer to physician.

       h. Burping gently accomplished

       i. Satisfaction: Baby sleeps for 2 hours after feedings

       j. Formula with vitamins, iron, and fluoride per office protocol

B. Sleep

    1. One or two sleep periods of 5–6 hours per 24 hours (individual pattern depends on temperament and energy level)

    2. Awake for feedings every 3 hours (more or less)

    3. Awake only short periods and seldom awake without fussing

    4. Sleeps through household noises; turns off stimuli, so quiet environment is unnecessary

C. Elimination

    1. Stools

       a. Breast-fed baby: Stools with every feeding, not formed, yellow

       b. Formula-fed baby: Stools less frequent, less loose, and stronger in odor than if on breast milk; light brown

    2. Urine: Light in color, no odor; wet diaper at each feeding

IV. Growth and development

A. Physical

    1. Central nervous system: Most important and fastest-growing system, as brain cells are continuing to develop in both size and number. Effects of nutritional deprivation at this time cannot be reversed.

       a. Holds head up when prone, to side when supine

       b. Hands in fist; palmar grasp

       c. Intense startle reaction

       d. Vision: At 2 weeks, baby is alert to moving objects and is attracted to light objects and bright color. Convergence and following are jerky and inexact.

       e. Movements are uncoordinated but smooth.

       f. Lusty cry

    2. Cardiovascular system: The efficiency of this system is identified by the following:

       a. Good color of body and warmth of extremities

       b. Energy and vigor of activity

       c. Increase of color during stress

    3. Respiratory system: Breathing is still rapid and irregular.

    4. Immune system

       a. Antigen–antibody response is present by 2 weeks, so immunization program can be started then.

       b. Maternal antibodies, which help protect baby from infection, are present.

B. Emotional development—Erikson: Basic trust versus mistrust. Quality of care provided can form the basis for baby's feelings and attitudes toward self and the world.

    1. Parents

       a. Obtains gratification from child care

      b. Feels adequate to care for baby

      c. Adequate support system; basic needs being met

    2. Baby

      a. Adequate physical development

      b. Searching for mother's face; making eye contact

      c. Contented baby

  C. Intellectual development—Piaget: Sensorimotor response. Stimuli to the five senses are the tools through which baby responds to environment.

    1. Parents: Understand crying as instinctive response to other discomforts besides hunger

    2. Baby: Individuality of response pattern becoming evident. Innate reflex responses guide spontaneous behavior.

  D. Risk factors

    1. Mother

      a. Overload of responsibilities, no adequate support system

      b. Low energy level and health problems

      c. Distressed by child care

    2. Baby

      a. Poor feeding habits, possible dehydration

      b. Lags in physical development

      c. Cannot be comforted

      d. Low weight gain

V. **Physical examination**

  A. Growth

    1. Weight gain 1 oz/day

    2. Fontanelles: Measure and record

    3. Developing consistent growth curve

  B. Appearance and behavior

    1. Movements uncoordinated but vigorous

    2. Intensity of startle reaction, with easy quieting

    3. Alert when awake; falls asleep easily

    4. Good color, rapid change in color with activity and crying

  C. Specific factors to note during routine physical examination

    1. Head: Configuration and smooth movement, bulging or depressed anterior fontanelle, seborrhea

    2. Eyes: Red reflex, discharge, reaction to light

    3. Mouth: Thrush (unremovable white spots on tongue). Tongue should be able to protrude beyond lips.

    4. Chest: Respirations—abdominal, irregular rate

    5. Heart: Refer to physician if abnormal sounds are present that have not been previously diagnosed. Sinus arrhythmia continues to be present; normal rate 100–130/min.

    6. Abdomen: Navel, liver, spleen, femoral pulses, hernias

    7. Extremities: Range of motion. Hips: Check for leg folds and abduction.

      8. Skin: Rashes, hemangiomas (measure and record)

  D. Parent–child interaction

      1. Parent: Expression of fatigue and nervousness in handling baby; ability to quiet baby

          a. Referrals or home visit

      2. Baby: Positive response to attention

      3. Referrals to help parents develop positive attitudes toward their new roles

VI. Assessment

  A. Physical

  B. Developmental

  C. Emotional

  D. Environmental

VII. Plan

  A. Immunization per office protocol

  B. Fluoride, vitamins, and iron per office protocol

  C. Problem list (devised with parent); SOAP (Subjective data, Objective data, Assessment, and Plan) format for each

  D. Appropriate timing for office, home, or telephone visits

NOTES

OVERVIEW

Anticipatory Guidance for the Period of 2–8 Weeks

I. **Parents**
   A. Becoming aware of baby's reactive pattern and interactive relationship with baby
   B. Check Breast-Feeding Guidelines.

II. **Baby**
   A. Physical
      1. Smoother muscular movement
      2. Hands reaching out
      3. Settling in to a feeding and sleeping schedule
   B. Emotional
      1. Responding appropriately to type of care being given
      2. Fussy baby needs careful investigation; see guidelines.
   C. Intellectual
      1. Curiosity shown by searching with eyes and reaching out with hands
      2. Responding by smiles and eye contact
         a. Stimulation: See guidelines

III. **Watch for:**
   A. Family realizes this is an adjustment period and coping with new problems.
   B. Baby sleeps and feeds without difficulty.
   C. Baby progresses from innate reflex movements of sucking and grasping to kicking and crying.
   D. Baby repeats purposeful actions, such as grasping objects (but not letting go at will), reaching out with arms when being picked up, and crying more selectively.
   E. Baby turns to localize sound and quiets to pleasant music (still startled reaction to loud, sudden noise).
   F. Baby accepts new experiences.
      1. Expect fussing, but will eventually accept a different crib
      2. Supplemental bottle for breast-feeding baby
      3. Change of caregiver
   G. Baby's observation of caregiver
      1. Eye contact: Baby's facial expression changes on attempting to vocalize.

NOTES

NOTES

ANTICIPATORY GUIDANCE FOR THE PERIOD OF 2–8 WEEKS

This is a quiet period of settling into a scheduled daily routine. It is also a time for parents to become sensitive to the individuality of the baby's reactive pattern and to the interactive relationship that is being established between the mother and baby and the baby's special response to the father's or partner's attention.

I. **Expectations of this period**
   A. Parents
      1. Developing confidence in ability to interpret baby's needs
      2. Enjoying and satisfied with new role
      3. Understanding and coping with own physical and emotional status
   B. Baby
      1. Still settling in to pattern of sleeping, feeding, and wakefulness
      2. Quieting easily when needs are met

II. **Family status**
   A. Basic needs being met; referrals as needed with follow-up
   B. Parents adjusting to their new roles
   C. Appropriate support systems available. Father or partner takes on some of the childrearing role.
   D. Identify sexual abuse of or by any family members.

III. **Health patterns**
   A. Nutrition
      1. Formula or breast milk the only food necessary due to immaturity of gastrointestinal tract and slow development of digestive enzymes
      2. Supplements of vitamins, iron, and fluoride per office protocol
   B. Elimination
      1. Stools continue to be loose.
      2. Urine light in color and odorless. If this changes, identify the cause, as this change can be an early indication of dehydration. Call the office if it continues.

IV. **Interpreting baby's signals**
   A. Crying after feeding and diapering
      1. Physical discomfort
         a. Bowel movement: It is helpful to have something for the infant's feet to push against. Hold the baby over the shoulder with one hand, and place the other hand on the soles of the feet.
         b. An air bubble in the stomach takes up space, is uncomfortable, and prevents the baby from eating as much as desired. Lay the infant across the parent's folded knees with head resting on the adult's arms. Hold one hand on the baby's abdomen and gently rub back in an upward motion.
         c. Diaper rash
            (1) Leave diapers off as much as possible.
            (2) Try another brand, if using disposables.

(3) If using cloth diapers, change soaps, rinse well, and use vinegar in the final rinse.

(4) Call the office if there is no improvement, and report any vaginal irritation.

2. Missing physical contact and sounds heard in utero

   a. Warmth and snugness: Wrap blankets tightly around baby and provide body support.

   b. Music: Lullabies are important; tapes and recordings make it easy to supply music.

   c. Rocking: Cradles and rocking chairs have proved effective over the years.

3. Need for stimulation

   a. Fussing can be a way for baby to say he or she is not ready to go back to sleep.

   b. Use a baby chest carrier; baby enjoys parent's heart sounds and motion.

   c. Take a bath with the baby.

   d. Air baths allow freedom of movement; change baby's position from back to stomach.

   d. Take baby outdoors for a change of colors, sounds, and temperature.

   e. A car ride is often used by harassed parents.

   f. Change of caregiver to hold and talk to baby is helpful.

B. Continued fussing

1. Clothes may be uncomfortable; baby may be too hot or too cold.

2. Colic

   a. Breast-feeding baby: More frequent feedings for smaller amount at each feeding

   b. Mother's diet: Restrict to simplest foods; no colas, coffee, tea; no medications or vitamins; add one food back at a time and see if there is any change in behavior

   c. Formula-fed baby: Smaller and more frequent feedings; eliminate vitamins and fluoride for a few days

   d. Return for medical check if no improvement

   e. Obtain extra caregivers so mother can get adequate rest.

V. **Stimulation**

A. Stimulation depends on baby's energy level and individuality.

B. Baby reacts to stimulation of all the senses—taste, touch, smell, sight, and hearing.

C. Caregiver interprets baby's signals for rest and quiet, such as:

1. Overactive

2. Turning away

3. Fussing

D. Caregiver can provide proper stimulation by spending time feeding, holding, and rocking baby, changing baby's position, establishing eye contact, and talking and singing to baby.

E. Suggested crib toys

1. Noisy clocks, music (radio or tapes)

    2. Paint a happy face on a paper plate and hang it about 10″ from the baby's face, or attach it to side of crib.

VI. Safety

A. Accidents happen most frequently:
1. When routine changes (holidays, vacations, illness in the family)
2. After stressful events for caregivers
3. When caregivers are tired or ill
4. Late in the afternoon

B. Accident prevention
1. Crib: Slats no more than 2″ apart; firm mattress; no plastic used as mattress cover
2. House: Fire alarm system; fire escape plan; no smoking in nursery or house. Baby should never be left alone in house for even 1 min.
3. Carrying: Football carry, with baby on hip with hand holding and protecting head; other hand free to prevent caregiver from falling
4. Car: Approved baby carrier in back seat
5. Baby seat: Sturdy, broad-based; place in safe, protected spot

C. Not all injuries are accidents. Investigate possible child abuse and neglect.

D. Babysitters

E. Emergency telephone numbers posted

VII. Asking for help

A. Appreciate importance of establishing a good working relationship with baby

B. Concerns and problems need to be evaluated.

C. Telephone contact available with pediatric nurse practitioner; home visits, office visits, referrals made as needed

D. Resources
1. Support group of relatives, friends, community group
2. Information on child care: Library can provide reading list.

VIII. Mother's plans to return to work

A. See Breast-Feeding Guidelines.

B. Caregivers

C. Referrals as needed

NOTES

NOTES

OVERVIEW

2-MONTH WELL CHILD VISIT

I. **Parents**
   A. Evaluation of new role
   B. Identify baby's developing skills and reactive patterns
   C. Identify any abuse of family members

II. **Baby**
   A. Physical
      1. Growth pattern, eating, and sleeping schedule evaluated
         a. Health problems identified
   B. Emotional
      1. Contented baby: Reacting to caregiver with enthusiasm
   C. Intellectual
      1. Responding to caregiver with smiles and vocalizing
      2. Watching more intently
      3. Reaching out to feel and touch

III. **Risk factors**
   A. Fussy or apathetic baby needs further investigation.
   B. Mother's fear of abuse of self and baby

IV. **See Injury Prevention Guidelines.**

INJURY PREVENTION

I. **Review safety protocol.**
   A. Age-appropriate precautions
      1. From cradle to crib as baby's size indicates
         a. Cradle in safe area, siblings supervised
      2. Crib
         a. Away from windows with cords from blinds and curtains or drapes that could fall into crib
      3. Sleeping on side or back, not sleeping in bed with adult
      4. Siblings and pets supervised when near baby
      5. Baby not left alone on changing table, bed, couch, bean bag, or floor
      6. Limited use of swings and car seats—too much pressure on lower spine
      7. Supervised exercise on floor or in tub
         a. Water safety: Baby can drown in 1″ of water.
      8. Choking: Good habit to begin keeping small objects out of baby's area. Cords from toys and cradle gyms should be secured.
      9. No smoking in house; check other caregivers.
      10. Prevent caregiver from falling by keeping stairs and floors clear of clutter.
          a. Carry baby so caregiver has one hand free to catch self if he or she trips.

      11. Use chest packs carefully; follow manufacturer's instructions.

      12. Appropriate car seats

II. **See protocol for special at-risk caregivers.**

III. **See protocol for frequency of accidents.**

    A. All injuries are not accidents; check for abuse.

CHILD ABUSE

I. **Age-specific concerns for safe environment**

II. **Physical identification**

    A. Failure to thrive; burns, bruises, apathetic, difficult to comfort

    B. Family presenting with unnecessary visits

    C. Any injury with delayed office visit or unreliable history

III. **At-risk baby**

    A. Difficult to care for, continuing physical problems

IV. **Identify:**

    A. Caregivers, adults, and siblings with at-risk patterns of behavior.

    B. Abuse of other family members

NOTES

| 2-MONTH WELL CHILD VISIT

The continued close symbiotic relationship of parents and baby is character-ized by the stabilization of physical systems and feelings of contentment and pleasure for parents and baby.

I. **Developmental process**
   A. Parents
      1. Deriving pleasure and satisfaction from care of baby
      2. Developing confidence in ability to understand and fulfill baby's needs
      3. Establishing consistent schedule
   B. Baby
      1. Normal developmental pattern
      2. Cries appropriately and quiets easily

II. **Family status**
   A. Lifestyle: Adequate housing and finances to meet needs
   B. Parental roles: Establishing responsibilities; feeling gratification and pride in new roles
   C. Siblings: Parental understanding of siblings' reactions to changes
   D. Concerns and problems: Ability to identify problems and to cope; referrals as needed
   E. Parents
      1. Physical status: Energy level, postpartum examination, family planning
      2. Emotional stability: Satisfactory support system, pride and pleasure in baby
      3. Appropriate plans for returning to work: continuing breast-feeding, sup-plemental feedings, breast pump available; reliable caregiver
      4. Identifying if any member of family is being abused

III. **Health habits**
   A. Nutrition
      1. Mother
         a. Breast-feeding: Understanding of dietary requirements
         b. Weight control
         c. Establishing a feeding schedule
      2. Baby
         a. Formula or breast milk continues to be adequate nutrition, as immatu-rity of gastrointestinal tract and slow development of digestive enzymes can cause difficulties if other food is added.
         b. 0.25 mg of fluoride per office protocol
         c. Check with physician about vitamin D supplementation at 3 months.
         d. Feedings: Showing satisfaction, sucking strength; beginning to establish a schedule
         e. Requirement: 50 cal/lb/day or 110 kcal/kg/day, so a 10-lb baby needs 10 $\times$ 50, or 500 cal, per day; a 4.54-kg baby needs 4.54 $\times$ 110, or 500 cal, per day.

    f. Standard formulas and breast milk have 20 cal/oz.

    g. $\dfrac{500 \text{ cal}}{20 \text{ cal/oz}} = 25$ oz or 750 ml of formula per day

B. Sleep

  1. Mother needs at least one sleep period of 6 hours for sufficient deep sleep.

  2. Baby

    a. Has one sleep period of 6–7 hours and sleeps a total of 14–16 hr/day

    b. Filters out household noises

    c. Awake for longer periods without fussing

C. Elimination

  1. Bowel movements at each feeding; continue to be loose

  2. Urine: Light in color, little odor; strong odor and dark color indicate need to investigate for dehydration.

IV. Growth and development

A. Physical

  1. Central nervous system

    a. Head not held at midline

    b. Arms have random movements

    c. Hands are held in fists, thumbs inside

    d. Startle reflex less intense

  2. Gastrointestinal system

    a. Sucking reflex continues to be strong.

    b. Satisfaction is important; if not met by frequent feedings, pacifier is helpful.

    c. Swallowing from a spoon is difficult because tongue thrust still occurs.

    d. Drooling and taste buds are not present until 3 months of age.

    e. Stomach somewhat larger; now holds 4–6 oz and empties every 3–4 hours

    f. Frequent watery stools continue because intestinal tract is immature and cannot absorb fluids well.

  3. Excretory system

    a. Immature kidney structure affects stability of fluid and solute balance.

    b. Wet diaper at each feeding

    c. Urine: Light in color

  4. Immune system

    a. Antigen–antibody response present by 2 months of age; immunization program per office protocol

    b. Maternal antigens still present in bloodstream

B. Emotional development—Erikson: Basic trust. Close symbiotic relationship of parents and child continues to envelop baby in an environment without stress. Needs of food, warmth, and human contact must be met to continue the establishment of security and trust in baby's new world.

  1. Parents

    a. Able to quiet baby

    b. Make eye contact with baby

      c. Respond to and appreciate baby's developing activities

  2. Baby

      a. Consistent physical growth

      b. Self-quieting

      c. Cries appropriately

C. Intellectual development—Piaget: Baby is learning through sensorimotor response to bodily needs. Eye contact and a responsive smile or irritability are early indications that baby is taking in the world around him or her.

  1. Parents

      a. Understand that crying is instinctive response to discomfort

      b. Take time and interest to understand baby's signal of distress

      c. Spoiling is not an issue at this age; a crying baby needs attention.

  2. Baby

      a. Low patience level; cannot postpone need satisfaction; does not anticipate, so cannot "wait"

      b. Language begins with random vocalizing other than crying.

      c. Begins to make different crying sounds for different needs, such as whimpering for unhappiness and cooing for contentment

D. Risk factors

  1. Parents

      a. Lack of pride in baby

      b. Unresponsive or overresponsive to baby

      c. Low energy level

      d. Inadequate support system

  2. Baby

      a. Poor feeding habits; weak sucking reflex

      b. Lethargic

      c. Cannot be comforted

      d. Stops crying and fussing only with difficulty

      e. Does not respond to soothing music but stops at loud unpleasant noises (such as vacuum cleaner) to shut out the world around him or her

  3. Child abuse indicators

      a. Parents

         (1) Cannot quiet baby

         (2) Overwhelmed by child care and dissatisfied with parental role

         (3) Mother's fear for her own safety

         (4) Isolated from friends and relatives

         (5) History of child abuse in their own lives

         (6) Drug abuse

V. **Physical examination**

A. Growth

  1. Length and weight: Coordinate within two standard deviations on growth chart.

        a. Weight gain 1 oz/day

        b. Length increase 1"/month

    2. Fontanelles: Measure and record.

B. Appearance and behavior

    1. Alertness: Eye contact, responsive smile

    2. Activity level: Smooth, uncoordinated movement with less vigorous movements in legs than in arms

    3. Color: Pink; color changes quickly with activity level and temperature of environment.

C. Specific factors to note during routine physical examination

    1. Head: Configuration and smooth movement; bulging or depressed anterior fontanelle; seborrhea

    2. Eyes: Smooth tracking, reaction to light, dacryostenosis, discharge; tears present from 2–3 months of age

    3. Mouth: Check for thrush (unremovable white spots on tongue). Tongue should be able to protrude beyond lips.

    4. Chest: Respirations: abdominal; irregular rate

    5. Heart: Shunts closed. Refer to physician if abnormal sounds are present that have not been previously diagnosed.

    6. Abdomen: Navel, femoral pulses, hernias, distention

    7. Extremities: Range of motion, smooth movements. Hips: Check leg folds and abduction.

    8. Skin: Rashes, hemangiomas (measure and record), bruises, burns

    9. Neurologic: All reflexes present but less intense

D. Parent–child interaction

    1. Parent: Expression of fatigue and nervousness in handling baby; ability to quiet baby; referrals or home visit as indicated

    2. Baby: Responsive to parent's attention

VI. Assessment

    A. Physical

    B. Developmental

    C. Emotional

    D. Environmental

VII. Plan

    A. Immunization series per office protocol; discuss importance of completing and recording series

    B. Problem list (devised with parent); SOAP for each

    C. Appropriate timing for office, home, or telephone visits

| OVERVIEW

ANTICIPATORY GUIDANCE FOR THE PERIOD OF 2-4 MONTHS

I. **Parents**

    A. Understanding and keeping records of development, description of baby's moods, and reactions to care

II. **Baby**

    A. Physical

        1. Increase in activity level and strength; muscular movements becoming more refined

        2. Reaches out and holds on but does not let go at will

        3. Eating and sleeping schedule being established

    B. Emotional

        1. Becomes upset when mother goes out of sight (see this guideline for details)

        2. Importance of a primary caregiver

    C. Intellectual

        1. By 4 months, the baby's crying when the mother goes out of sight is the beginning of memory development and the baby's striving to control his or her world. Parents must understand that this is a necessary step toward reaching out of self and must not hinder this development with overindulgence.

III. **Risk factors**

    A. No consistent caregiver with whom baby can develop a relationship

IV. **See Injury Prevention Guidelines.**

V. **Watch for:**

    A. From innate reflexive movement to purposeful activity

    B. Repeating activities to create results, such as hitting mobile to cause it to move

    C. Body movements more vigorous but still uncoordinated

    D. Head held at midline so baby can follow moving objects

    E. Finds hands and watches them intently

    F. Arms held out to be picked up

    G. Watches mother intently, follows her, responds to her with vigorous arm and leg movements, attempts to vocalize to her, and turns to her voice

    H. By 4 months, reacts to mother's going out of view

    I. Parents becoming aware of and appreciating the baby's wonderful developmental strides

NOTES

NOTES

|ANTICIPATORY GUIDANCE FOR THE PERIOD OF 2–4 MONTHS

A responsive smile is one of the first important signs that the baby is beginning to take the outside world into account. As babies' physical systems stabilize and mature, their energies are freed, enabling them to become aware of what is going on around them. Although they continue to respond instinctively, they are developing a reactive pattern to the world. They react joyfully and energetically to care that is consistent and loving, but they react with crying and irritability when their basic needs are not met. By 4 months of age, their reactions are less instinctive, and they begin to respond in a manner that will best serve their own purpose.

I. **Expectations of this period**
   A. Parents
      1. Responsive to baby's rhythms and signals
      2. Can define and appreciate baby's individuality
      3. Safety for self and family—fear of abuse
   B. Baby
      1. Responds to primary caregiver with responsive smile, extended eye contact, turning to voice
      2. Comforted and quieted easily
         a. Increased awareness of separation from mother causes distressful crying because object permanence is not yet present.
         b. Parents must understand and appreciate this first clash of wills.
         c. Playing music and keeping baby around family activities may help dispel this feeling of desertion.
         d. Too-frequent changes of caregivers may inhibit the development of this first important step toward attachment.

II. **Family status**
   A. Basic needs being met
      1. If referrals are made, follow up to be sure appropriate help is received.
      2. Adequate support system available
   B. Parents
      1. Adjustment to and enjoyment of new roles
      2. Understanding of symbiotic role of mother and baby and that both will have a broadened emotional base by 4 months
      3. Knowledge and appreciation of childhood developmental tasks
   C. Child abuse indicators
      1. Maladjustment to new roles and responsibilities by parents
         a. Fatigue and poor health in parents
         b. Crankiness in baby
      2. Unrelieved social and emotional pressures
      3. Aggressive pattern of behavior by those in contact with baby
      4. Caregivers abused in their own childhood

III. **Health patterns**
   A. Nutrition

1. Formula or breast milk continues to be adequate nutrition.
2. Do not substitute with cow's milk.
3. Offer water between feedings, particularly in warm weather, because baby loses fluids quickly; color and odor of urine indicate state of hydration.
4. Baby begins to develop pattern of eating five or six times a day. Night feedings continue until larger amount is taken during the day. Stomach has 4- to 6-oz capacity.
5. Hold baby when bottle-feeding to continue development of close parent–baby relationship. Never give baby a bottle in bed: Baby will fall asleep with bottle in mouth, which can lead to tooth decay due to prolonged exposure to lactose, the sugar in milk.
6. If baby continues fussing after and between feedings, investigate other areas of need satisfaction. Schedule office visit if problem continues.

B. Sleep

1. Sleeps for longer periods (8 hours); total of 14–16 hr/day
2. Night feedings discontinued when able to take larger feedings during day
3. Sleeps through family noises; being kept within family activity area or having music played during naps continues ability to sleep through normal sound levels.
4. By 4 months of age, baby is aware of separation from mother and may have difficulty falling asleep. Continued music may help.

C. Elimination

1. Stools: Maturation of gastrointestinal tract allows better fluid absorption, so stools are firmer and less frequent.
2. Urine: Kidneys do not function at mature level until 4 months of age, so dehydration is still a concern.

IV. Growth and development

A. Physical

1. Central nervous system
   a. Myelination continues in a cephalocaudal direction.
   b. Fastest-growing system; adequate nutrition essential for maximum development
   c. Head: From resting on crib to being held at midline
   d. Arms: From random to purposeful movements
   e. Hands: Baby opens and closes hands; thumbs held in grasping position
   f. Extremities: Legs more vigorously active, held off crib
   g. Vision: Bifocal vision develops when head held at midline; mother observes "finding" hands, scrutiny of faces, attraction to colors
   h. Hearing: Sound discrimination (recognizing voices)—mother observes baby turning toward sound of her voice

B. Emotional development

1. Basic trust continues to be established.
2. Primary caregiver provides consistent loving care. Too many different caregivers can interfere with the establishment of basic trust.
3. Baby responds to caregiver by vocalizing, making eye contact, and smiling.

C. Intellectual development

1. Reactive patterns becoming more stable and consistent—quiet or noisy, energetic or passive, joyful or somber

2. Awareness of and attachment to primary caregiver established, but object permanence (memory) not yet present, so there are distress signals if baby observes mother or primary caregiver leaving

3. Language: Experimenting with making sounds; pays close attention to mother's mouth as she talks

D. Risk factors

1. No loving primary caregiver

2. Cranky, inconsolable baby

E. Childrearing practices

1. Consistent schedule; few changes for visits or visitors

2. Touching, rubbing, rocking needed in addition to food and sleep

3. Early intervention for concerns and problems

F. Stimulation

1. Communication and sounds

    a. Sing to child.

    b. Encourage smiling and laughing.

    c. Use music and rhythms only as a quiet background.

    d. Introduce sounds—running water, rattles, household noises.

2. Touch and smell

    a. Cuddling, holding, kissing, stroking

    b. Feed and change from both sides.

3. Sight

    a. Place a single bright object such as a mobile 12″ from eyes; change it frequently.

    b. Move objects in arcs and circles for eyes to follow.

4. Gross motor

    a. Exercise arms and legs while bathing.

    b. Place baby on stomach on a firm surface (preferably the floor, if safe from siblings and animals).

    c. Help baby roll over, first from stomach to back.

    d. Use bounce chair to increase leg strength and enjoyment of body movement.

5. Fine motor

    a. Give baby objects of various textures to handle.

    b. Bring hands together around bottle or toy.

    c. Provide bright objects for eyes to follow.

6. Feeding: Make feeding a relaxed and pleasant time, staying within scheduled time of every 3 or 4 hours.

7. Schedule: A consistent daily routine helps establish body rhythms and anticipatory responses.

8. Watch for baby's cues of overstimulation.

G. Safety

1. Accidents happen most frequently:
   a. When usual routine changes (holidays, vacations, illness in the family)
   b. After stressful events for caregivers
   c. When caregivers are tired or ill
   d. Late in the afternoon

2. Accident prevention
   a. Crib away from window and curtain cords
   b. Fire: Never leave baby in house alone; install smoke alarms.
   c. Always use proper car seat; never hold baby in adult's lap while riding in car; all adults should use seat belts.
   d. Baby seat: Baby strapped in, seat set in safe, protected area
   e. Keep all objects smaller than 2″ out of baby's reach.
   f. Do not leave baby alone on bed or couch. Developing strength makes it possible to roll over or hitch self to edge and roll off.

3. Not all injuries are accidents. Investigate possible child abuse and neglect.

4. Instructions to babysitters

5. Emergency telephone numbers posted

NOTES

OVERVIEW

4-MONTH WELL CHILD VISIT

I. **Parents**
   A. Can describe effects of new baby on all family members
   B. Show appreciation for baby's increasing physical skills, individual temperament, and way of reaching out and getting attention
   C. Identifying any abuse of family members

II. **Baby**
   A. Physical
      1. Increase in weight and height continues on previous pattern on growth chart.
      2. Holding head in midline: Purposeful reaching out
   B. Emotional
      1. Turning to mother when distressed
      2. Fussing when mother goes out of sight
   C. Intellectual
      1. Purposeful repetition of activities
      2. Stimulated to activities by caregiver and bright objects and sounds in environment

III. **Risk factors**
   A. Dissatisfaction by parent with new role
      1. Lacking confidence in ability to provide adequate care
      2. Cannot spend extra time with baby
      3. Fearful of safety for self and baby
   B. Baby difficult to comfort

IV. **See guidelines for specific factors to be noted in physical examination.**

INJURY PREVENTION

I. **Review safety protocol.**
   A. Age-appropriate precautions need special attention as baby increases in strength and activity.
      1. Can push off bed, changing table, couch, etc. to head or foot of crib; gets tangled in blankets
      2. Beginning to get hand to mouth, so all small objects within reach are dangerous
      3. Crib gyms and toys must be removed if baby can reach them.
      4. Reaching out and hitting hot drink of caregivers
      5. Riding backwards in front seat; positioned in back seat if there is an air bag in passenger side of front seat
   B. Put baby in safe place, such as crib or playpen, when left alone, even for a few minutes.
   C. No baby walkers or jumpers

II. See protocol for special at-risk caregivers.

III. See protocol for frequency of accidents.

CHILD ABUSE

I. **Age-specific concerns**

A. Falls: Seldom broken bones at this age in fall from moderate height

II. **Physical identification**

A. Shaken baby syndrome indicated if other family members abused; may have abnormal respiratory pattern and bulging fontanelles

B. Failure to thrive

III. **At-risk baby**

A. All bruises and burns need investigation.

B. Difficult baby to care for, physical problems continue, physical abnormalities

IV. **Identify:**

A. At-risk caregivers

B. Abuse of other family members

NOTES

4-MONTH WELL CHILD VISIT

The close symbiotic relationship of mother and child is changing in the direction of individualization for both of them.

I. **Developmental process**

A. Mother

1. Return to prepregnant health pattern (weight and energy level)
2. Coping with family responsibilities
3. Relating to other family members
4. Developing or returning to outside interests
5. Appreciation of importance to baby of one primary caregiver
6. Returning to work, finding a satisfactory caregiver
7. Able to continue breast-feeding

A. See Breast-Feeding Guidelines.

B. Baby

1. Schedules for feeding and sleeping being established
2. Investigating environment: Reaching out with arms, grasping with hands, searching with eyes
3. Social awareness: Smiling and vocalizing for reaction from parent, crying at separation from family

II. **Family status**

A. Concerns and problems: Ability to identify problems and to cope; understanding of problem-solving techniques; referrals as needed
B. Siblings: Parents' understanding of siblings' adjustment to family changes

1. Time allotted for continuing involvement with them

C. Adequate support system for all members
D. Abuse of any family members identified

III. **Health habits**

A. Nutrition

1. Mother

a. Breast-feeding: Understanding of dietary requirements
b. Weight control: Adequate diet
c. Use of drugs, cigarettes, stimulants

2. Baby

a. Breast milk or formula with iron per office protocol; five feedings daily; amount depends on weight and correlation of weight with length (as shown on growth chart); no other foods needed
b. Water offered between feedings if strong odor and color of urine indicate need for more fluids

B. Sleep

1. One long sleep period of 6–8 hours; total of 15 hr/day
2. Awake for roughly 2-hour periods with less fussing
3. Crying when put to bed, as baby is aware of separation from parent

C. Elimination
   1. Bowel movements are not formed but are less frequent.
   2. Urine Important to note color, odor, amount

IV. **Growth and development**
   A. Physical
      1. Central nervous system: Increased myelination
         a. Holds head at midline while prone; lifts head and chest while supine
         b. Body: Rolls from front to back
         c. Extremities: Arms beginning purposeful reaching; hands open, beginning to grasp; legs held off crib, vigorous kicking
      2. Vision: Bifocal, staring, searching
      3. Speech: Experimenting with sounds; attempting to imitate
      4. Hearing: Localizing sound; quieted by pleasant sounds (voice and music)
   B. Emotional development—Erikson: Basic trust—adaptation through experience. An environment providing adequate physical care and consistent, loving attention fosters the feeling that the world is a safe and dependable place.
      1. Appropriate physical growth
      2. Baby relaxed, easily quieted
      3. Baby turns to caregiver when distressed
   C. Intellectual development—Piaget: From 4–6 months of age, automatic and random reactions are progressing to purposeful repetition of activities to form patterns of intentional action. Baby begins to adapt behavior through the following experiences:
      1. Anticipating and waiting (for feeding, to be picked up)
      2. Fascinating caregivers with sparkling eyes, vigorous body activity, gurgles, and smiles as repetitive response to loving care, or fussing, crying, poor sleeping if this is the only way to have needs met
      3. Repeating activities but cannot instigate them at will
   D. Risk factors
      1. Parents
         a. Dissatisfaction with role; unsure of ability to provide adequate child care
         b. Unresponsive or overresponsive to baby
         c. Cannot tune into baby's signals
         d. Fear of abuse to self or baby
      2. Baby
         a. Feeding problems; failure to thrive
         b. Excessive activity and crying
         c. Difficult to comfort; unresponsive
      3. Child abuse indicators: Parents
         a. Inability to quiet baby; feeding problems
         b. Fatigue; overload of responsibilities
         c. Inadequate support system
         d. Aggression as a reactive pattern

V.   Physical examination
  A. Growth
   1. Length commensurate with established pattern
   2. Weight varying with caloric intake, energy level, and illnesses: Weight within two standard deviations of length
   3. Genetic factors should be considered.
  B. Appearance
   1. Color still easily affected by environment and activity
   2. Movements becoming smooth and coordinated
   3. Legs: Alternate flexing
  C. Specific factors to note during routine physical examination
   1. Anterior fontanelle measurements: Bulging, depressed
   2. Skin: Seborrhea, rashes, bruises, burns
   3. Heart sounds: Refer to physician if murmur present.
   4. Hips: Equal leg folds, full abductions
   5. Extremities: Forefoot adduction
   6. Reflexes: Still present but of diminished intensity; check for head lag and poor muscle tone.
  D. Caregiver–child interaction
   1. Caregiver: Holds baby close to body, makes eye contact when baby responds; able to quiet baby
   2. Baby: Responsive to caregiver's attention
VI.   Assessment
  A. Physical
  B. Developmental
  C. Emotional
  D. Environmental
VII.   Plan
  A. Immunizations
  B. Screening: Laboratory tests and developmental screening as indicated
  C. Problem list (devised with parent); SOAP for each
  D. Appropriate timing for office, home, or telephone visits

NOTES

NOTES

OVERVIEW

ANTICIPATORY GUIDANCE FOR THE PERIOD OF 4–6 MONTHS

I. **Parents**
   A. Responsive to baby's needs
   B. Understanding and appreciating baby's developmental strides
   C. Asking for help if concerned

II. **Baby**
   A. Physical
      1. Increased vigorous body movements
      2. Appropriate weight and height gain
      3. Eating and sleeping with schedule established
   B. Emotional
      1. See guidelines for discussion of separation anxiety.
      2. Responding to attention with smiles, gurgles, reaching out
   C. Intellectual
      1. Beginning of object permanence (memory): Will begin to accept that caregiver's absence is not permanent
      2. Beginning to initiate purposeful activities

III. **Risk factors**
   A. Low growth rate
   B. Apathetic; difficult to comfort
   C. No loving primary caregiver
   D. Not turning outward to investigate environment

IV. **See guidelines for specifics of child-rearing practices and accident prevention.**

V. **Watch for:**
   A. Wonderful period of contented, energetic, healthy baby
   B. Increase in body activity; attempting to roll over
   C. Random activity to purposeful behavior; repeating activity to get desired results
   D. Fussing to get mother back in view
   E. Developing self-quieting routine
   F. Follows moving object but still does not follow if object goes out of line of vision
   G. Coordination of hand–eye movement improving
   H. Positive response of caregiver helps develop baby's confidence in ability to control world and begins building self-esteem.

NOTES

NOTES

ANTICIPATORY GUIDANCE FOR THE PERIOD OF 4-6 MONTHS

This is a delightful period of a now physically well-organized baby who is turning outward to his or her caregivers and environment and finding that his or her activities can influence the outside world.

I. **Expectations of this period**
   A. Parents
      1. Respond to baby's overtures for approval and attention
      2. Concerned at negative behavior; investigate and ask for professional help if unsuccessful in understanding and coping
      3. Provide loving, approving primary caregiver
   B. Baby
      1. Gurgles, smiles, vigorous body movements, and sustained eye contact get responses of approval and attention.
      2. Increased fussing, wakefulness, and poor feeding also get attention and will become a pattern of response if that is the only way attention is obtained.
   C. Separation anxiety: Baby has increased awareness of primary caregiver, and object permanence (memory) is not sufficiently developed for baby to realize that disappearance of caregiver is not permanent.
      1. Parents: Understand problem of separation anxiety; keep crib in family area; family noises not diminished for baby; voice contact and music may help this transitory problem.
      2. Baby: Fusses when left at bedtime; even mother's walking out of room causes tears of anguish.

II. **Family status**
   A. Parents provide adequate environment for each family member.
   B. Parents understand developmental needs of each child.
   C. Sufficient support system exists for parents' needs; not using children as only means of gratification.
   D. Identify sexual abuse to or by any family member.

III. **Health patterns**
   A. Nutrition
      1. Baby continues to require 50 cal/lb or 100 kcal/kg daily.
      2. Breast milk or formula is only food needed until roughly 6 months of age.
      3. Vitamins and fluoride continued per office protocol.
      4. A consistent growth pattern is one of the indicators of the state of nutrition.
      5. Continued fussing or crying after feeding: Investigate reasons other than hunger (discomfort, unsatisfied sucking instinct, need for comfort or cuddling). Schedule office visit if problem continues.
   B. Feeding
      1. Stabilizing schedule: Sleeping through the night (8 hours); as size of stomach increases, larger feedings possible during the day
      2. Tongue thrust diminishing
      3. Taste buds mature; taste discrimination present
      4. Solid foods not needed for proper nutrition; add rice cereal with iron only per office protocol

       5. Be alert to overfeeding. A healthy baby is best able to regulate when and how much to eat. Parents should pay attention to signals and not force extra formula or cereal.

  C. Drooling

      1. Increased activity of salivary glands, not an indication of teething

      2. Up to 2 years before automatic swallowing is present

  D. Sleep: Fussy at bedtime

      1. Try leaving dim light or music on.

      2. Keep baby in crib, but bring to where family is; baby is self-quieting with the security of being near others.

  E. Elimination

      1. Bowel movements are better formed as gastrointestinal tract matures.

      2. Distention caused by undigested foods or illness: Limit diet by eliminating all foods but formula; if it continues, dilute formula with water; call office if no improvement.

      3. Urine: Watch color and amount; if there is a change, increase fluids; call office if no improvement.

IV. **Growth and development**

  A. Physical

      1. Central nervous system still the fastest-growing system; adequate nutrition mandatory for its development

      2. Gross motor skills: Able to sit with support; rolling over; putting weight on feet; enjoying bounce chair

      3. Fine motor skills: Reaching out and grasping; bringing hand to mouth at will

  B. Speech

      1. Experimenting with making sounds; trying to repeat them

      2. Paying attention to mouth action of caregiver; attempting to imitate

      3. Listening to own sounds; attempting to repeat

  C. Emotional development—Erikson: This period is the beginning of the baby's establishment of trust in self. By their beguiling ways, babies enchant their caregivers into providing attention, and they learn to repeat the activities that bring them this attention.

      1. Smiling, vocalizing, making good eye contact

      2. Has a loving, approving primary caregiver with whom a positive response pattern can be developed

  D. Intellectual development—Piaget: Developing object permanence (memory) by finding consistent results from own activities and from those of others

      1. Beginning to realize that if mother leaves, she will return

      2. Anticipating events of daily routine

      3. Spends much time repeating simple activities

         a. Reaching out and touching: Has awareness of sizes, shapes, textures

         b. Listening: Shows recognition of familiar voices and sounds; responds to rhythms

         c. Looking: Is fascinated by faces (even own reflection), varied colors and shapes

    d. Large muscle development: Enjoys free activity, bounce chair, and swing; hitches body to reach out and grasp toys

    e. Body confidence: Enjoys being tossed, swung high (caution: swinging or lifting by arms can dislocate elbows)

  4. Language: Parents respond to baby's vocalizing; baby attempts to imitate and repeat sounds

E. Risk factors

  1. Parents

    a. Inability to cope with problems

    b. Lack of pleasure and satisfaction in child care

    c. Not understanding importance of child development principles

  2. Baby

    a. Physical developmental lag

    b. Nutritional deprivation and inadequate growth pattern

    c. Emotional immaturity: Unresponsive; no eye contact; dominant mood of fussiness

    d. Inadequate child care; no one significant person as caregiver

F. Childrearing practices

  1. Regular schedule with as few interruptions as possible; baby's learning to anticipate events is helped by consistency of schedule.

  2. Demanding of attention: Respond within reason; provide other stimulations, such as variety in toys, sounds, things to look at (for instance, put crib in another part of house).

  3. Weaning: Separation awareness at 4–5 months is a difficult period for baby, so weaning is more easily accomplished at 3 months or at 6 months.

  4. Day care centers: Ratio of caregivers to infants 1:3; visual and auditory stimulation provided; opportunity to exercise (not kept in crib all the time); time for caregiver to hold and cuddle

  5. Babysitter: Careful selection; know personally or get references; set up job description, pay schedule, telephone contacts; spend time with family before left alone with them

G. Stimulation

  1. Communication and sounds

    a. Call child by name.

    b. Tell child what you are doing; name objects.

    c. Point out various sounds—whispering, the wind, cars, animals.

    d. Keep background of soft music: music that is too loud prevents learning from usual sounds of environment.

  2. Touch and smell

    a. Rub baby with different textures—silk, feather, wood, yarn.

    b. Play touching games such as "this little piggy."

    c. Point out various odors—flowers, clothes, foods.

  3. Sight

    a. Move crib around room; move infant to different rooms and near windows.

    b. Use bright sheets, blankets, clothing.

      c. Hold baby up to a mirror to see reflection.

  4. Gross motor

      a. Sitting position for short periods

      b. Sits up on a mat on the floor

      c. Time spent on protected area on floor for large muscle activity

  5. Fine motor

      a. Colorful plastic keys on a ring

      b. Cradle gym

H. Safety

  1. Accidents happen most frequently:

      a. When usual routine changes (holidays, vacations, illness in family)

      b. After stressful events for caregivers

      c. When caregivers are tired or ill

      d. Late in the afternoon

  2. Accident prevention

      a. Crib should be away from open window and curtain cords.

      b. Fire: Never leave baby in house alone. Install smoke alarms.

      c. Never take baby in car without proper car seat. Do not hold baby in adult's lap in car. All adults should use seat belts.

      d. Baby seat: Baby strapped in; seat set in safe, protected area

      e. Keep objects smaller than 2″ out of baby's reach.

      f. Be alert to baby's developing ability to become self-propelled.

  3. Not all injuries are accidents. Investigate possible child abuse and neglect.

  4. Instructions to babysitters

  5. Emergency telephone numbers posted

NOTES

OVERVIEW

6-MONTH WELL CHILD VISIT

I. **Parents**
   A. Appreciation of baby's developing personality and skills
   B. Providing safe environment for increased mobility of baby
   C. Identifying any abuse of family members

II. **Baby**
   A. Physical
      1. Sits without support
      2. Transfers objects from one hand to the other
      3. Teething
         a. Makes for a cranky baby
         b. Increased incidence of upper respiratory infection
   B. Emotional
      1. Keen observer of what is going on around him or her
      2. Responds to music and motion
      3. Turns to caregiver for support and comfort
   C. Intellectual
      1. Random activities replaced by purposeful actions
         a. One of first such actions as teeth erupt is learning not to bite nipple when breast-feeding

III. **Risk factors**
   A. Poor weight gain
   B. Frequent illnesses
   C. Check safety guidelines

IV. **See guidelines for specific factors to be noted in physical examination.**

INJURY PREVENTION

I. **Review safety protocol.**
   A. Age-appropriate precautions
      1. Increased activity of creeping, rolling over, sitting up, reaching out, and ability to get hands to mouth make constant supervision necessary.
      2. Time to baby-proof house—see protocol.
      3. Crib
         a. When baby can pull self to sitting, kneeling, standing position, have mattress low enough so he or she cannot fall out.
         b. Remove bumpers that baby could climb on.
         c. Remove toys on strings or cords to avoid choking.
         d. Keep sides of crib up and securely locked.
         e. Have crib in safe area, away from drapes and cords from blinds.
      4. Have safe place to put baby when he or she must be left alone, even for a few minutes.

     5. Baby needs freedom to investigate world around him or her; gates and doors keep baby in safe area.

     6. Cover electrical outlets with protectors; pad sharp edges of furniture; keep cords, such as lamps and telephones, out of reach.

     7. Developmentally, baby cannot remember "no" or "don't touch" to prevent repeating activity.

       a. Begin using a particular tone of voice that means "no" or "stop."

       b. Behavior control not yet established

     8. Use appropriate car seat.

II. **See protocol for special at-risk caregivers.**

III. **See protocol for frequency of accidents.**

    A. Not all injuries are accidents; check for abuse.

CHILD ABUSE

I. **Age-specific concerns**

II. **Physical identification**

    A. Injuries with delayed treatment and confused history of accident

    B. All bruises and burns investigated

    C. Fearful child, uncontrolled crying during examination

    D. Sudden infant death syndrome: investigate, as family members may be abused.

III. **At-risk baby**

    A. Difficult to care for; physical disabilities

    B. Overactivity—difficult to feed and to get to sleep

    C. Poor sleeping pattern

    D. Frequent illnesses

IV. **Identify:**

    A. At-risk caregivers

    B. Abuse of other family members

NOTES

6-MONTH WELL CHILD VISIT

Children of this age have a less vibrant personality and are becoming students, concentrating on what is going on around them. Repetitive activities replace random movements.

I. **Developmental process**
   A. Parents
      1. Understand developmental principles and appreciate baby's accomplishments
      2. Developing a philosophy of childrearing practices
      3. Provide adequate stimulation and safe environment
   B. Baby
      1. Sits propped up or in baby seat, scrutinizing all that can be touched and seen (particularly primary caregiver)

II. **Family status**
   A. Basic needs being met
   B. Marital stability
   C. Single parent
      1. Needs being identified and goals established
      2. Referrals: Provide with follow-up
      3. Visits scheduled to provide support and help in establishing healthy childrearing practices
      4. Reporting fear of abuse
   D. Parents
      1. Concerns and problems: Ability to identify problems and to cope
      2. Realistic assessment and appropriate expectations of baby's development
      3. Deriving satisfaction and pleasure from parental role
      4. Mother's interests defined as student, working, special interests
      5. Child care arrangements: day care center, babysitters
      6. Fear of abuse identified

III. **Health habits**
   A. Nutrition—diet history
      1. Breast-feeding: Supplementary formula, weaning
      2. Formula: Number of feedings and amount
      3. Vitamins and fluoride per office protocol
      4. Other foods: Rice cereal with iron the first food
   B. Sleep
      1. Sleeps for 8-hour period at night
      2. Awake for 4-hour periods
      3. Less fussing when put to bed; self-quieting routine being established
   C. Elimination
      1. Bowel movements less frequent, better formed; distention and flatulence with diet change
      2. Urine better concentrated; color and odor used as indicators of hydration

IV. **Growth and development**

    A. Physical

        1. Central nervous system

           a. Vertical position possible, with ability to sit and hold head erect

           b. Puts weight on legs; stands with support

           c. Grasps with both hands; transfers from one hand to another

        2. Teething

           a. Usually the first teeth cause physical discomfort and succeeding eruptions are less difficult; chilled pacifier is helpful.

           b. Importance of night bottle syndrome understood

        3. Period of low immunity, causing susceptibility to infections

        4. Vision: Improved distance vision and depth perception; staring at objects or movement at distance

        5. Speech

           a. One-syllable babbling; attempts to imitate sounds

           b. Watches intently the mouth of someone speaking to him

    B. Emotional development—Erikson: Establishment of basic trust is evident by baby's turning out to explore environment. Baby is eager to touch, feel, and taste all within reach. Baby watches caregivers in particular. Establishing a close attachment to one person who can give support to explorations is a preliminary step toward the next developmental task of beginning the path toward independence.

        1. Eager to touch, feel, and mouth all things within reach

        2. Watches results of activity with surprise and pleasure

        3. Responds to mood of caregiver

        4. Keen observer of activities of caregiver

    C. Intellectual development—Piaget: Development of object permanence (memory). Repetition of activities and finding consistency of results replace random movements with purposeful activity. Baby attempts to repeat the kind of activity that affects the care and attention he or she receives.

        1. Daily schedule important

        2. Responding to familiar voices and sounds

        3. Crying and fussing more selectively

        4. Delight at return of primary caregiver

        5. Language: May be less vocal, as main concern is observing environment and caregivers

    D. Risk factors

        1. Parents

           a. Unresponsive to baby's cues

           b. Restless at confinement of parental role

           c. Overprotective: Keeping as "baby"; giving little stimulation or opportunity for physical activity or new adventure

           d. Not providing one consistent caregiver

2. Baby
    a. Not attempting to reach out
    b. Lack of body confidence; rigid body movement
    c. Unsatisfied needs; whiny
    d. Restless sleep
    e. No loving, approving primary caregiver
  E. Child abuse indicators: Parents
    1. Low self-esteem; lack of confidence and competence in managing their world
    2. Rigid response pattern
    3. Marital conflict
    4. Fatigue; overload of responsibilities
    5. Inadequate support system
    6. Child abuse in parent's childhood

V. Physical examination
  A. Growth: Continues on established pattern; check for excess or inadequate weight gain
  B. Appearance and behavior
    1. Chubby
    2. Sits with support
    3. Good head control
    4. Happy, bright-eyed; delightful member of the family; not generally fussy or fearful
  C. Specific factors to note during routine physical examination
    1. Anterior fontanelles: Bulging, depressed
    2. Skin: Seborrhea, rashes, bruises, burns
    3. Eyes: Equal tracking
    4. Teeth: May be erupting; gums swollen
    5. Heart sounds: Refer to physician if murmur present.
    6. Hips: Equal leg folds, full abductions
    7. Extremities: Forefoot adduction
    8. Reflexes: Disappearance of tonic neck reflex, Moro reflex; sucking and rooting (when awake), palmar grasp still present
  D. Parent–child interaction
    1. Mother holds baby less closely; is willing to have others care for baby.
    2. Baby responds to others but still turns to mother for comfort.

VI. Assessment
  A. Physical
  B. Developmental
  C. Emotional
  D. Environmental

VII. Plan
  A. Immunizations and laboratory tests as needed

B. Problem list (devised with parent); SOAP for each
C. Appropriate timing for office, home, or telephone visits

NOTES

| OVERVIEW

ANTICIPATORY GUIDANCE FOR THE PERIOD OF 6–8 MONTHS

I. **Parents**
   A. Understand physical changes
   B. Ask for help as needed
   C. Show pride in and affection for baby
II. **See guidelines for specifics of stranger anxiety.**
III. **Baby**
   A. Physical
      1. Increased activity, losing chubbiness
      2. Rolls over and reaches out to obtain what he or she wants
      3. Teething and illnesses less a problem by 8 months
      4. See guidelines for introduction of new foods and homemade baby food.
   B. Emotional
      1. Illnesses, new activities, and adventures broadening emotional responses
      2. Needs primary caregiver for comfort and support
   C. Intellectual
      1. Watch persistence in trial and error to accomplish new skills. Frequent failures can cause frustration and fussiness.
IV. **Risk factors**
   A. Safety
   B. Frequent illnesses
V. **See guidelines for specifics of child-rearing practices and safety protocols.**
VI. **Importance of understanding tone of voice**
   A. Baby responds to caregiver's tone of voice.
   B. Baby's behavior control not established
VII. **Watch for:**
   A. Cranky, fussy periods caused by:
      1. Teething
      2. Illnesses—ear infections, upper respiratory infections
      3. Introduction of solid foods (stomach ache, distention)
      4. Increased mobility (cuts, bruises)
      5. Less able to be distracted from desired quest
   B. Turns to caregiver for comfort

NOTES

NOTES

ANTICIPATORY GUIDANCE FOR THE PERIOD OF 6–8 MONTHS

I. **Expectations of this period**

    A. Baby

        1. Increased awareness; insatiable desire to investigate, reaching out to touch, taste, scrutinize

        2. Baby is increasingly fussy. He or she wants to reach out and experiment and is frustrated when unable to do so.

    B. Parents

        1. Positive reinforcement of baby's accomplishments

        2. Provide stimulating but safe environment

    C. Stranger anxiety

        1. By 8 months of age, object permanence (memory) is present. Baby can identify from whom he or she most often receives attention and comfort and appears to concentrate attention on this one person. Other adults seem to interfere with his or her efforts to form a close attachment to this primary caregiver and so are rejected.

        2. This attachment is the beginning of the baby's forming the emotional capability for future relationships of trust and love.

        3. Lack of stranger anxiety can indicate that the baby has no one significant caregiver.

        4. Critical caregiver misunderstanding of this crying can hinder baby's trust in environment.

II. **Family status**

    A. Basic needs being met; assess coping ability; referrals as needed

    B. Problem-solving techniques used

    C. Parents

        1. Appreciate and evaluate child's developmental progress

        2. Understand individuality of each child

    D. Identify sexual abuse to or by any family member.

III. **Health patterns**

    A. Nutrition

        1. Breast-feeding: Solids should be introduced by 6 months; breast milk is low in iron and may not contain enough protein for the baby's needs.

        2. Weaning: There is no right time for weaning; it depends on the mother's schedule and feelings and the baby's cues. Delay if the baby is fussy from teething or ill. Do it slowly, over a week or more. Follow office protocol for change from breast milk to formula.

        3. Vitamins and fluoride continued per office protocol

    B. Introduction of new foods

        1. Add one new food at a time (per week) so any allergic reaction can be identified.

        2. Cereal is the first new food; start with iron-fortified rice cereal, which is the least allergenic cereal. Use dry cereal mixed with apple juice, formula, or breast milk. Begin with 1–2 tbsp once a day, increasing gradually to a third or a half cup total, fed twice a day. If this is tolerated, barley or oatmeal can be tried.

3. Vegetables or fruits are the second food; 1 tsp at a time, working up to 3–4 tbsp of fruits and vegetables by 1 year of age.

   a. Vegetables should be introduced first, because they are harder to learn to like than fruits, which are sweeter. Begin with green ones, then yellow.

   b. Fruits: Bananas and applesauce are constipating; pears, peaches, and prunes are bowel softeners.

4. Egg yolk can be given at 6 months of age; hard-boil and strain over foods. Delay introduction of egg whites until all other foods have been introduced.

5. Meats: Introduce last. Try all kinds. Buy jars of meat; mixed dinners have only small amounts of meat.

6. Do not feed from the jar unless the whole jar is to be used, because saliva from the spoon stays in the jar and can cause spoilage. Refrigerate any food not used.

7. Most commercially prepared baby foods contain no preservatives and are acceptable. Do not season with salt or sugar: these are unnecessary and can lead to poor eating habits.

C. Homemade baby foods

1. Equipment needed

   a. Electric blender, food processor, or food mill

   b. Clean pans for cooking

   c. Utensils: Vegetable brush, spatula, peeler, knife

   d. Ice cube trays, preferably with separate "pop-out" cubes

2. Freezing and serving

   a. After food is prepared and pureed, pour into ice cube trays.

   b. Freeze quickly.

   c. Pop out frozen cubes and put into plastic freezer bags; label and date.

   d. Each cube contains about 3 tbsp.

   e. Before a meal, take out food cubes and thaw in the refrigerator or warm in a warming dish or in an egg poacher over hot water.

   f. Cubes travel well for short trips; they defrost quickly.

3. Food preparation

   a. Fruits

      (1) Fresh fruits retain the best nutritional value, but juice-packed canned or frozen fruits may also be used.

      (2) Cooked fresh or canned fruits blend very well into a fine puree.

      (3) Do not add sugar; babies prefer the natural sweetness in fruits.

      (4) Pureed fruits can be added to cottage cheese or plain yogurt (a good source of protein, calcium, and riboflavin).

   b. Vegetables

      (1) Fresh vegetables have the best nutritional quality; frozen vegetables are more convenient; canned vegetables are already cooked and need only be pureed.

      (2) Use canned vegetables that have no salt.

    c. Meats, poultry

        (1) Meats tend to shred in the blender rather than purée; if ground first, they are easier to purée; add 1 cup of liquid per pound of ground meat.

        (2) Chicken livers purée very well.

        (3) Meats should be cooked by braising or roasting, not frying; no seasoning is necessary.

    d. Fish

        (1) Should be poached or baked; preferably cod, haddock, or flounder

        (2) Do not give shellfish to infants (can cause allergies).

        (3) One pound of fish yields about eight food cubes.

    e. All foods can be combined to make stewlike dinners. Meat, potato, and vegetable, for example, can be puréed together; seasoning is unnecessary.

  4. Freezer life of home-prepared baby foods

    a. Temperature must be 0°F or below; use a true freezer or a separate-door freezer/refrigerator combination; freezer compartment inside refrigerator does not stay cold enough.

    b. Timetable for keeping foods

        (1) Fruits: 6 months

        (2) Vegetables: 4 months

        (3) Meats: 3 months

        (4) Liver: 1 month

        (5) Fish: 1 week

        (6) Poultry: 3 months

        (7) Dried beans, peas, etc.: 3 months

        (8) Combination dinners: 2 months

  5. Suggested reading

    a. Castle S. *The Complete Guide to Preparing Baby Foods at Home.* New York: Bantam, 1992.

    b. Lansky V. *Feed Me! I'm Yours:* New York: Bantam, 1994.

    c. Satter E. *Child of Mine: Feeding with Love and Good Sense.* Palo Alto, CA: Bull, 1991.

D. Establishing good eating habits

  1. Baby will take sufficient food for needs. When satiated, he or she does not take food from spoon and pulls back. Do not force food.

  2. Babies are messy and will spit out food, throw food, upset dish, not sit still.

  3. Always use a quiet, matter-of-fact manner.

  4. Nutritional patterns established during infancy can have lifelong effects.

    a. Feeding is a learned experience; each child develops at his or her own rate.

    b. Food preferences are acquired.

    c. Ethnic patterns influence food preferences.

E. Sleep

  1. Less fussing at bedtime; may need favorite toy or blanket

       2. Sleeps through the night; awakes early, does not cry; can amuse self for a short period

       3. Still needs two naps

  F. Elimination

       1. New foods are usually no problem if added slowly; if a problem does occur, eliminate the new food and try again later in small amounts.

       2. Urine: Continue to check amount, color, and odor for indication of hydration.

IV. Growth and development

  A. Physical

       1. Teething: Baby's first experience with pain; usually the first tooth is the most bothersome (Table 1-1). Reduce gum swelling and pain by providing a cold, wet cloth to chew on or a chilled pacifier.

       2. Low immunity: Susceptible to infections; immune system still immature and protection from maternal antigens diminished

       3. Gross motor skills: Progressing from immobile to self-propelled; sitting to creeping to crawling to standing is a long period of trial and error.

       4. Fine motor skills: Use of hands to reach out, grasp, and let go at will; touching as means of investigating; reaching out as a perceptual motor skill

       5. Speech

          a. Attempts to duplicate sounds; repeats syllables such as dada, mama

Table 1-1. Schedule of teeth eruption

Teeth	Age
Primary	
Lower central incisors	5–10 months
Upper central incisors	8–12 months
Upper lateral incisors	8–12 months
Lower lateral incisors	12–14 months
Lower & upper first molars	12–14 months
Lower & upper canines	16–22 months
Lower & upper second molars	24–30 months
Secondary	
First molars	5–7 years
Central incisors	6½–8 years
Lateral incisors	7–9 years
First bicuspids	9–11 years
Second bicuspids	10–12 years
Canines	10–12 years
Cuspids	11–14 years
Second molars	11–13 years
Third molars	16–21 years (or later)

      b. Babbles contentedly to self on waking

B. Emotional development—Erikson: Establishment of basic trust gives baby assurance to investigate environment. This is done tentatively, with looking back at or returning to caregiver for reassurance. A significant caregiver is needed to provide encouragement for these new adventures.

  1. Increased awareness of movement, color, sounds

    a. Keen observer of movement, color, sounds

    b. Reaching out to touch and hold

    c. Fascinated by looking at and picking up small objects

  2. A dangerous period, because baby can physically get to more places and cannot be trusted not to "do it again"

C. Intellectual development—Piaget: Object permanence (memory) is becoming better developed, and baby uses repetitive actions to establish purposeful activity.

  1. Repetitive actions are building up memory of cause and effect.

  2. Develops control by persistent trial and error; gets to sitting position unaided; manages to crawl in the right direction and around obstacles. Frequent failures cause increase in frustration and fussiness.

  3. Increase in watching and studying caregiver

  4. Sitting up improves depth perception, so studies things in motion carefully

  5. Language

    a. Enjoys being talked and sung to; responds to rhythms

    b. Attention to goings on in environment supersedes concentration on vocal development.

    c. Responds to caregiver's tone of voice

D. Risk factors

  1. Parents

    a. Cannot cope with baby's periods of frustration

    b. Fail to provide stimulating environment; baby given no opportunity to move about freely

    c. Child abuse indicators present

  2. Baby

    a. Physical developmental lag

    b. Passive—does not attempt to reach out and investigate

    c. Lack of loving, approving, consistent caregiver

E. Childrearing practices

  1. Increased fussy periods can be due to frustration at not being able to get at or have what he or she wants.

  2. The baby's being persistent and difficult to distract makes life more complicated for caregivers and baby.

  3. Use tone of voice to show approval or disapproval of baby's activities.

  4. Environment important

    a. Area large enough to satisfy new skill of crawling

    b. Safety the main factor

      (1) Baby cannot be trusted to control behavior.

        (2) Eliminate all small objects, because everything possible is put in mouth.

        (3) Almost constant surveillance is necessary; siblings and babysitters need careful instructions.

F. Stimulation

  1. Communication and sounds

    a. Praise language attempts, but do not overemphasize.

    b. Provide toys that make noise or music.

    c. Sing and talk to baby; demonstrate rhythms.

  2. Touch and smell

    a. Provide various motions, such as swinging, water play, dancing.

    b. Tickling and touching games

    c. Textured and patterned objects to handle

    d. Identify different odors.

  3. Sight

    a. Alternate toy selection—divide into groups, change groups frequently.

    b. Mirror play

    c. Indicate outdoor objects in motion—trucks, cars, birds, airplanes.

  4. Gross motor

    a. Rock back and forth on beach ball on stomach.

    b. Support while sitting; sitting alone

    c. Water play

    d. Rides on adult's shoulders

    e. Jumper swing—feet supported

    f. Open, safe area for crawling

  5. Fine motor

    a. Blocks, lids, pans to bang

    b. Various-sized containers to fill and empty

    c. Small objects of various shapes to handle (too large to be swallowed)

  6. Feeding

    a. Offer cup.

    b. Finger foods: Crackers or hard toast (zwieback), especially when teething

    c. Baby dips fingers into foods and brings them to mouth.

G. Safety

  1. Accidents happen most frequently:

    a. When usual routine changes (holidays, vacations, illness in family)

    b. After stressful events for caregivers

    c. When caregivers are tired or ill

    d. Late in the afternoon

  2. Accident prevention

    a. Baby-proof house

    b. Mobility: Be prepared for unexpected mobility of baby; new skills make constant surveillance necessary.

    c. Be aware that all objects picked up go into the mouth.

    d. Choking: First-aid instruction per office protocol

    e. Water safety: Never leave baby alone in tub or wading pool.

    f. Provide safe spot for baby when caregiver is out of sight (playpen, crib).

    g. Use proper car seat at all times.

3. Investigate possibility of child abuse and neglect if many bruises or burns are present, if child is extremely resistant to strangers, or if child has rigid body and movements.

4. Instructions to babysitters

5. Emergency telephone numbers posted

NOTES

OVERVIEW

8-MONTH WELL CHILD VISIT

I. **Parents**

A. Understand baby's new needs of a safe environment to explore and investigate

  1. Understand the baby's frustrations and anxiety from these new adventures

B. Baby rejects all other adults and turns only to primary caregiver for comfort.

C. Primary caregiver needed to provide safety and encouragement

D. Identify any abuse of family members

II. **Baby**

A. Physical

  1. Increased mobility: Persistent in exploring

  2. Increased interest in food

  3. Difficulty falling asleep

B. Emotional

  1. Developing confidence in own capabilities

  2. Finding ways to gain control of world, such as refusing food, crying at parents' leaving, staying awake at night

C. Intellectual

  1. Increase in memory, helping him or her to rely on world and repeat activities, either positive or negative, that get attention

III. **Risk factors**

A. Parents' unrealistic expectations of baby

B. Lack of primary caregiver for baby to rely on

IV. **See guidelines for specific factors to be noted in physical examination**

INJURY PREVENTION

I. **Review safety protocol.**

A. Age-appropriate precautions

  1. Toddlers cannot be trusted.

  2. Consistent behavior control is not established.

  3. Natural curiosity and energy lead to unexpected activities.

B. Caregivers

  1. Constant supervision necessary

  2. Reaction to injury is imitated by child.

    a. Calmly and reassuringly take care of situation; promotes confidence in child's world

    b. Overresponse can also be imitated.

  3. Begin to establish off-limit areas.

  4. Provide a safe place where child can be placed in an emergency or when left alone.

C. Most common accidents
   1. Poisons
      a. Put all poisons in house in locked cupboard.
      b. Pocketbooks can contain dangerous pills.
   2. Falls
      a. Toddlers tumble and fall easily, but refer if child has fallen on head or does not respond to voice.
      b. Gates, doors, window screen guards necessary
   3. Burns
      a. Avoid carrying hot liquid or food near child.
      b. Stoves, wall heaters, floor heaters, cooking utensils, wood stoves protected
   4. Fires
      a. Test batteries in smoke alarms monthly.
      b. No smoking in house
      c. Fire drills established
D. Safety checks
   1. Lead paint, if in older house or apartment
   2. Gates on stairs: Give child time to climb stairs under surveillance.
   3. Electrical outlets capped
   4. Cleaning fluids, soaps, medicines behind secured doors
   5. Appropriate car seat used at all times
   6. Safe place to put baby while not in caregiver's sight, such as playpen or crib

CHILD ABUSE

I. **Physical identification**
   A. Broken bones not usual in toddler's frequent falls and tumbles
   B. Bruises and burns may be caused by careless caregiver, but investigation is important.
II. **At-risk child**
   A. Difficult child to care for
   B. Unsafe environment
   C. Inadequate medical care
III. **Identify:**
   A. At-risk caregiver
   B. Abuse of other family members

NOTES

NOTES

8-MONTH WELL CHILD VISIT

This is a watershed period in which the physical and emotional patterns developed over the past 8 months provide new skills. With increased physical abilities and the establishment of basic trust, infants begin, in their own way, to test out and develop their capabilities. Erikson defines this process as moving from the stage of basic trust to the new stage of autonomy.

I. **Developmental process**

    A. Parents

        1. Understand baby's new needs

            a. Provide adequate, safe environment for exploring

            b. Accept baby's periods of frustrations and anxiety caused by new adventures

            c. Develop a philosophy of childrearing to promote positive behavior patterns

            d. Report abuse to self or family

    B. Baby

        1. Eager to move about; frustrated at confinement

        2. Persistent, less distractible

II. **Family status**

    A. Parental concerns and problems: Ability to identify problems and to cope

    B. Parental and sibling roles redefined to accommodate the increased activity and safety needs of baby

    C. Child care arrangements adequate to provide safety and promote development

III. **Health habits**

    A. Nutrition

        1. Diet history; tolerance and acceptance of new foods. Minced foods (including meat), enriched breads, potatoes, rice, and macaroni should be introduced, as well as cottage cheese, soft cheese, and egg yolks.

        2. Eating habits can be a battleground between parents and baby; parents should accept and outwit an uncooperative, independent baby.

        3. Nutritional needs: Decrease amount of breast milk or formula to 12–16 oz/day; introduce cup.

    B. Sleep

        1. Difficulty "turning off" to fall asleep

        2. Awake for periods during the night

        3. Fretful sleep—carryover from daytime activities

    C. Elimination

        1. General curiosity includes curiosity about feces

        2. Parents should understand the physical and emotional components of toilet training (see anticipatory guidance for the period of 14–18 months).

    D. Dental care

        1. Importance of night bottle syndrome understood

        2. Teething: Number of teeth; problems during eruptions

IV. **Growth and development**
   A. Physical
      1. Central nervous system: Myelination to extremities (giving strength and control)
      2. Immune system: Maternal antigens decreased; baby developing own immunity; particularly susceptible to upper respiratory infections
      3. Hematopoietic system: Maternal red blood cells decreased; baby now developing sufficient red blood cells for own needs; iron-fortified foods per office protocol
      4. Vision: Eye–hand coordination and depth perception improving
      5. Hearing: Reacts to whisper test; localizes sounds
   B. Emotional development—Erikson: With the security of basic trust, baby is free to:
      1. Become aware of the differences in people and sense their importance to him or her. For babies with strong support from a specific adult, other adults do not provide the same feeling of security—hence, stranger anxiety.
      2. Move physically out into the environment, eager to use new physical skills to explore
      3. Develop a sense of own capabilities
      4. Expand emotional responses to new experiences
         a. Frustration in the long process of learning new skills
         b. Anxiety at leaving the safety of physical and emotional supports— walking without mother's hand, watching mother put on her coat to leave baby with someone else
         c. Affection: Returning to parent for encouragement and support
   C. Intellectual development—Piaget: Progressing from equilibrium to disequilibrium as new physical and emotional development produces new challenges
      1. Intentional behavior replaces random responses with increasing ability to form patterns of behavior.
      2. Persistent repetition practicing new skills
      3. Language
         a. Repeats definite sounds; begins to understand the meanings of a few words (although unable to use them), such as no, good, bye-bye
         b. Regularly stops activity when name is called
   D. Risk factors
      1. Parents
         a. Unrealistic expectations of baby's control of behavior: over- or underprotective; coerces baby to perform desired behavior
         b. Dissatisfied with role of parenting in this new phase (end of baby's complete dependency)
         c. History of child abuse in own family
      2. Baby
         a. Not exhibiting drive to investigate surroundings
         b. A "too-good" baby—shallow emotional responses
         c. Dull personality; irritable; unloving
         d. No primary caregiver with whom to form loving relationship

V.   Physical examination
   A. Growth: Continuing on established pattern; length, weight, and head circumference within two standard deviations
   B. Appearance and behavior
      1. Less rotund; beginning to lengthen out
      2. Activity level: Difficult to keep baby lying down on examination table, quieter on mother's lap
      3. Serious scrutiny of strangers; difficult to establish eye contact
   C. Specific factors to note during routine physical examination
      1. Skin: Excessive bruising or burns, carotenemia
      2. Eyes: Equal tracking without strabismus
      3. Teeth: Central incisors present
      4. Ears: Mobility of tympanic membrane, ability to locate sound
      5. Musculoskeletal: Bearing weight on legs; hips—Ortolani's click, equal gluteal folds; tibial torsion, genu varum, externally rotated hips; stance, gait
      6. Genitalia: Female—irritation, discharge; male—phimosis, descended testes
      7. Reflexes: Presence of parachute reflex; sucking and rooting no longer present
   D. Parent–child interaction
      1. Baby turns to parent for support when frightened
      2. Cheerful, pleasant rapport between parent and child
VI.   Assessment
   A. Physical
   B. Developmental
   C. Emotional
   D. Environmental
VII.   Plan
   A. Screening: Hematocrit, lead, urine, developmental as indicated
   B. Problem list (devised with parent); SOAP for each
   C. Appropriate timing for office, home, or telephone visits
      1. Continued close contact during this critical period
      2. Visits planned according to needs of family and developmental and physical needs of baby
      3. Home visits to assess environment as indicated

OVERVIEW

ANTICIPATORY GUIDANCE FOR THE PERIOD OF 8–14 MONTHS

I. **Parents**

    A. Must learn the importance of this period so they can continue their appreciation and understanding of their baby's free-wheeling activities. During this period, a quiet, consistent schedule is important.

II. **Baby**

    A. Physical

        1. Needs safe environment but with opportunity to investigate, examine, and use stored-up energy

    B. Emotional

        1. Slowly beginning to accept behavior control for kind support and gentle reinforcement of appropriate behavior

    C. Intellectual

        1. Recall of previous results of a particular activity

        2. Responds to caregiver's voice; upset by disapproval

III. **Risk factors**

    A. Parents lack understanding and have unrealistic expectations.

    B. Baby lacks energy and curiosity in his or her environment.

IV. **See guidelines for specific factors on caregiving arrangements.**

V. **Watch for:**

    A. Baby is less cranky; usually no problem with teething and developing immune system helps prevent illnesses.

    B. Development of speech decreases as baby concentrates on new physical activities.

    C. Broader emotional reactions, such as affection, stubbornness, fear, anger

    D. Reaction to positive or negative reinforcement as a good kid versus a naughty one

    E. Improved memory: Will look for object when taken away and hidden

    F. Strong attachment to mother; other adults, even usual caregiver or grandmother, causes outburst of crying.

NOTES

NOTES

ANTICIPATORY GUIDANCE FOR THE PERIOD OF 8–14 MONTHS

These 6 months are a critical period for both parents and baby, because it is during this time that a cooperative working relationship between parent and child needs to be established. Babies, with their new skills of moving about, are eager to investigate their surroundings in their own way, at their own pleasure, without any interference. Parents must protect the baby during these adventures and must help him or her learn that only acceptable behavior will receive rewards and praise. In turn, the baby is learning that his or her need for approval and affection may be worth the effort of accepting these constraints. It is through this willingness to compromise that the baby experiences the wonderful feelings of self-worth and self-confidence.

I. **Expectations of this period**

  A. Parental tasks

   1. Provide a safe environment that gives baby the opportunity to use new motor skills of crawling, climbing, and walking and that also satisfies baby's need to investigate by touching, tasting, and manipulating

   2. Provide a reliable and consistent caregiver who will be aware of the baby's activities at all times and who will provide positive reinforcement for appropriate behavior

   3. Provide a routine schedule that the baby can anticipate; this will help baby accept daily events and develop a sense of consistency in the world.

   4. Provide freedom of activity within this environment and schedule so that there is as little opportunity for rebellion and frustration as possible

   5. Understand the developmental stages so that unattainable tasks are not expected (such as toilet training, table manners, sharing, reliable behavior control)

   6. Understand that attention given to a particular activity will cause this activity to be repeated. Rewards and praise for a behavior will help establish this behavior as a pattern. Unacceptable behavior will also be repeated if that is the only way that attention is gained.

   7. Provide a primary caregiver who will give encouragement and comfort and who will accept the baby's attempts to express affection

  B. Baby's developmental tasks

   1. Master the physical skills of walking and using the hands to carry and manipulate objects

   2. Use new physical skills and self-confidence to investigate surroundings

   3. Learn by repetition of an activity to anticipate its result

   4. Develop a close relationship with and affection for someone outside self through consistent interaction with that person

  C. The nurse practitioner can now plan extended office visits, or preferably home visits, so as to be a resource for and support to the parents in understanding and coping during this critical period of growth.

II. **Family status**

  A. Basic needs being met

   1. Referrals: If made, follow up to ensure appropriate help is received.

   2. Adequate support system available

B. Family unit
  1. Mother
    a. Satisfied with lifestyle; confident, cheerful, energetic
    b. Support system intact; outside interests present
    c. Maturation level: Own needs being met; can view baby objectively and not as the only means of satisfying her needs
    d. Coping with confusion of women's role in today's society—women's rights, career planning, divorce, separation, men's changing role
  2. Working mother
    a. Satisfied with child care arrangements
    b. Adjusting to physical stress of two jobs
    c. Able to express and work through emotional reactions, such as guilt at leaving home, distress if going to work is a necessity, and satisfactions from new role
  3. Single parent
    a. Needs identified and goals established
    b. Referrals: Provide follow-up.
    c. Visits scheduled to provide support and help in establishing healthy childrearing practices
    d. Fear of violence and abuse identified
  4. Mother and father
    a. Developing a unified philosophy of childrearing
      (1) Evaluating their own upbringing as to disciplinary practices and cultural influences
      (2) Identifying how these influence their childrearing practices
      (3) Gaining knowledge of developmental principles
    b. Interactive patterns and communication skills
      (1) Reactive pattern when under stress
      (2) Knowledge and application of problem-solving techniques
  5. Siblings: Goal is to develop positive feelings toward each other.
    a. Each child should have the opportunity to develop at his or her own pace without interference.
    b. Separate planning for each child (bedtimes, activities, play, schools)
    c. Playing together and sharing takes about 6 years to develop. Children need to learn to respond to disagreements with positive behavior patterns.
    d. Parents reinforce positive behavior and demonstrate gentleness.
    e. Parents appreciate children's attempts to show concern for one another.
C. Identify sexual abuse to or by any family member.

III. Health patterns
A. Nutrition
  1. Baby showing less interest in food; too busy investigating world
  2. Growth rate slowed, so smaller intake normal
  3. Anemia: Be sure hematocrit is done.
    a. High-iron diet

      b. Cut back formula intake to 12–16 oz.

   4. Balanced diet to include:

      a. Finger foods—fruit, vegetables, meat

      b. Protein—eggs, fish, whole-grain cereals, meat

      c. Milk: 12–16 oz, per office protocol

      d. Water—offer frequently. Avoid soda pop. Give diluted fruit juices, not "fruit drinks."

B. Sleep

   1. Baby often needs help slowing down. Establish bedtime routine, with quiet time with reading or music; not a time for roughhousing.

   2. Waking during the night; needs reassurance often; when further along in establishing autonomy, will sleep soundly all night

      a. Develop routine for these periods such as diapering, playing soft music, singing from parents' room; use night-light.

      b. Part of developmental pattern; needs careful consideration and consistent response

   3. Watch carefully for attempts to climb out of crib; safety is the prime consideration.

      a. If baby is climbing out, leave sides down so he or she can get out without a serious fall.

      b. Put a mattress on the floor or get a regular bed.

      c. Baby-proof room, particularly ensuring that window screens are secured and bureau drawers hooked closed.

      d. Put gate on baby's room door so he or she cannot roam the house while parents sleep.

C. Elimination

   1. Muscle control of sphincters not sufficiently developed to begin toilet training

   2. Bowel movements and urinary output can help in evaluation of dietary and liquid intake.

   3. Constipation (cow's milk can cause problems); to prevent, include in diet large amounts of water, whole-grain cereals, dried fruits; ask for professional help if problem continues

IV. Growth and development

  A. Physical

   1. Motor development

      a. Gross motor: Joys and perils of learning to creep, crawl, walk, and finally climb; getting direction straightened; moving forward or backward at will; negotiating obstacles; pulling to standing and learning to get back down; hands and arms used as balancing pole; need to carry something in hands

      b. Fine motor: Manipulating objects; turning knobs; pulling, opening, poking; pincer grasp

   2. Reaction to pain

      a. Inability to locate

      b. Continues activity level

      c. Irritability the usual indicator

3. Reaction to illness
   a. Skill development halted
   b. Return to earlier developmental stage
   c. Separation from primary caregiver overwhelming

B. Emotional development—Erikson: Progression from basic trust to stage of autonomy. This is a transitional period that, if successful, shows the amazing progress from a stationary, happy baby to a mobile, impatient, energetic investigator. Babies begin to realize, through the encouragement of caregivers, that they have the ability to be alright—most of the time—out on their own.

1. Affection: Returns hugs and kisses
2. Joy: Excitement at parent's return, at accomplishing a task, at rhythm of body movement
3. Ambivalence of feeling: Returning to earlier behavior patterns when tired, distraught, or ill
4. Obstinate: Persistent in solving problems by trial and error
5. Anger: At body constraint, at interruptions during play
6. Fear and anxiety: Natural response to new adventures, so reassurance from primary caregiver important
7. Distress: Irritable, apathetic, unlovable (risk factor if this is dominant mood)

C. Intellectual development—Piaget: Development of causality. Baby is progressing from random activities to intentional activities by observing and recalling previous results of a particular activity.

1. Steps in learning self-control
   a. Watches response of caregiver to efforts to conform
   b. Delayed gratification: Waiting for meals to be served; waiting to be picked up when first awake
   c. Amuses self for longer periods
   d. Comforts self
2. Memory
   a. Recognizes self in mirror (reaches up to touch something on self seen in mirror)
   b. Anticipates sequence of daily routine
   c. Object permanence: Will search for an object after it is out of sight
   d. Recognizes sounds—car or footsteps; individual voices
   e. Repeats actions: Plays pat-a-cake, waves bye-bye
   f. Recognizes foods and demonstrates likes and dislikes
3. Language
   a. Word development: Repeats definite sounds (dada, mama)
   b. Understands words before being able to use them (commands, names, body parts)
   c. Listens to own voice
   d. Attends as caregiver names objects
   e. May subordinate language development while attending to new motor skills

D. Risk factors
   1. Parents
      a. Dissatisfaction with role
      b. Own experiences of abuse
      c. Emotional poverty (low self-esteem, rigid response patterns, marital conflict)
      d. Fear of violence and abuse
   2. Baby
      a. Developmental and physical lags
      b. Irritable, apathetic, overly cautious
E. Childrearing practices
   1. Parents have confidence in coping with spontaneous feelings of frustration, boredom, anger; appreciate the need for ingenuity, patience, and positive ways of expressing these emotions
   2. Honest responses: Baby soon learns which behaviors bring hugs and which bring unpleasant feelings.
   3. Reinforce positive behavior; set up environment so few opportunities for negative behavior
   4. Identify individuality of baby's capabilities and reactive patterns
   5. Provide cheerful, fun-loving environment
   6. Let baby try to solve own problems; help only when necessary
F. Caregiver arrangements
   1. Babysitter
      a. Able to be regular caregiver
      b. Cheerful and energetic but gentle
      c. Responsible: follows daily schedule; takes safety precautions; responds appropriately to baby's cues; enjoys child care
   2. Day care center
      a. Parents should investigate and observe several centers before choosing one.
      b. State-approved, with professional, educated personnel
      c. Environment: Attractive, quiet; sufficient space for activities; sufficient equipment for stimulation; safety precautions observed
      d. Caregiver: Consistency in baby's caregiver; responds to individual needs, has time to give individual attention
      e. Health services
         (1) Safe, sanitary conditions
         (2) Nutritious food
         (3) Identification of sick child: appropriate plans for care
         (4) Health education services to parents—group meetings, regular health bulletins to families
      f. Evaluation of facility
         (1) Observe children enrolled (relaxed, happy children).
         (2) Watch responses of caregivers to children's requests.
         (3) Get assessment from other parents.

G. Stimulation

   1. Communication and sounds

     a. Provide toy phone; let baby listen to real phone.

     b. Use single names for toys, foods, names, animals.

     c. Name and point to body parts.

     d. Play blowing games: Bubbles, horns.

     e. Provide noisy push-and-pull toys.

     f. Read books with simple, repetitive themes and rhymes.

   2. Touch

     a. Encourage baby to return affection by hugs and kisses.

     b. Bathtub toys: Boats, various-sized containers, colored sponges

   3. Sight

     a. Texture pictures: Encourage touching; change often.

     b. Change of environment: Trips to the store, out in the car; point out distant objects such as birds, planes, clouds.

   4. Gross motor

     a. Removing clothes

     b. Fetching and carrying

     c. Opportunity to climb up and down stairs, with supervision

     d. Walking backward

     e. Walking on variety of surfaces: Grass, mattress, sidewalk.

     f. Using wading pool, with supervision

   5. Fine motor

     a. Puts things in boxes and takes them out

     b. Plays in sand box with spoons, cups, cars, strainer

     c. Transports objects

     d. Builds tower with cubes

     e. Opens, shuts cupboard doors

   6. Feeding

     a. Feels food: Raw, cooked, dough, vegetables, liquid

     b. Splashes, stirs, pours

     c. Feeds self; uses cup

     d. Can use mealtime to demonstrate he or she can get own way

H. Safety

   1. Accidents happen most frequently:

     a. When usual routine changes (holidays, vacations, illness in family)

     b. After stressful events for caregivers

     c. When caregivers are tired or ill

     d. Late in the afternoon

   2. Accident prevention

     a. Increased mobility: Baby needs freedom to investigate but must also have constant surveillance.

     b. Safe place to put baby while caregiver is out of sight

    c. Falls and burns: First-aid instructions per office protocol
3. Investigate frequent injuries for possible child abuse and neglect.
4. Instructions to babysitters
5. Emergency telephone numbers posted

NOTES

| OVERVIEW

14-MONTH WELL CHILD VISIT

I. **Parent**
   A. A quieter period with a more relaxed, cooperative toddler. A more consistent schedule can be established with new activities and outside excursions. giving the toddler a wider view of the world.
   B. Identify any abuse of family members

II. **Baby**
   A. Physical
      1. Eating and sleeping habits improve.
      2. Improving coordination and large muscle strength
   B. Emotional
      1. Shows more confidence in using new skills, reflecting caregiver's attitude toward child of acceptance and affection versus disapproval and mistrust
   C. Intellectual
      1. Concentrates on one thing at a time. Language interest but may be subordinated to improving physical capabilities.

III. **Risk factors**
   A. Unresponsive or overactive
   B. Frequent illness or accidents
   C. No consistent caregiver

| INJURY PREVENTION

I. **Review safety protocol.**
   A. Age-appropriate precautions
      1. Constant activity, insatiable curiosity, poor coordination, and lack of body awareness necessitate constant surveillance.
      2. Child-proofing house related to child's new physical ability
      3. Safe area needed for play and investigation
      4. Curiosity leads to putting everything in mouth.
         a. Ipecac in home; poison center number available
         b. Ipecac used only after identifying what has been swallowed and on direction from health professional
      5. Behavior control not yet reliable; beginning to notice "no" or "stop"
         a. Certain tone of voice used for emergencies
         b. Praise given when attention paid

| CHILD ABUSE

I. **Physical identification**
   A. Tumbles and falls rarely cause broken bones, so any broken bone needs a detailed history and investigation—also, burns, bruises, and bites.

    B. Delayed visit for care and unreliable history

II. **At-risk child**

    A. Fearful, unresponsive, or overreacting to being touched

    B. Continued illnesses—parents making seemingly unnecessary visits

    C. Physical disabilities, retardation, and difficult to care for

III. **Identify:**

    A. At-risk caregivers

    B. Unsafe environment

    C. Abuse of other family members

NOTES

14-MONTH WELL CHILD VISIT

This is a period of consolidation. New-found physical skills are being refined, and the progression from dependence toward independence is becoming a smoother path, although frequent backsliding is still seen. The excitement of mastering physical skills and the courage to "do it myself" make for a happier and more relaxed toddler.

I. **Developmental process**
   A. Parents
      1. Show pride and pleasure in each new step of baby's growth and development
      2. Establish consistent family schedule
      3. Set realistic limits for acceptable behavior
      4. Abuse of any family member identified
   B. Baby
      1. Behavior characterized by playfulness and good humor
      2. Testing own power by frequent use of "no"
      3. More selectivity and control in activity

II. **Family status**
   A. Parental concerns and problems: Ability to identify problems and to cope
   B. Baby now meshed happily into family circle
   C. Adequate child care arrangements

III. **Health habits**
   A. Nutrition
      1. Diet history
         a. Being offered and accepting a balanced diet. Servings should be small: A good rule is to offer a measuring tablespoon of each food for each year of age, or one quarter of an adult serving.
         b. Accepting new foods; high-protein and high-iron foods essential
      2. Eating habits
         a. Self-feeding of finger foods
         b. Drinking from cup, attempting to use spoon
         c. Mealtimes are short and matter-of-fact
         d. No forcing of unwanted foods
         e. Food never used as reward or punishment
   B. Sleep
      1. Sleeps total of 10–15 hr/24 hr
      2. Improvement in sleeping all night
      3. Falling asleep more quickly
      4. Long afternoon nap; morning nap short or discontinued
      5. Crib: Attempts to climb out; safety factors assessed
   C. Elimination and toilet training
      1. Baby developing awareness of soiling
      2. "Catch" bowel movements in potty chair if consistent pattern established

    3. Potty chair used only if baby cooperates to sit on it at time of bowel movement

    4. Avoid praise or threat; a matter-of-fact attitude to prevent putting too much importance on something baby may not yet be able to control

IV. Growth and development

A. Physical

    1. Smooth, coordinated movements

    2. Gross motor: Increase in strength; climbs stairs on hands and knees; throws ball overhand

    3. Fine motor: Good pincer movement; improving eye–hand coordination

    4. Speech

        a. Uses phrases but cannot use individual words out of the phrases

        b. Uses about seven true words

        c. Has developed phrasing and sounds into jargon talk

    5. Vision

        a. Smooth ocular movements

        b. Good eye–hand coordination being established

        c. Improved depth perception: Dropping and watching objects fall

    6. Hearing

        a. Reacts to soft sounds (likes to be whispered to)

        b. Traces source of sound

        c. In a loud, shouting, noisy environment, baby "turns off" sounds; this decreases natural response from stimuli and can result in undeveloped language skills.

B. Emotional development—Erikson: Completing the passage from basic trust to autonomy is to work toward establishing self-esteem and independence. Babies' improving physical skills push them to new and daring feats. They turn from such adventures to those around them for admiration and from these responses learn that they are special. Without this response, they learn nothing positive about themselves.

    1. Cheerful and playful versus irritable and destructive

    2. Energetic and curious versus apathetic and fearful

    3. Eye contact with strangers

C. Intellectual development—Piaget: Period of consolidation or equilibrium. Toddler is comfortable with new skills and beginning to appreciate own competencies. This confidence allows him or her to take the next step of observing the consequences of actions, called causality.

    1. General mood of self-satisfaction

    2. Attends specifically to one toy rather than being distracted by other toys

    3. Attempts to solve a problem before turning to parent for help

    4. Language

        a. Development may still be subordinated while baby is attending to new motor skills and explorations.

        b. Attends to objects and people named by caregiver

D. Risk factors

    1. Parents

      a. Lack of pride in baby, reflected in attitude and actions toward baby

      b. Lack of confidence in child care ability

      c. Unrealistic expectations of baby, such as behavior control and successful toilet training

      d. Overwhelming personal problems

  2. Baby

      a. Frequent health problems

      b. Not settling into family circle

      c. Distractible, tense

      d. Not moving out to investigate surroundings

V. Physical examination

  A. Growth: Continuing on established pattern; if parent states baby is not eating, use growth chart to help parent understand he or she is eating enough to maintain normal growth.

  B. Appearance and behavior

    1. Has lost roundness of babyhood

    2. Energetic but better able to sit still and concentrate on one toy

    3. Less fearful of strangers

  C. Specific factors to note during routine physical examination

    1. Skin: Excessive bruising, burns, scratch lines

    2. Teeth: Central incisors present

    3. Ears: Mobility of tympanic membrane

    4. Hair: Texture, nits

    5. Musculoskeletal: Bearing weight on legs; hips—Ortolani's click, equal gluteal folds; check for tibial torsion, genu varum, externally rotated hips; stance, gait

    6. Reflexes: Presence of parachute reflex

  D. Parent—child interaction

    1. Parents understand child's behavior patterns.

    2. Baby shows recognition of parents' commands.

    3. Cheerful, pleasant rapport between parents and child

VI. Assessment

  A. Physical

  B. Developmental

  C. Emotional

  D. Environmental

VII. Plan

  A. Screening: Hematocrit, lead, urinalysis as indicated

  B. Problem list (devised with parent); SOAP for each

  C. Appropriate timing for office, home, or telephone visits

    1. Continue close contact during this critical period.

    2. Visits planned according to needs of family and developmental and physical needs of baby

    3. Home visits to assess environment as needed

OVERVIEW

ANTICIPATORY GUIDANCE FOR THE PERIOD OF 14–18 MONTHS

I. **Parents**

    A. Understand toddler's progress and appreciate new skills and needs. Both parents' roles are important to give toddler broader experiences and support.

II. **Toddler**

    A. Physical

        1. Decreased appetite as growth rate slows

        2. Falls asleep more easily

        3. Increased strength; needs opportunity to use large muscles

        4. Toilet training—see guideline

    B. Emotional

        1. Attempts to set balance between doing things his or her way and accepting necessary constraints on behavior; uses "no" as an experimental tool

        2. See guidelines for specific factors of development of self-esteem, temper tantrums, and childrearing practices

    C. Intellectual

        1. Returns to fascination with language

        2. Needs a listener but not one who overcorrects

III. **Risk factors**

    A. See safety protocols.

    B. Frequent illnesses with slow recovery

IV. **Watch for:**

    A. Increase in physical strength and activity

    B. Curious and persistent in new adventures

    C. Gives single-word commands, uses "no" and observes its effect on caregiver

    D. Enjoys quiet periods of watching and listening

    E. Responds to caregivers' authority when needed

NOTES

ANTICIPATORY GUIDANCE FOR THE PERIOD OF 14–18 MONTHS

Review the previous outlines to identify the parental and toddler tasks that have been accomplished. Development is such an individual process that the stages cannot be closely related to a specific age period. Office or home visits still need to be set up on an individual basis.

The baby has now become a toddler, and with this new title comes, fortunately for the family, the skills to settle down. Physically, the child has better coordination and muscle control, and his or her energy is now not wasted on random activities but can be used to accomplish specific tasks. The child is better able to pay attention to caregivers and more willing to respond with the type of behavior that gets the most attention. Continuing to satisfy the need for attention and approval through behavior control, he or she is becoming a more cooperative member of the family.

I. **Expectations of this period**

   A. Parental tasks

      1. Encourage with attention and reward (love pats, not food) the type of behavior expected.

      2. Continue to provide a safe environment and regular schedule.

      3. Stimulate new activities and then allow toddler to carry on (but without pressure to complete activity).

      4. Provide a loving, caring caregiver.

   B. Toddler tasks

      1. Settling into household routine

      2. Developing positive behavior pattern that receives the most attention from primary caregiver

      3. Turning to caregiver for encouragement and affection

II. **Family status**

   A. Basic needs being met

      1. Adequate finances, secure environment, stable lifestyle

      2. Knowledge of where to obtain aid

   B. Parents

      1. Good interactive pattern; problem-solving skills

      2. Cooperation in establishing childrearing practices

   C. Working mother

      1. Adequate child care arrangements

      2. Acceptance of sharing child care with others

      3. Communicating philosophy of childrearing practices to caregiver

      4. Health maintenance

   D. Single parent

      1. Adequate support system

      2. Good health habits

      3. Career goals being implemented

   E. Father important to child's well-being

      1. Broadens emotional response of toddler

2. Serves as role model for boys

3. Helps girls develop ability to form close relationship with opposite sex

F. Siblings

1. Independent activities and separate schedules

2. Positive behavior patterns established toward toddler

G. Identify sexual abuse to or by any family member.

III. **Health patterns**

A. Nutrition

1. Emotional and physical factors may increase difficulty of maintaining adequate nutrition.

a. Physical factors: Slower growth rate; appetite and need for food decrease

b. Emotional factors: Distractibility and negativism; using refusal to eat as means of showing power

2. Eating habits: Will sit still longer; enjoys feeding self finger foods; still a poor family dinner companion

B. Sleep

1. By 18 months of age, falls asleep more easily

2. Can amuse and talk to self; will turn off outside stimuli

3. Sleeps through the night; awakens early and can amuse self for longer period

4. Naps: Changing from two naps to one longer one during the middle of the day

5. Regular daily schedule important

C. Elimination

1. Regular pattern established; new foods less irritating

2. Distention and flatulence: Return to simpler diet.

3. Dry for longer periods, as bladder is larger

4. Toilet training

a. "Catch" bowel movement if pattern established.

b. Have toddler practice sitting on potty chair (regular toilet too frightening) with diaper on, then finally with it off.

c. Do not expect success too early; pressure to comply only adds to confusion for toddler.

d. Girls train earlier than boys, small children more easily than big ones.

e. Play it cool; toddlers who realize they can get a lot of attention from this will prolong the process.

IV. **Growth and development**

A. Physical

1. Able to get to most places; practices getting back down

2. Increased strength: Needs to use large muscles; pushes or carries around large objects

3. Fine motor: Established pincer movement; delights in handling small objects, poking, pushing, turning

4. Grasping and releasing at will—if well established, may indicate the time to begin toilet training

   5. Spatial relations: Spends much time working this out, doing things such as putting toys in and out of boxes, dropping and throwing objects, climbing up and down, steering self around obstacles
B. Emotional development—Erikson: Development of autonomy. Toddler is setting a balance between the drive for independence and the need to become a member of society. This means being able to accept constraints on self-will and impulses, which he or she will learn to do through the expectations and approval of caregivers.
   1. Development of self-esteem established through:
      a. Negativism: Testing power to affect others
      b. Challenging physical activities: Climbing higher, carrying heavier objects
      c. Taking initiative for actions: Self-amusement
      d. Demanding attention by showing off, being mischievous and joyful
      e. Attempting more than he or she has the ability to do
      f. Absorbing attitudes and feelings shown by others toward him or her; beginning to select behavior that fits into these expectations
      g. Childrearing practices
         (1) Treat child with respect; attempt to see the world from his or her perspective.
         (2) Avoid battles over "no" when possible, and do not try to win them all.
         (3) Provide enough freedom for toddler to try new activities.
         (4) Constructively reinforce accomplishments.
   2. Development of self-control
      a. Identified by:
         (1) Accepting and anticipating daily routine; being less impulsive; fitting into family plans more easily
         (2) Learning that behavior has consequences; parental reaction teaches what is right and what is wrong.
      b. Childrearing practices
         (1) Control of impulses will continue to take time and much reinforcement.
         (2) Provide a safe environment, as a toddler of this age cannot be completely trusted not to act on impulse.
   3. Development of aggression
      a. Frustrations from too many commands and unrealistic expectations lead to stored-up energy; toddler has few ways of releasing this energy constructively.
      b. Frustrations also caused by siblings, fatigue, hunger, illness, and changes in routine, in caregiver, etc.
      c. Stored-up energy can be released in a way destructive to child and others, such as temper tantrums, breath-holding, biting, hitting.
      d. Childrearing practices
         (1) Temper tantrums
            (a) Provide firm but soothing restraints (hold under arm); do not leave alone, as child is frightened by loss of control.

       (b) Keep record of events preceding the incident, intervention, and results.

       (c) Seek professional help if such destructive behavior continues.

       (d) Provide a quiet, gentle, consistent environment.

    (2) Negativism

       (a) "No" used as a means of learning which behaviors are acceptable. Caregiver must demonstrate that acceptable behavior has more power to get attention and approval than unacceptable behavior.

       (b) Avoid opportunities for toddler to use negative response. Do not ask him or her to make a choice; state what is to be done, such as, "This is what we will have to eat" or "Now it is time for bed."

       (c) Set limits; do not give in to unreasonable requests.

       (d) Maintain a cheerful, fun-loving, well-organized daily routine.

       (e) Provide a large, stimulating, safe environment.

4. Risk factors

   a. Parents: Demanding coercive behavior that is beyond toddler's developmental ability to comply

   b. Toddler: Excessive negativism; frequent temper tantrums; dominant mood of irritability or apathy; frequent illnesses

C. Intellectual development—Piaget. Toddler is learning intuitively about the environment with the increase in physical agility and memory development. He or she is also taking the first steps in symbolic thinking but needs concrete symbols first (drink for teddy bear requires a cup).

  1. Independent actions; beginning to observe actions of others and to imitate caregivers, siblings, peers

  2. Studying

   a. Experimenting (things in motion, difference in weights)

   b. Varying a pattern and observing the results

   c. Varying response to an activity and observing the results

  3. Language

   a. Returns to fascination with words; is word-hungry

   b. Articulation lags behind vocabulary; carries on "jargon" conversations with self and toys

   c. Experiments with using words to affect those around him or her

   d. Childrearing practices

    (1) Talk and sing to child; name objects, feelings, odors, textures, sounds.

    (2) Listen; pay particular attention as child attempts to talk to you.

    (3) Accept child's strivings to express self; do not overcorrect and do not overload; let child take the lead in how much he or she wants.

    (4) Look at pictures and name things, but do not expect the child to sit still for story hour.

D. Stimulation

1. Communication and sounds: Parents
   a. Read short, simple stories.
   b. Give simple directions.
   c. Say words for objects child desires.
   d. Provide books with cardboard pages, simple colorful pictures, rhymes, songs.
2. Touch: Water tubs, sandboxes
3. Sight: Bulletin board in child's room, using large single picture; point at things at a distance.
4. Gross motor
   a. Walks up and down stairs
   b. Balances on one foot
   c. Jumps
   d. Rides kiddie car
   e. Does somersaults
5. Fine motor
   a. Uses paper and crayons to scribble; provide large paper such as old newspapers.
   b. Enjoys finger paints
   c. Puts on shoes
   d. Washes and dries hands

E. Safety

1. Accidents happen most frequently:
   a. When usual routine changes (holidays, vacations, illness in family)
   b. After stressful events for caregivers
   c. When caregivers are tired or ill
   d. Late in the afternoon
2. Accident prevention
   a. Most dangerous age, because child is mobile but has little ability to control behavior and poor depth perception (for instance, may step off high step)
   b. Child-proof house, yard, porches.
   c. Constant surveillance necessary
   d. Insist that child remain in car seat.
3. Investigate possibility of child abuse and neglect.
4. Instructions to babysitters
5. Emergency telephone numbers posted

| OVERVIEW

18-MONTH WELL CHILD VISIT

I. **Parents**
    A. Understand toddler's self-centered world and growing willingness to conform by controlling behavior. Child does this for the return of support and affection; if misbehavior is the only behavior that gets attention, child will continue that behavior.
    B. Identify any abuse of family members
II. **Toddler**
    A. Physical
        1. Walks alone
        2. Manipulates small objects
        3. Slower growth rate
        4. Falls asleep more easily
    B. Emotional
        1. Struggle toward independence can lead to excessive use of "no." Child is a keen observer of how this word affects caregivers.
    C. Intellectual
        1. Increased interest and use of language can begin the development of pretending or symbolizing.
III. **Risk factors**
    A. Parents who let the use of "no" develop into battleground of wills
    B. Whiny child needs investigation.
    C. Illness becoming a way to gain attention

| INJURY PREVENTION

I. **Review safety protocol.**
    A. Age-appropriate precautions
        1. Toddler's increase in physical ability and boundless energy, intense curiosity, persistence in endeavors, and minimal behavior control combine to make this a dangerous period.
    B. Safety standards that need to be carefully maintained
        1. House—safe environment
            a. Gates or doors on stairwells, kitchen, bathroom, bedroom
            b. Crib: If child is climbing out, use bed or mattress with gate on door so toddler does not roam the house while parents sleep.
            c. Bureau drawers with safety locks so toddler cannot climb into a drawer and have bureau topple over on him or her
            d. Windows and screens securely fastened, cords and drapes removed
            e. Bathroom—gate and toilet seat locked
        2. Car: Child in car seat at all times in back seat facing forward
    C. Caregiver
        1. Alert to toddler's ability to dash off into danger

   2. Carefully and quietly demonstrates what behavior is expected and pays particular attention to toddler's steps toward behavior control

CHILD ABUSE

I. **Age-specific concerns**
   A. Toddler's activities often lead to injuries, so it is important to differentiate between injury and abuse.

II. **Physical identification**
   A. Investigate unusual burns and injury, and broken bones.
   B. Consider corporal punishment and shaken child syndrome.

III. **At-risk child**
   A. Overactive, impulsive
   B. Cranky, whiny, angry
   C. Continuing health problems

IV. **Identify:**
   A. Careless caregiver
   B. Unsafe environment
   C. Abuse of other family members

NOTES

⎮ 18-MONTH WELL CHILD VISIT

For the last few months, the toddler has been concentrating on mastering and perfecting physical skills. Now that physical skills take less concentration and energy, the child turns to the next developmental task: language acquisition.

I. **Developmental process**
   A. Parents
      1. Listen to toddler's expostulations
      2. Talk to child about child's world
   B. Toddler
      1. Attends to speech of others
      2. Assertive; gives two-word commands
      3. Physical agility and coordination

II. **Family status**
   A. Basic needs being met
   B. Stable family structure
   C. Siblings receiving appropriate care and age-specific activities; relationships evaluated and referrals given as needed
   D. Parental concerns and problems: Ability to identify problems and to cope

III. **Health habits**
   A. Nutrition
      1. Diet history
         a. Variety of foods
         b. Amount of milk
         c. Adequate caloric intake; relate to pattern on growth chart
      2. Eating habits
         a. Self-feeding, manages spoon
         b. Reasonable time spent on meals
         c. Atmosphere pleasant; no attention given to rejected foods
   B. Sleep
      1. Sleeps total of 10–15 hr/day
      2. Contented in crib for longer periods; practicing jargon and new words
      3. In a bed if able to climb out of crib; gate on door of room; windows, screens fastened securely
      4. Room unstimulating to promote restfulness
      5. Accepting bedtime routine
      6. Daytime naps: Parents aware of type of behavior child will display when he or she runs out of steam
      7. Able to turn off stimulation and relax
   C. Elimination
      1. Toilet training not usually accomplished by 18 months (see protocol)
      2. Parents understand principles of toilet training

      3. Regularity of bowel movements established

      4. Longer periods between urinating

  D. Dental

      1. Teeth cleaned with soft brush

      2. See tooth eruption schedule.

IV. Growth and development

  A. Physical

      1. Gross motor: Testing strength; pushes and carries heavy and large objects

      2. Fine motor: Handedness; scribbling

      3. Speech

         a. Uses two- or three-word phrases but cannot use the words separately

         b. Gives two-word commands

         c. Follows one-step directions

         d. Perfects inflections and rhythms of speech in jargon

  B. Emotional development—Erikson. Feelings of autonomy and self-esteem continue to grow through child's mastery of physical control of body and activities. Language acquisition continues to add to self-esteem by giving child a new tool with which to understand and control the environment.

      1. Physical agility, good coordination, high energy level

      2. Plays with putting together a string of sounds

      3. Experiments with words and observes their effect on caregiver

      4. Content to play by self for longer periods

      5. Instigates own activities

  C. Intellectual development—Piaget. Sensorimotor learning is progressing to the beginning of preoperative or intuitive learning, which is the ability to store mental images (as in memory) and to symbolize (as in words being substituted for the actual object, feeling, or event).

      1. Attends carefully to activities of peers but does not play interactively

      2. Shows interest in names of things and people

      3. Remembers where possessions belong

      4. Simple pretending

  D. Risk factors

      1. Parents

         a. Too helpful; fearful of providing physical challenges

         b. Too busy or uninterested to spend time listening to or talking with child

         c. Unhappy, frustrated

      2. Toddler

         a. Physically cautious

         b. Does not initiate activities for self; sits doing nothing for long periods

         c. Clings to caregiver; whiny or irritable

         d. Does not attempt to use words to get what he or she wants

V. Physical examination

  A. Growth: Continues on established pattern; periods of illness will affect the pattern, but growth should be made up within a period of months.

    B. Appearance and behavior
        1. Good physical coordination
        2. Energetic, playful
        3. Cautious in relating to strangers, but more trustful than at previous visit
        4. Eye contact possible
    C. Specific factors to note during routine physical examination
        1. Skin: Excessive bruising, burns
        2. Head: Anterior fontanelle usually closed
        3. Eyes: Smooth tracking; no strabismus
        4. Teeth: Lateral and central incisors present; first and second molars may be present.
        5. Cardiovascular system: Heart rate 90–100/min
        6. Musculoskeletal: Coordination, gait
    D. Parent–child interaction
        1. Parent understands child's behavior patterns.
        2. Toddler shows recognition of parents' commands.
        3. Rapport between parent and child appears cheerful, pleasant.
VI. Assessment
    A. Physical
    B. Developmental
    C. Emotional
    D. Environmental
VII. Plan
    A. Immunizations per office protocol
    B. Screening: Hematocrit, urinalysis as indicated
    C. Problem list (devised with parent); SOAP for each
    D. Appropriate timing for office, home, or telephone visits; continue individual scheduling

NOTES

OVERVIEW

ANTICIPATORY GUIDANCE FOR THE PERIOD OF 18–24 MONTHS

I. **Parents**

    A. Able to discuss understanding of discipline versus punishment and the establishment of realistic goals for toddler

    B. Parents who cannot provide such support need referrals, more frequent visits, or home visits.

II. **Child**

    A. Physical

        1. Better able to concentrate on meals. Milk intake should be no more than 16 oz, as too much milk will curb appetite for other foods.

        2. Enjoys strenuous activities; needs appropriate and safe environment

        3. Toilet training—see guidelines.

    B. Emotional

        1. Increased feeling of competence so has less need for using "no"; continues to be egocentric (selfish, stubborn, assertive)

        2. See guidelines for child-rearing practices and risk factors.

    C. Intellectual

        1. Learns words important to him or her first. Careful listening by caregiver encourages use of language.

        2. Able to symbolize a thing by using words, so can begin to pretend

    D. Social development

        1. Egocentric: Unable to share

        2. Amoralistic: Will show signs of guilt if found doing something wrong

III. **Risk factors**

    A. See safety protocol.

    B. Frequent illness

    C. No interest in using language

    D. No primary caregiver to help establish behavior control through positive reinforcement

IV. **Watch for:**

    A. Happy, healthy, energetic child

    B. Accepts daily routine

    C. Uses language to make wishes known

    D. Shows guilt if found doing an established behavior wrong

    E. Begins to accept behavior control for attention and approval

NOTES

NOTES

ANTICIPATORY GUIDANCE FOR THE PERIOD OF 18–24 MONTHS

Review previous guidelines to serve as a reference point for the toddler's developmental level. It is important to identify a family environment that does not support or facilitate optimal development, as proper intervention at this time can be of lasting benefit.

These months continue the long road toward establishing a balance between the individual's needs and society's expectations. A very tentative beginning has been made by the toddler's experiencing and anticipating the results of controlling behavior. However, the toddler's impulses and drive for independence rule most of his or her activities. It is the caregiver's task to persuade him or her, through attention and affection, that it is worth the effort to conform. The acquisition of language is an added tool that can make this development easier.

I. **Expectations of this period**
   A. Parental tasks
      1. Continue to provide a safe environment
      2. Provide opportunities to develop physical strength and agility
      3. Provide a variety of experiences
      4. Provide a caring adult to encourage and praise child's efforts, to talk with him or her, and to listen to his or her efforts to use language
   B. Toddler tasks
      1. Bargains for behavior control
      2. Attempts to use language to control activities
      3. Increasing socialization; delights in being with and watching others

II. **Family status**
   A. Basic needs being met; referrals providing needed help, with follow-up of these referrals
   B. Parents
      1. Health and resources sufficient to maintain satisfactory lifestyle
      2. Appreciate importance of this age period
      3. Wholesome childrearing practices established
      4. Derive satisfaction and pride from role
      5. Content with lifestyle
   C. Working mother
      1. Health and energy level sufficient for daily schedule
      2. Satisfactory child care arrangements
      3. Arranges some time each day to be alone with toddler
   D. Single parent
      1. Receives satisfaction from child care but does not depend on this care for only emotional support
      2. Adequate parenting skills developed
      3. Adequate support system
      4. Career goals being implemented

   E. Siblings

      1. Older siblings demonstrate caring and gentleness with toddler.

      2. New baby in family

         a. Toddler will show crude reactive patterns to hold parents' attention; regressive behavior understood and not punished

         b. New emotion of jealousy; toddler must learn another step in coping with world.

   F. Toddler

      1. Basic physical and emotional needs being met

      2. Learning that needs, but not all wants, are met

   G. Risk factors

      1. Reaction of parents to children during divorce or separation: Lack of attention, overprotection, use as emotional crutch, broken routine, abandonment

      2. Siblings: Teasing or aggressive acts; frustrating toddler into destructive action toward self or others

   H. Identify sexual abuse to or by any family member.

III. Health patterns

   A. Nutrition

      1. Sufficient calories for high energy level; include high-value food (potatoes, dark bread, peanut butter, yogurt, honey, molasses).

      2. Avoid junk food (if such foods are not bought, they will not be available).

      3. Food variety: Keep menus and seasoning simple; add new foods in small amounts.

      4. The following foods must not be given to toddlers: Potato chips, coconut, nuts, popcorn, whole kernel corn, hot dogs, raw carrots, and peanut butter on a cracker. They are difficult to chew and swallow and can cause choking or aspiration.

      5. Eating habits

         a. Improved attention to food, as now less distractible

         b. Expects to feed self, so finger foods best

         c. Offer simple, bland foods; no substitutes offered, no snacks between meals if food refused at mealtimes

         d. Watch milk intake, and offer only after or between meals.

         e. Keep mealtime a short, matter-of-fact event; give no attention to rejected food.

         f. Do not offer food as a reward or withhold it as a punishment.

   B. Sleep

      1. Sleeps 12–15 hr/day

      2. Definite schedule and routine at bedtime continued

      3. Now better able to "turn off" stimulation around him or her, so falls asleep more easily

      4. Enjoys talking to self and wants a bedtime companion such as a teddy bear

      5. Returns to sleeping through the night

      6. Naptime: One long nap in middle of day

      7. Fatigue: Watch for behavior when tired; help child establish a quiet place

C. Elimination: Toilet training

  1. Girls train earlier than boys, small children earlier than big children.

  2. Treat as a matter-of-fact event; special attention encourages delaying the training for continued attention.

  3. Attempt training if:

    a. Regular pattern of bowel movement established

    b. Toddler connects physical awareness of bowel movement and parental request to use toilet (heads for potty at time of bowel movement)

    c. Toddler willing to sit still on potty chair

  4. Bladder control usually not accomplished until at least 3 years of age

D. Risk factors

  1. Frequent illnesses

  2. Divergence from expected growth pattern

  3. Child irritable, whiny, distractible

  4. Exaggerated feeding or elimination problems

E. Dental

  1. Clean teeth with soft brush.

  2. No extreme discomfort with teeth eruption

IV. Growth and development

A. Physical

  1. Improved coordination and agility

    a. Needs large area to expend energy

    b. Improved agility; running and jumping

  2. Spatial relations: Exploring possibilities by climbing up and down, crawling in and out, dropping toys over and over again; fascination with balls rolling and bouncing

B. Emotional development—Erikson. Continued development of self-esteem. Language is a new tool that can be used to increase self-worth by helping toddler control activities and influence environment.

  1. Less negativism; developing feeling of competence, which diffuses need for testing power

  2. Shallower mood swings; words help others understand needs and wishes

  3. Continues to demonstrate affection

  4. Fewer frustrations since learning to put problems into words

  5. Continues to be egocentric (selfish, stubborn, assertive)

  6. Destructive feelings of defiance, willfulness, and combativeness need careful investigation of what is wrong in the child's environment.

  7. Childrearing practices

    a. Overexaggerated praise can be detected as insincerity.

    b. Expect compromises to be accepted.

    c. Provide different environments for toddler to observe.

    d. Play games (hide and seek, for example) to use memory skills.

    e. Avoid putting toddler in situations where more is expected of him or her than he or she can perform.

    f. Overstimulation can reduce desire to learn.

      g. Provide a regular, quiet schedule most of the time.

      h. Provide a caring adult to listen.

      i. Begin to identify learning style (an observer, a toucher, a talker).

  8. Risk factors

      a. Temper tantrums, breath-holding, irritability, crying (see protocol)

      b. Problems with eating, sleeping, elimination

      c. Developmental lag; continues characteristics of 14-month-old (distractible, no interest in naming objects, extreme negativism)

      d. Overdependent; lack of initiative

      e. Excessive crying; whining; appears lazy (be sure no physical problem exists)

C. Intellectual development—Piaget. Language allows for use of words to symbolize actions, objects, and feelings. This skill develops by repetition of activities, object permanence, and vocabulary development.

  1. Language opens a new world; labeling and categorizing the world is a difficult job. "What's that?" is toddler's favorite question—needs a simple answer, no long explanation.

  2. Improved problem-solving techniques; works out alternative solutions

  3. Increase in memory; knows own possessions and where they belong

  4. Spends time observing the world around him or her; increased interest while looking out the window, riding in the car, going shopping

  5. Mimics actions of others—tone of voice, facial expressions, mannerisms

  6. Periods of apparently doing nothing—taking time to "catch up" (a risk factor if this becomes a dominant mood)

  7. Language

      a. Toddlers learn best what they need to know when they need to know it and remember first the words that are important to them, such as:

         (1) Words that gain attention (me do, watch)

         (2) Words that express feelings (tired, hungry)

      b. Uses own name and "I," which indicates increased awareness of self

      c. Reaction of caregivers to efforts of toddler to express self gives or takes away motivation to acquire language.

  8. Childrearing practices

      a. Minimal instruction and correction; toddler turned off if expectations are beyond his or her capacity

      b. Interesting to watch errors, as they demonstrate method of learning

      c. Caregivers should describe in simple terms what they are doing, their reactions, and their emotions; this helps the child develop appropriate vocabulary.

      d. Caregivers should maintain eye contact when toddler is attempting to tell them something.

      e. Books: Simple action books; toddler has short attention span and cannot be expected to sit still and listen to a story.

      f. Fascinated with rhymes and music; enjoys nursery rhymes, recordings; have toddler sing with caregiver.

      g. Listening: Identify various sounds and point out new ones; observe if child can pick up faint sounds.

      h. Handle toddler's commands with gentleness, humor, and diversion.

  9. Risk factors

      a. Failure to respond to speech with speech

      b. Lack of primary caregiver to listen to and talk with toddler

D. Social development

  1. Autonomy: Uses own name; is possessive about own things; if pressure by older siblings or peers, shows hostility and fights back; is bossy with younger siblings

  2. Self-control: Less impulsive; beginning to comprehend effect of actions

  3. Egocentric: Unable to share; sees the world only from his or her perspective

  4. Amoralistic: Beginning to appreciate what is acceptable behavior through caregivers' teaching; will eventually accept cultural and moralistic code of parents in return for security, respect, and love

      a. Will show signs of guilt if found doing something he or she knows is wrong

  5. Childrearing practices

      a. Provide opportunity for toddler to observe other children.

      b. Do not expect toddler to share or play cooperatively with others.

      c. Emphasize acceptable behavior through attention and affection.

      d. Ignore unacceptable behavior as far as safety will allow.

E. Stimulation

  1. Communication and sounds

      a. Child fills in words of stories and rhymes.

      b. House and small people dolls

      c. Naming games

      d. Listening—naming sounds; music, poetry

      e. Books—nursery rhymes

  2. Sight

      a. Identifies colors

      b. Identifies shapes

      c. Points out and identifies things at a distance

  3. Gross motor

      a. Dresses with help

      b. Walking games—well-defined track to follow

      c. Large riding toys

      d. Wooden blocks

  4. Fine motor

      a. Busy board

      b. Clay

      c. Simple puzzles

      d. Play to enjoy, not to accomplish a task

      e. Parents interact in enjoyment

F. Safety

  1. Accidents happen most frequently:

    a. When usual routine changes (holidays, vacations, illness in the family)

    b. After stressful events (either for caregivers or for toddler)

    c. When caregivers are tired or ill

    d. Late in the afternoon

2. Accident prevention

    a. Negativistic period makes toddler seem disobedient.

        (1) Save severe tone of voice for emergency.

        (2) Develop a method for emergency compliance (use of whistle, hand clap); practice and use rewards.

    b. Do not trust child's training; lack of behavior control and little memory will not stop child from dangerous activity.

3. Investigate frequent injuries as possible child abuse and neglect.

4. Instructions to babysitters

5. Emergency telephone numbers posted

NOTES

OVERVIEW

24-MONTH WELL CHILD VISIT

I. **Parents**
   A. Understand and appreciate toddler's personality and capabilities.
   B. Provide a safe, stimulating, varied environment.
   C. Identify physical or emotional abuse of any family member.

II. **Child**
   A. Physical
      1. Continues on usual growth curve; short illnesses will not affect this.
      2. Needs a quiet place of his or her own to use during the day
      3. Walks with confidence
      4. Uses hands to carry toys while walking
   B. Emotional
      1. Dominant mood of cheerfulness and cooperation
      2. Attempts new activities
      3. Responds to parents' tone of voice and will act sorry if found doing something wrong
   C. Intellectual
      1. Enjoys experimenting with language and using it to get what he or she wants
      2. Can symbolize words for things so can now enjoy pretending

III. **Risk factors**
   A. Not attempting to use speech
   B. Using aggressive behavior to get what he or she wants

IV. **See guidelines for specific factors to be noted in physical examination**

INJURY PREVENTION

I. **Review safety protocol.**
   A. Toddler still needs constant surveillance but is becoming less impulsive in activities and is also better able to attend to vocal commands.
   B. Safe environment
      1. Needs constant review as toddler's physical ability increases
      2. Voice commands and tone of voice
      3. Continue to establish simple command for use in emergency; may take time and a great deal of positive reinforcement.
   C. Acting out and continued negativism may indicate that this behavior may be the best way for toddler to get attention.

CHILD ABUSE

I. **Physical identification**
   A. Frequent injuries or injuries more severe than history indicates

    B. Corporal punishment accepted by parents as means of behavior control

II. **At-risk child**

    A. Overly submissive, shy, fearful

    B. Extreme negativism, aggressiveness

    C. Overactive, impulsive

    D. Continued illness and disabilities

III. **Identify:**

    A. At-risk caregivers

    B. Assessment of all adults with access to child

    C. Abuse of other family members

NOTES

24-MONTH WELL CHILD VISIT

The acquisition of a few important words has given the toddler a new sense of power. It is of great help to be able to name what he or she wants and tell how he or she feels. With amazing rapidity, the toddler is labeling and categorizing the world. This makes for an easier and more pleasant rapport between toddler and family.

I. **Developmental process**
   A. Parents
      1. Give simple, concise, gentle commands, but still do not attempt to reason with child
      2. Demonstrate understanding of toddler's capabilities
   B. Toddler
      1. Vocabulary of about 25 words
      2. Half of speech intelligible to other than family members
      3. Responds to parents' requests

II. **Family status**
   A. Basic needs being met
   B. Parental concerns and problems: Ability to identify problems and to cope
   C. Illness in family since last visit; course; resolution
   D. Parental assessment of child's development
   E. Fear of violence and abuse identified

III. **Health habits**
   A. Nutrition
      1. Diet history: Food intake, including snacks; balanced diet being offered
      2. Eating habits, appetite: Regular schedule of meals and snacks; self-feeding; pleasant atmosphere at mealtime; limited time for eating; no attention paid to unwanted foods; food not used as reward or punishment
   B. Sleep
      1. Well-established bedtime routine
      2. Sleeping all night
      3. Danger of climbing out of crib: Put child in a bed or leave sides of crib down; make room safe and put a gate on bedroom door; windows and screens securely fastened; unable to open bureau drawers
      4. One nap period
      5. Quiet place for rest periods
   C. Elimination
      1. Regular bowel movements; effects of new foods; periods of constipation or diarrhea
      2. Urinating less frequently as bladder capacity increases
      3. Color of urine indicator of state of hydration
      4. Toilet training only if bowel movements regular (see toilet training protocol)
         a. Practicing with potty chair with or without diapers on

   b. Too much pressure on toilet training can be seen by regressive behavior patterns such as eating problems, waking during the night, and increased negativism.

IV. **Growth and development**

   A. Physical

   1. Gross motor

   a. Improved coordination and agility

   b. Increased muscle strength

   c. Rides kiddie car

   2. Fine motor

   a. Improved hand–eye coordination

   b. Observes and handles small objects such as pebbles and crumbs

   c. Traces patterns and designs

   B. Emotional development—Erikson. Toddler is reaching a plateau of physical and emotional development for first period of growth. Language acquisition will lead to next developmental task of using words to help control environment and own actions. Toddler is now willing to accept compromises in behavior for affection and attention from important adults. Without this positive reinforcement, child will reflect the negative feelings of discouragement and shame. Positive and negative reinforcements are the origin of the basic values of optimism and pessimism.

   1. Physical well-being

   2. Dominant mood of cooperation and cheerfulness

   3. Uses words appropriately

   C. Intellectual development—Piaget. Being able to symbolize thoughts and actions through words opens up a new world of imagination and fantasy.

   1. Vocabulary development

   2. Pretending without actual object present (can pretend to give teddy bear a drink without needing an actual cup)

   D. Risk factors

   1. Parents

   a. Unrealistic demands on child for self-control

   b. Harsh vocal commands

   c. Too busy or distracted for a quiet, gentle approach to child

   2. Toddler

   a. Frequent illnesses

   b. Failure to respond to speech with speech

   c. Exhibits behavior of earlier period (distractible, unobservant, pronounced negativism)

V. **Physical examination**

   A. Growth: Continuing on established pattern; use this as a guide for parents for toddler's continued growth and caloric intake.

   B. Appearance and behavior

   1. High energy level, but a degree of ability to control actions (sit still, follow directions)

   2. Losing cherubic look; taller and thinner

C. Specific factors to note during physical examination
1. Skin: Excessive bruising, burns; birthmarks fading
2. Eyes: Equal tracking; no strabismus
3. Teeth: Complete set of 20 teeth by 2.5 years of age
4. Musculoskeletal: Smooth coordination and gait; check hips
D. Parent–child interaction
1. Child turns to parent for support
2. Parent's ability to quiet child after painful experience such as immunization or blood test
3. Child's ability to separate from parent

VI. **Assessment**
A. Physical
B. Developmental
C. Emotional
D. Environmental

VII. **Plan**
A. Immunizations per office protocol
B. Screening: Hematocrit, urinalysis as indicated
C. Problem list (devised with parent); SOAP for each
D. Appropriate timing for office, home, or telephone visits; continue individual scheduling.

NOTES

OVERVIEW

ANTICIPATORY GUIDANCE FOR THE PERIOD OF 24–36 MONTHS

I. **Parent**

    A. Some characteristics of the "terrible twos" can be eliminated if parents can appreciate the toddler's attempts to give up comfortable baby ways to accept a new world of playing with peers, going off without parent to play school, completing toilet training, and often coping with a new baby in the family. This is a time of great fluctuation between independence and overdependence.

II. **Child**

    A. See guidelines for expectations of this period for toddler and family.

    B. Physical

        1. Increased agility and eye–hand coordination

        2. Diet: Provide various foods, but no pressure to eat; do not use food as a reward.

        3. Sleep: Change of pattern needs investigation.

        4. Speech: Two- or three-word sentences intelligible to family

    C. Emotional

        1. Greater range of emotional responses; see guidelines for development of personality traits.

    D. Intellectual

        1. By 3 years, can symbolize, using words for objects; world of pretend becomes part of play.

        2. Listening carefully to toddler is a way to understand how he or she is beginning to see the world and the things that are important to him or her.

    E. Social

        1. Separates from family easily; enjoys being with peers

        2. Needs external controls for being good

        3. May have an imaginary friend he or she uses as scapegoat

        4. Sexual identify

            a. Selects type of behavior that society has accepted for each sex

        5. See guidelines for childrearing practices and risk factors.

III. **Risk factors**

    A. Fails to use speech as a tool

    B. Regresses to earlier behavior patterns

    C. At-risk caregivers

    D. Any family member being abused

IV. **Watch for:**

    A. Attitude of confidence and good will

    B. Cooperative most of the time

    C. Willing to control behavior for positive response

    D. Negative response by caregiver reinforcing negative behavior

    E. Toilet training first big step in behavior control (see protocol)

    F. Beginning of self-fulfilling prophecy—"I am a good kid" versus "I am a bad kid"

G. Whining, fussy child who has not established these positive, cooperative behaviors is at risk.

NOTES

ANTICIPATORY GUIDANCE FOR THE PERIOD OF 24–36 MONTHS

Review previous guidelines for a reference point as to the toddler's developmental level, and schedule future visits as needed. In this most important year, the toddler completes the tasks of the first period of growth. By 3 years of age, successful completion of these developmental tasks can be expected.

I. **Expectations of this period**
  A. Stability of bodily processes and mastery of physical skills
  B. Toddler learns to see self as an individual with ability and value
  C. Appears confident in activities and curious to investigate world
  D. Uses language as a tool to influence own actions and affect environment
  E. Can compromise activities for attention from a meaningful caregiver
  F. Shares affection with a primary caregiver

II. **Family status**
  A. Basic needs being met; self-direction in coping with problems
    1. Able to discuss if abuse present
  B. Parents
    1. Stable lifestyle; family routine established that allows child to predict what is going to happen and gives child a feeling that life has some consistency
    2. Cooperate in and understand their childrearing practices
    3. Understand that child will begin to move away from them and become interested in peers and outside world
    4. Identify and implement a plan for own life goals
    5. Appreciate their role as family coordinators and standard-bearers for the family's behavioral patterns, mores, and spiritual foundation
    6. Set example of a gentle, caring attitude
    7. Understand importance of child spacing
    8. Abuse of any family member identified
  C. Working mother
    1. Adequate health practices and satisfaction with lifestyle
    2. Schedules sufficient time with toddler to ensure implementation of her philosophy of childrearing
    3. Counseling available for career goals and personal support
  D. Single parent
    1. Able to assess childrearing practices of caregivers and to coordinate with own
    2. Support system intact; does not use child as only means of emotional satisfaction
    3. Fear of being abused
  E. Siblings
    1. Parents provide opportunity for each child to pass through each developmental stage without undue interference from siblings.
    2. Identify whether one child is overly dominant or submissive.
    3. Prohibit teasing; teach alternative ways of interacting.

4. Older siblings seen as role models

5. Initiate use of communication skills as a way of expressing feelings and resolving conflicts.

III. Health patterns

A. Nutrition

1. Good appetite; will eat most foods offered

2. Adequate diet being offered

   a. Adequate nutrients and calories can be supplied by simple, easily eaten finger foods; rely on foods of high caloric concentration, such as bread, potatoes, peanut butter, cheese.

   b. Sufficient intake of fluids can be identified by color and odor of urine. Avoid sweetened drinks such as chocolate milk, drinks containing colored sweeteners, and sodas; encourage frequent drinks of water and diluted fruit juice.

   c. Periods of crankiness and fatigue need to be investigated.

      (1) Offer quickly absorbed foods such as fruit juice and a cookie.

      (2) If food is helpful, attempt to avoid such periods by scheduling meals and snacks at more frequent intervals.

3. Eating habits: There are so many developmental tasks going on in this period that putting too much attention on food and eating can become an unnecessary burden to the toddler.

   a. Asking what the child wants to eat or giving him or her a choice can be too confusing to a toddler busy experimenting with the things around him or her and learning a language.

   b. Using food as a reward can begin establishing the need for oral satisfaction throughout life—as seen in obese people, chain-smokers, and those who have inverted the process and have difficulty eating and enjoying food.

   c. Children mimic the world around them and will adopt the attitudes and habits about foods and the use of food of those around them.

B. Sleep

1. Regular pattern

   a. Sleeps 10–12 hr/night; one nap period

   b. Falls asleep quickly

   c. Sleeps all night

2. Disturbances in pattern indicate health or emotional problems.

   a. Review previous anticipatory guidance outlines to identify unaccomplished tasks by age 3 years. By 3 years, nightmares may occur.

   b. Identify environmental changes.

   c. Check physical examination and laboratory tests.

3. Safety

   a. Out of the crib and into a bed

   b. Room and windows checked for safety; gate placed on bedroom door to keep toddler from roaming the house while the rest of the family sleeps

C. Elimination

1. Regular pattern; little effect with new foods; continued problems need investigation.

2. Toilet training: Expectation of control of bowel movements and daytime wetting by 3 years of age

    a. Schedule regular periods for sitting on potty.

    b. Clothing should be easy to remove; use training pants.

    c. Carefully watch child's reaction to training.

        (1) If using as a means of getting attention, look for dissatisfaction in other areas.

        (2) Successful training provides a feeling of self-control and adds to feeling of self-worth.

D. Risk factors

   1. Frequent illnesses; overattention to illnesses by parents

   2. Poor appetite; inadequate nutrition

   3. Regressive behavior

IV. **Growth and development**

A. Physical

   1. Gross motor: Good coordination, smooth movements, agility, increased muscle strength

   2. Fine motor: Improved eye–hand coordination; can fasten large buttons; scribbles with some intent

   3. Enjoys physical activity; has body confidence—enjoys being tossed in the air, rolling down a hill, splashing in water, etc.

   4. Stability of body systems

   5. Growth rate leveling off

     a. Grows 3"/year in length

     b. Gains 5 lb/year in weight

     c. Legs grow faster than rest of body; head slows in growth rate.

     d. Child loses top-heavy appearance.

   6. Speech

     a. Vocabulary development of about 50 words; discards jargon

     b. Articulation

        (1) Half intelligible to people outside family

        (2) Omits most final consonants

        (3) Uses all vowels

     c. Sentence structure

        (1) Two- or three-word sentences, grammatically correct

        (2) Uses pronouns and prepositions correctly

        (3) Uses simple adjectives (big, little, short, long)

        (4) Verb tense denotes sense of time—not always used correctly until 5 years of age

B. Emotional development—Erikson. By 36 months, autonomy—or self-worth—has been established and child is ready to move on and use physical abilities to learn new skills and interact with others. Without this confidence, the child turns inward, feeling guilty and shameful. However, the period from 2–3 years of age is a time of great fluctuation between independence and overdependence. Personality traits that come into focus during these years are:

1. Temperament
    a. Assertiveness: Accomplishing tasks without using destructive acts toward self or others
    b. Aggressiveness: Child has inadequate controls for the pressures put on him or her.
        (1) Substitutes actions such as bedwetting, temper tantrums
        (2) Watch to whom child is aggressive, and identify the reasons.
    c. Stubbornness: Ascertain whether caused by giving up a pleasure or being overcome by some fear—an expected reaction to child's drive for autonomy and egocentric outlook.
2. Fears and anxiety
    a. These develop now because memory and fantasy are working well enough to distort reality.
    b. Demand for impulse control provides fear of failure; child copes by projecting failure on others or on things and can even conjure up an imaginary friend to take the blame.
    c. Help needed if fears interfere with normal functions of age
3. Affection
    a. Forms attachment to others besides parents
    b. Fond, helping relationship with siblings; constant aggression or teasing between siblings needs investigation.
4. Ambivalence
    a. Despite urge to "do it myself," turns frequently to parents for reassurance
    b. Changes in environment and periods of illness cause regression to earlier behavior patterns.
5. Cooperation: Continues to develop ability to postpone gratification and accept compromise
6. Competence: Wants to try new activities and shows pride in accomplishments
7. Wariness: Keen observer of surroundings
8. Joy: Good health, combined with the feeling of the value of self and others, can make joyfulness the child's dominant mood.
9. Childrearing practices
    a. Continue to converse with child; help child express feelings and ideas.
    b. Provide opportunities for companionship of peers.
    c. Careful supervision necessary to avoid one child's becoming overly dominant or submissive
    d. Variety of friends gives child opportunity to observe wide range of behaviors.
    e. Playing, at 3 years of age, consists of enjoying being with and watching each other, with little interchange. When they talk, each talks about a different topic with little relevance to the other.
    f. Adult needed as referee
    g. As much as possible, provide a consistent, gentle environment.
    h. Begin enlarging the environment for wider experiences.

    i. Stretch expectations, but with an understanding of the child's individual developmental patterns and capabilities; be aware of regressive reactions.

C. Intellectual development—Piaget. Progression from sensory to intuitive learning continues, as shown by the development of memory and symbolic play. Memory is used to recall what has happened in previous incidences and to predict the outcome of the present situation. In symbolic play, by using symbols (words) for actual objects, the child frees him- or herself from reality and can take off into fantasy or can take reality apart and put it together in a different manner. By 3 years of age, the following characteristics are present:

1. Uses toys to represent different things (blocks become bridges)
2. Anticipates consequences of actions; expects parental reaction when caught doing something wrong and is more cautious in attempting new physical activities
3. Symbolizes and pretends; make-believe becomes part of play
4. Dramatic play, usually imitating those around him or her
5. Concentrates on projects but keeps an eye on what is going on around him or her
6. Understands time—before, after, yesterday
7. Language
       a. Increased vocabulary; perfects sentence structure and grammar
       b. Continues labeling and categorizing
       c. Can make most of wants known verbally
       d. Makes statements about feelings ("I like you" or "I hate you"; "I'm mad at you")
       e. Understands most of what is said to him or her
           (1) Learning what world is like and what its values are
       f. Follows three-step directions
       g. Can relate experiences from recent past
8. Childrearing practices
       a. Stimulation
           (1) Play equipment for large muscle use and agility—climbing gyms, balance beam, swings
           (2) Fine motor: Scribbling, puzzles, variety of textures to handle, toys of various shapes and sizes
           (3) Spatial relations: Sandboxes, water tubs
           (4) Language: Simple stories and picture books; being listened to, talked with, and given minimal instruction and correction; child is turned off if expectations are beyond his or her capacity.
           (5) Not burdened with choices and reasoning
       b. Anticipating consequences
           (1) Talk about plans for the day.
           (2) Have child take as many plans forward as possible ("After breakfast"; "After Daddy comes home").
           (3) Discuss "if I do this, then I will have to do that."
           (4) Expect and insist on occasional delayed gratification.

(5) Get child started on projects, but let him or her carry on as he or she wishes.

(6) Show approval when child plans out an activity; also help him or her anticipate the results and consequences.

   c. Dramatic play

     (1) Simple make-believe helps stretch the imagination.

     (2) Help child act out and talk about areas of pressure (sibling rivalry, dominating peers, toilet training, fear of abandonment, punishment, abuse).

   d. Needs individual attention for personal rewards and exchange of affection

9. Risk factors

   a. Poor motor coordination

   b. Delayed speech development (investigate possible hearing loss); inability to use language as a tool

   c. Inability to initiate activities for self; play is random, without plan or make-believe

   d. No primary caregiver to turn to for help, comfort, and positive reinforcement

D. Social development

  1. Shows initiative to go off on own

   a. Most of the time, separates from parent easily

   b. Enjoys being with peers, but can play by self and initiate own activities

  2. Can show affection to others

  3. Practices self-control; learns to accept realistic limits

  4. Continues to need external controls for being good

   a. Approval and affection of parents is the incentive, but child needs consistent limit setting before self-control is dependable.

   b. Shows guilt only if found doing something wrong

   c. Accepting self-criticism and responsibility for actions takes much gentle insistence on behavior standards.

   d. Will blame others and even use an imaginary friend as a scapegoat

  5. Confidence in turning to adults; good eye contact

  6. Cooperative, affectionate; eager to please

  7. Enjoys small group of peers; keenly observant of their behavior; little sharing; no conversation—each talks about own interest

  8. Sexual identity established

   a. Ability to look beyond self; observes physical differences

   b. Selects type of behavior society has accepted for each sex

     (1) Girls: Given positive reinforcement, indulgence, and protectiveness

     (2) Boys: Given negative reinforcement and less sympathy; toys and play of aggressive nature

   c. Role model of female caregiver: Girls rewarded for following role model and boys punished for it; approved behavior is a trial-and-error situation for boys, demanding ingenuity and creativeness

     d. Masturbation: Natural result of increased body awareness; a concern if used as major form of self-satisfaction

  9. Childrearing practices

     a. Safety is greatest concern; caregivers' expectations of impulse control can be unrealistic.

     b. Stretch expectations, but be aware of signs of too much pressure.

     c. Provide friends; watch and listen to interaction; be available as a referee.

     d. Attempt to equalize sex behavior expectations.

        (1) Treat boys positively and gently.

        (2) Treat girls with greater expectations of independence and self-assertiveness.

     e. Accept masturbation as normal; ask for help if concerned.

     f. Discipline consists of positive actions toward promoting self-control, in contrast to punishment, which consists of aggressive actions by caregivers, leading to self-degradation of child.

     g. Limit setting: Provide consistent routine and safe environment; pay attention to any and all acceptable behavior; correct unacceptable behavior with as little attention and show of emotion as possible.

     h. Parental role: Setting exemplary standards with which child can identify

  10. Risk factors

     a. Limit setting does not provide establishment of impulse control.

        (1) Overindulgence: Child does not lose parents' affection, so has no motive to bargain appropriate behavior for approval and attention.

        (2) Overstrictness: Child fears rejection by parents, so does not admit naughtiness done by self—blames others or a mythical friend. Child becomes unsure he or she can control behavior in a new situation, so refuses to try.

     b. Child identified as mean and cruel to others—cannot feel or give affection. In other words, child cannot understand the feelings of others, so feels no remorse for actions toward others.

        (1) Needs referrals and home visits

     c. Parents

        (1) Too anxious, strict, or permissive

        (2) Exacting standards above child's ability to conform

        (3) Cannot accept child's sex; foster inappropriate behavior

     d. Child

        (1) Immature behavior of negativism; distractible and impulsive

        (2) Cannot relate to adults or peers with affection; appears furtive, aggressive or shy, unhappy

E. Safety

  1. Accidents happen most frequently:

     a. When usual routine changes (holidays, vacations, illness in family)

     b. After stressful events (either for caregivers or for child)

     c. When caregivers are tired or ill

     d. Late in the afternoon

2. Accident prevention
   a. Increased energy and curiosity with little behavior control continue to make this a dangerous period.
   b. When in car, child should always remain in car seat.
   c. Accidents—check environment.
   d. Constant surveillance
3. Investigate possibility of child abuse and neglect.
4. Instructions to babysitters
5. Emergency telephone numbers posted

V. Suggested reading

A. Eyre L, Eyre R. *Teaching Your Children Values.* New York: Simon & Schuster, 1993.

B. Freedman B, Brooks A (eds). *On Base.* Kansas City, MO Base Systems Publishing (a division of Westport Press), 1989.

C. Satter E. *How to Get Your Kid to Eat—But Not Too Much.* Palo Alto: Bull Publishing Company, 1987.

NOTES

OVERVIEW

3-YEAR WELL CHILD VISIT

I.   **Special visit**
  A. Review accomplishments of 3 years.
  B. Health and personality patterns well established
  C. Investigation of any concerns or problems will have better results now than ever again.

II. **Parents**
  A. Assessment and appreciation of child's accomplishments
  B. Identify any abuse of family members

III. **Child**
  A. Physical
    1. Following growth chart pattern
    2. Accepting simple balanced meals
    3. Sleep: Dreams and nightmares may frighten child from wanting to follow usual bedtime routine.
    4. Toilet training accomplished: Girls earlier than boys
    5. Systems review: See guidelines.
  B. Emotional: Increasing confidence and independence
  C. Intellectual: Using language for things important to him or her
  D. Social
    1. Enjoys peers: Carefully watches their activities but little interaction
    2. Plays equally well with either sex

IV. **Risk factors**
  A. Frequent illnesses and slow recovery
  B. Impulsive behavior or excessive shyness
  C. No eye contact
  D. No primary caregiver to help establish behavior control

INJURY PREVENTION

I.   **Review safety protocol.**
  A. Memory sufficiently established so that recent past activities and their consequences can be used to restrict behavior. Increased language ability also aids in behavior control. Reasoning with toddler is ineffective; setting consistent limits is imperative.
    1. 3–4 years: Child still in dangerous world of make-believe
    2. 4–5 years: Child more realistic in behavior, but often needs to try out some new activity without being able to predict the outcome
    3. 5–6 years
      a. Child's language skills and behavior control make it more likely that he or she will act carefully.
      b. Child can begin to take some responsibility for own safety.

    c. Child's widening environment needs careful assessment—playground, school, bus, crossing streets, strangers.

CHILD ABUSE

I. Age-specific concerns

    A. Increased physical ability may lead to injuries that are not the result of abuse. Detailed history is important.

    B. Corporal punishment may be a pattern of abuse by caregivers to attempt to establish behavioral control.

II. At-risk child

    A. Insufficient impulse control

    B. Overly passive or aggressive

    C. Health problems

    D. Fearful or aggressive when touched during physical examination

    E. Other members of family being abused

    F. Assessment of all adults with access to child

III. Verbal and psychological abuse needs to be identified.

NOTES

3-YEAR WELL CHILD VISIT

This visit can be planned as a special review session to assess the growth and development that have taken place during the past 3 years. Identifying both accomplished and unaccomplished tasks will provide a guide for the next critical period of growth: the preschool years, ages 3–6.

I. **Review outline.**
   A. Parents
      1. Provide basic physical and emotional needs
      2. Self-direction in identifying and coping with problems
      3. Appreciate their role in setting standards for family's behavioral and cultural patterns
      4. Abuse to any member of family identified
   B. Children
      1. Each child has the opportunity to pass through own developmental stage without undue interference from siblings.
      2. Caring, cooperative, interactive pattern of behavior
   C. Toddler
      1. Stability and maturation of physical systems
      2. Sees self as a person of worth and competence; self-confident, cheerful, cooperative attitude
      3. Identifies sexual identity
      4. Begins to use language as a tool

II. **Health habits**
   A. Nutrition
      1. Accepts simple, balanced menus
      2. Pleasure in eating, but not emphasized as a way of gaining attention or a substitute for emotional needs
   B. Sleep
      1. Accepts bedtime as another pleasant part of daily routine
      2. Sleeps 10–12 hours at night, with one nap or rest period
      3. Dreams are beginning to become real, as the ability for magical thinking develops; inaccurate assessment of reality can be frightening.
   C. Elimination
      1. Daytime control usually by 3 years of age
      2. Nighttime control accomplished later
      3. Takes pride in accomplishment of this control
   D. Speech
      1. Adequate vocabulary to express needs
      2. Not all consonants articulated
      3. Labeling and categorizing

III. **Review of systems**
   A. Growth
      1. Growth pattern consistent with genetics, nutrition, and illnesses

    2. Rate of growth decelerating—height 3″/year, weight 5 lb/year

    3. Weight four times birth weight; length half of adult size

    4. Head 80% of adult size; rate of growth slowing

    5. Legs growing faster than other body parts

B. Skeletal

    1. Bones become stronger as ratio of cartilage to bone decreases; long bones are the first to be ossified, joint bones last.

    2. Craniofacial development gives facial features more definition.

    3. Skeletal age can be used as an indication of overall body maturity.

    4. Bone functions as a reservoir for calcium and bone marrow, providing adequate production of red blood cells.

C. Muscle

    1. Muscle tissue development influenced by hormones, nutrition, and exercise.

    2. Muscle strength depends on amount of tissue, age, and exercise.

    3. Because endurance relates to maturation of cardiac and respiratory systems, which supply oxygen to the muscle tissue, children often have less endurance than expected.

D. Teeth

    1. Complete set of 20 deciduous teeth present; important for mastication and prevention of malocclusion; dental care important

    2. Permanent teeth being formed in jaw

    3. Dental age an indication of overall body maturation

E. Skin

    1. Functioning more efficiently to maintain temperature control

        a. Number of sweat glands developing

        b. Maturity of function of capillaries

        c. Development of adipose tissue, which decreases evaporation of body fluids

    2. Increased acidity of skin aids in resistance to infection.

    3. Increase in melanin production provides better protection from sun's rays.

    4. Sebaceous glands are less active, so skin may become dry.

    5. Subcutaneous fat decreases until about 6 years of age.

F. Vision

    1. Normal acuity at 2–3 years 20/80

    2. Hyperoptic until about 8 years

    3. Astigmatism may still be present because of immaturity and distortion of lens.

    4. Depth perception incomplete until about 6 years

G. Hearing

    1. Acuity at adult level

    2. Aware of pitch and tone

H. Central nervous system

    1. Continuation and refinement of myelination gives increasing neuromuscular coordination.

2. Intellectual abilities increasing because of continued development of cerebral cortex
3. Location of sensations possible; better able to locate and describe pain

I. Cardiovascular
1. Body temperature, pulse, and blood pressure more stable
2. Heart size increasing
3. Sinus arrhythmia still present; heart murmur in 30% to 50% of children

J. Respiratory
1. Increasing lung capacity, as number and size of alveoli increase and muscles of chest are stronger
2. Diaphragmatic breathing still present until about 6 years of age

K. Digestive
1. Digestive juices all present and functioning; all types of simple foods can be digested.
2. Peristalsis less sensitive, so assimilation and absorption of food more efficient
3. Less frequent and firmer stools
4. Habit of swallowing saliva established; drooling no longer occurs.

L. Excretory
1. Maturation of kidney function provides more stable solute levels and less danger of dehydration.
2. Increase in bladder size and sphincter control makes toilet training possible.

M. Immune
1. Ability to produce antibodies improving, but immunoglobulin levels unstable
2. Lymphoid tissues growing rapidly; provide protection from infection until immunoglobulin production is mature
3. Develops own set of antibodies as infections are overcome; slowly increasing resistance to infection

N. Endocrine
1. Growth hormones well developed
2. Pituitary gland regulating growth rate
3. Thyroid gland involved in regulating metabolism and skeletal and dental growth
4. Adrenal gland regulating blood pressure, heart rate, and glucose metabolism
5. Islets of Langerhans regulating blood sugar levels. Immaturity of this system can cause periods of low blood sugar; nutrition and timing of food intake must be evaluated.

IV. Growth and development
A. Emotional
1. Sufficient confidence to participate in activities away from home and parents
2. Resourceful in managing to get own way
3. Can give and receive affection

    4. Dominant mood of cheerfulness and self-satisfaction

 B. Intellectual

    1. Begins to anticipate and verbalize consequences of actions

    2. Continues to attempt to solve problems through trial and error

    3. Distorts reality with make-believe

    4. Begins to use language as a tool

 C. Social

    1. Still separates from parent with some apprehension

    2. Enjoys being with peers but has little interaction with them

    3. Plays well by self

    4. Aware of sexual identity, but plays equally well with members of own and opposite sex

    5. Indicates awareness of right from wrong but shows guilt only if found doing something wrong; eager to please

 D. Risk factors

    1. Inadequate environment to provide basic needs

    2. Inconsistent growth pattern and poor coordination

    3. Health problems not under medical supervision

    4. Impulsive and aggressive or passive behavior patterns

    5. Inability to use language as a tool

    6. Inability to show affection or accept affection from others

    7. No primary adult with whom to establish a caring relationship

    8. Child abuse, physical or verbal, identified

V. **Physical examination**

 A. Growth: Continues on established pattern; "catch up" if there was severe or prolonged illness

 B. Appearance and behavior

    1. Color

    2. Posture

    3. Body proportion

    4. Energy level, alertness, attention to instructions, ability to control activity

    5. Good eye contact, confident manner, interaction with adults other than parent

 C. Specific factors to note during routine physical examination

    1. Skin: Bruising, burns

    2. Eyes: Strabismus

    3. Ears: Mobility of tympanic membrane

    4. Throat: Enlarged tonsil tissue

    5. Neck: Lymph nodes

    6. Chest: Increased breath sounds; diaphragmatic breathing

    7. Heart: Sinus arrhythmia; heart murmur—refer to physician if not previously evaluated.

    8. Abdomen: Muscle tone, femoral pulses, hernias

    9. Genitalia: Irritation, discharge; testes

      10. Musculoskeletal: Muscle development and tone; range of motion

      11. Central nervous system: Gait; more refined coordination; balance; stands on one foot; hops on one foot; buttons up; beginning control in using crayons

  D. Parent–child interaction

      1. Parent: Pride and affection evident

      2. Child: Attention to parent for support and control of activity

VI. Assessment

  A. Physical

  B. Developmental

  C. Emotional

  D. Environmental

VIII. Plan

  A. Immunizations: Complete schedule as needed

  B. Screening: Hematocrit, urinalysis as indicated; blood pressure; hearing and eye test; dental visit

  C. Problem list (devised with parent); SOAP for each

  D. Appropriate timing for office, home, or telephone visits; continue individual scheduling

NOTES

OVERVIEW

ANTICIPATORY GUIDANCE FOR THE PERIOD OF 3–6 YEARS

I. **Guidelines**
  A. Should be viewed as a continuum as each child passes through these developmental stages at own pace
  B. Chronological age may not be applicable.

II. **Parents**
  A. Parents' interest, support, and affection will help guide child from 3-year-old and his or her world of magic to a realistic 6-year-old ready for school and friends.
  B. Identify any form of abuse to family members

III. **Child**
  A. Physical
    1. Health
      a. Following growth pattern
      b. Frequent colds as associating with other children and slowly building up own immunity
      c. Eating
        (1) Selective and independent about food
        (2) Wide variety of foods offered with no choices or discussion
        (3) Food not used as threat or reward
      d. Sleeping
        (1) See guidelines.
        (2) Nightmares are common at 3–4 years of age, but investigation is needed if still frequent by 6 years.
  B. Emotional
    1. Continuing development of self-esteem and confidence to turn from security of home to outside world of peers and school
    2. May be a difficult path, with frequent regressive or aggressive behavior
    3. Child can maintain expected behavior with positive reinforcement.
    4. Beginning to distinguish right from wrong
    5. Consistent caregiver needed to turn to for guidance and encouragement
    6. See guidelines for childrearing practices of each age.
  C. Intellectual
    1. Learning through increased memory of experiences and their consequences
    2. Initiating own activities and creative play
    3. Television watching can inhibit these creative activities.
    4. See guidelines for each age's expectations.
  D. Social
    1. Enjoys being with peers, but watching each other rather than interactive play. Listening to children's conversations is a way to observe how each child is carrying on own independent conversation.
    2. Practices how to maintain own egocentric wishes
    3. Sexual identity

       a. Plays equally well with either sex

       b. See guidelines for each age's expectations and childrearing practices.

IV. **Risk factors**

    A. Poor health or serious illness

    B. Overly shy or overly aggressive behavior

    C. Poor language development

    D. No appropriate role model

V. **Watch for:**

    A. Cheerful, mischievous, energetic child

    B. Good eye contact with adults

    C. Shows pride and self-confidence in accomplishments

    D. Language understandable to others besides family members

    E. Gives directives to others but does not always accept suggestions from others

    F. Accepts behavioral standards; shows guilt if found doing something wrong

    G. Unhappy, aggressive, whining child needs special attention.

NOTES

ANTICIPATORY GUIDANCE FOR THE PERIOD OF 3–6 YEARS

These 3 years provide the time needed to expand physical and psychosocial skills. By age 6, the child will be a competent, self-assured, friendly first-grader.

I. **Expectations of this period**
   A. Physical maturity
      1. Increasing muscle strength and endurance
      2. Developing immunity to infectious disease
   B. Magic and fantasy give way to reality.
   C. Language skills developing. Child begins to attend to what others are saying; by 6 years, interactive speech is possible.
   D. Values of environment are being internalized, and actions are being guided by these standards.

II. **Family status**
   A. Parents
      1. Provide basic physical and developmental needs
      2. Responsible for adequate child care arrangements
      3. Household tasks scheduled and responsibilities for each family member defined
      4. Emergency planning—accidents, illness, fire, telephone contacts
      5. Family meetings to share experiences, plan activities, and give support to each other
      6. Abuse to any family member investigated
   B. Children
      1. Each developing according to own capabilities without being overpowered by parents or siblings
      2. Demonstrating tolerance, affection, and support for each other
      3. Developing interactive techniques without teasing or aggression
      4. Abuse identified

III. **Health patterns**
   A. Nutrition
      1. Child is selective and more independent about food.
      2. Encourage some involvement in food preparation and shopping.
      3. Encourage good breakfast habits in anticipation of school years.
      4. Offer small amounts of nutritious foods often during the day.
      5. Encourage eating of vegetables and fruits (children often prefer these raw) as snacks.
      6. Do not force child to eat; poor appetite needs investigation.
      7. Do not use food as a bribe, threat, or reward.
   B. Health
      1. Frequent colds expected because of child's associating with other children and still building up immunity to infections
      2. If recovery prolonged, evaluation of basic health pattern needed

C. Sleep
1. Regular pattern established (10–12 hours at night)
2. Naps: Help child become aware of periods of fatigue and provide a rest area.
3. Dreams can be frightening, as child is still learning to distinguish dreams from reality. Investigate overstimulation, anxiety, exhaustion.
4. Teeth grinding: Correlates with frequency of nightmares; can be a way of releasing unrelieved emotional pressures
D. Elimination
1. Regular pattern established; learning to manage self
2. Occasional accidents, usually due to illness, changes in world, or some traumatic experience
3. Continued soiling or return to bedwetting needs investigation.
4. Enuresis: See Enuresis in Part II.
E. Childrearing practices
1. No rewards for illness
2. Responsibility for wellness becoming part of child's learning
3. Provide openness to talk about unusual discomforts, body functions, and maltreatment.
F. Risk factors
1. Basic health patterns not becoming routine
2. Somatic complaints being used for emotional support

IV. **Growth and development**
A. Physical
1. Growth rate about 3″/year
a. Legs growing the fastest
b. Facial bones developing and fat pads disappearing; by age 5, child looks as he or she will as an adult.
c. Muscle development and strength increasing through activity; not sex-dependent
2. Gross motor: Improving coordination makes hopping, skipping, and dancing possible.
3. Fine motor: By 5–6 years, child can draw recognizable objects.
4. Speech
a. Vocabulary
(1) Increasing seemingly without any effort
(2) By 5–6 years of age, child uses verb tenses and plurals correctly.
b. Articulation
(1) Stuttering is occasionally present, as ideas come faster than words can be found.
(2) Lisping until 5–6 years is a matter of maturation.
B. Emotional development—Erikson: Initiative versus guilt. This stage sees the progression from activities motivated merely by responses to stimuli or imitative actions to purposeful activity. Initiating activity, both physical and intellectual, continues the development of competence and feeling of independence. Without the opportunity or the physical skills to explore, manipulate, and

challenge the environment, the competencies and independence that could have been attained are delayed or never developed. These experiences become the basic values determining the ratio of self-confidence to inferiority.

1. Emotions become more stable as the child develops.
   a. Feeling of competence in doing things for self
   b. Able to manage away from home
   c. Able to make friends and relate to adults other than parents
   d. Increase in intellectual capacity, so child understands world and can plan activities
2. Temperament
   a. Egocentric: Enjoys being with peers, but not until age 7–8 will he or she listen to another's point of view
   b. Innovative in activities
   c. Mischievous, joyful
   d. Affection: An egocentric reaction for approval and attention
   e. Assertive: Improving memory and language skills used to direct activities and influence others
   f. Aggression
      (1) Mode of behavior that continues through observing adult role models
      (2) Means of getting rid of unrelieved frustrations
      (3) Egocentric needs not met
   g. Cooperation: Continues to bargain appropriate behavior for approval and attention
   h. Fear: Expected reaction to world of fantasy and increase in physical daring
   i. Shyness
      (1) Lack of feelings of competency and independence
      (2) Personality characteristic
   j. Passivity: Overcontrol by adults can make child fearful to act on own. Lack of developed built-in behavioral controls can prevent child from attempting activity.
   k. So much is to be accomplished in these 3 years that occasional reversals to earlier behavior patterns can be expected.
3. Risk factors
   a. Fearful
   b. Explosive
   c. Inactive
   d. Withdrawn
   e. Insufficient language or unable to express self
   f. Poor sleep pattern
4. Childrearing practices
   a. 3–4 years
      (1) Short periods of peer companionship under adult supervision; child needs sufficient time by self to develop pleasure from initiating and accomplishing activities.

        (2) Open spaces and large equipment for play

        (3) Safe boundaries and consistent limits on behavior

        (4) Primary adult listener, confidant, and giver of attention and approval

  b. 4–5 years

        (1) More time with peers, but with continued supervision

        (2) Variety of activities and experiences to broaden response pattern

        (3) Learning to use language rather than aggressive acts to get own way

        (4) Give opportunities to take responsibility for behavior.

        (5) Primary adult listener, confidant, and giver of attention and approval

  c. 5–6 years

        (1) Opportunity to use increased skills for independent planning and performance of activities

        (2) Plan peer interaction and participation in simple group games.

        (3) Improve interaction by asking child to repeat ideas given by others.

        (4) Child still needs primary adult for attention and support.

C. Intellectual development—Piaget. These years continue the child's egocentric way of seeing the world. Learning intuitively through self-activity, having little concern for reality, and using increasing memory and language, children keep reconstructing their world to fit their needs. By 6 years of age, the influence of peers and their own experiences force children to take a more realistic view of the world around them.

  1. Expectations

    a. 3–4 years

        (1) Intuitive learning through free-wheeling activities

            (a) Pretending; trying on role activities of other

            (b) Increase in mental functioning and memory; learning cause and effect of activities

            (c) Investigating and manipulating everything that can be reached

            (d) Watching activities of others

            (e) Magical world: Limited experience gives incorrect explanations of events.

        (2) Memory continues storing up events and their outcomes.

    b. 4–5 years

        (1) Intuitive learning continues through the initiative to attempt new and creative ways to do things.

        (2) Magical world is giving way to reality as past experiences are used to predict the correct outcome, often causing an unhappy, rebellious child.

        (3) Logical reasoning is still a long way off.

    c. 5–6 years

        (1) Beginning to learn through language

        (2) Can maintain a single line of thought

        (3) Listens to others, but with little exchange of ideas

    (4) Integrates past experiences to form a more reliable version reality and time, making for a more contented, cooperative child

  d. Risk factors

    (1) Passive and cautious in activities

    (2) Magical thinking still dominating activity at age 4–5

    (3) Impulsive, quarrelsome behavior at age 4–5

    (4) No primary adult to provide support and affection

  e. Childrearing practices

    (1) Safe areas where high-level energy can be expended

    (2) Variety of activities with opportunity for some association with children slightly older

    (3) Play equipment: for large muscle activity, for perceptual learning; materials and opportunity for dramatic play

    (4) Discussion of activities; time for someone to listen to child

    (5) Primary adult to provide support and affection

2. Language

  a. 3–4 years

    (1) Makes declarative statements about own wants and feelings

    (2) Thinks out loud; cannot be expected to keep a secret

    (3) Conversations consist of each child talking only for self, not attending to or responding to ideas of others.

    (4) Enjoys being read to and memorizing nursery rhymes

    (5) Body language supplements these limited language skills.

  b. 4–5 years

    (1) A quarrelsome period of learning to interact with peers

    (2) Quarrels force child to express ideas and listen to the ideas of others.

  c. By 5 years

    (1) Listening skills are improving, but not until 7–8 years can child listen to others well enough to have an exchange of ideas.

    (2) Improving ability to use words in place of action; needs role model of people doing this and help in developing this skill

  d. Risk factors

    (1) Impulsive behavior; unable to use language as a controller of action

    (2) Too quiet; retreating into silence in confrontations

    (3) Continued baby talk and poor fluency

  e. Childrearing practices

    (1) Avoid correcting errors; child will make own corrections.

    (2) Pay no attention to stuttering; increased concern will add to problem.

    (3) Provide good speech and language role models.

    (4) Provide a patient listener to hear child express feelings and ideas.

3. School readiness by 6 years

  a. Able to manage away from home

    b. Able to accept behavior control expectations

    c. Able to interact with adults other than parents

    d. Language skills sufficient to express ideas

    e. Listening skills sufficient to attend to directions of others

    f. Sufficient self-esteem to be able to carry on independent activity

4. Television watching

    a. Passive activity; replaces important learning from self-initiated activity

    b. Child fascinated by color, sound, motion; energy put into watching, not taking in story

    c. Child cannot distinguish between fantasy and reality

    d. By age 5, child relates to characters as role models; aggressive behavior seen as appropriate

    e. Usurps family conversations and interaction

5. Television control

    a. Discuss as a family what programs are to be selected, each member having a limited choice.

    b. Discuss programs.

    c. Watch programs with child.

    d. Pay attention to snacks eaten while watching TV; often they are junk foods, high in calories and fat and low in nutrients.

    e. Set up play equipment near TV set as an alternative to watching.

    f. Set up definite times for TV watching and definite times when TV is turned off.

D. Social development

    1. Expectations: Sequential development in becoming a member of society; by the time child enters first grade, the following expectations must be met so that child is freed of egocentric needs and can reach out to learn and enjoy the companionship of others:

        a. 3–4 years

            (1) Managing away from home; sufficient ability to control behavior

            (2) Observant of what is going on around him or her; peer relationships consist of watching each other but playing independently

            (3) Instigating own activities

            (4) Turning to adults for help and support

        b. 4–5 years

            (1) Easily accepts expected appropriate behavior

            (2) Peer relationships are often quarrelsome, as each child attempts to argue for his or her own way

            (3) Eager to please primary caregiver, remorseful if caught doing wrong

        c. 5–6 years

            (1) Able to join peers in simple interactive games

            (2) Dogmatic; changes rules as needed to benefit self

            (3) Internalizing behavioral patterns; standards of family and peer group accepted

      (4) Sufficient self-esteem for independent activities without constant demanding of attention

  2. Sexual identity

    a. From 3–5 years, child is usually indiscriminate as to which sex he or she is with; will take on role of either sex in dramatic play

    b. By age 6, prefers company of own sex; this preference continues until adolescence.

    c. Social expectations of each sex are internalized.

      (1) Boys more combative and daring

      (2) Girls use words as weapons and coyness and guile to get their own way.

    d. Modification of sex-typing patterns

      (1) Boys: Gentleness, nonpunitive punishment

      (2) Girls: Develop feelings of competence and industry by devising more challenging physical activities and intellectual projects.

  3. Risk factors

    a. Parents with low self-esteem have difficulty enforcing consistent behavioral standards.

    b. Inadequate environment for active, curious child

    c. Few opportunities to be with other children; little supervision if with other children

    d. No primary caring adult

  4. Childrearing practices

    a. Promoting acceptable behavior

      (1) Safe environment with sufficient space and equipment for constructive activities

      (2) Consistent daily schedule; expected behavior defined and maintained

      (3) Caregivers understand child's ability to comply with demands put on him or her.

      (4) Child spends some time with older children; imitating is easiest way for child to learn.

      (5) Positive reinforcement, such as hugs and kisses; approval needed for each small step; be aware of things child is doing right.

      (6) Remember that logic and reasoning are not part of child's skills yet.

    b. Discipline

      (1) Expect child to control behavior for attention and approval.

      (2) Give positive reinforcement for all appropriate behaviors.

      (3) Harmful behavior to self and others must be stopped but must not be the only way for the child to get attention.

      (4) Frequent aggressive and uncontrolled behavior needs investigation into the child's role models, unrelieved pressures, and physical problems.

      (5) Punitive punishment feeds into anger and violence.

E. Safety

  1. Accidents happen most frequently:

   a. When usual routine changes (holidays, vacations, illness in family)
   b. After stressful events (for caregivers or for child)
   c. When caregivers are tired or ill
   d. Late in the afternoon
2. Accident prevention
   a. Child is beginning to understand consequences of actions.
   b. Responsibilities given as child demonstrates reliability
   c. Magical thinking makes child think he or she can do the impossible.
   d. Family rules established and discussed
      (1) Responsibilities outlined for each family member
      (2) Fire drills practiced and meeting place established
      (3) Emergency plans established and rehearsed
      (4) Telephone numbers posted and practiced
3. Investigate frequent injuries as possible child neglect or abuse.
4. Instructions to babysitters

V. Suggested reading
   A. Berenstain S, Berenstain J. *The Berenstain Bears Learn About Strangers.* New York: Random House, 1985.
   B. Lenett R, Crane B. *It's OK to Say No!: A Parent–Child Manual for the Protection of Children.* New York: Tom Doherty & Associates.
   C. Porett J. *When I Was Little Like You.* Washington DC: Child Welfare League of America, 1993.
   D. "Winnie the Pooh: Too Smart for Strangers." Walt Disney Home Video: Burbank, CA, 1985.

NOTES

| OVERVIEW

6-YEAR WELL CHILD VISIT

I. **Parents**
   A. Observing carefully child's ability to:
      1. Cope with long day away at school
      2. Maintain appropriate behavior and independence with new friends
      3. Talk about daily experiences, although child still has difficulty expressing ideas and feelings
   B. Identify abuse of any family member
II. **Child**
   A. Physical
      1. Slow growth rate for both sexes
         a. Enjoys food and accepts a well-balanced diet; family emphasis on physical fitness enjoyed
         b. Sleeps 10–12 hours; nightmares should be occurring less frequently
         c. Speech: Articulation of all sounds
         d. Loosing teeth in same order as eruption
   B. Emotional: Initiates own activities but has difficulty following activities of others; still attempts to control own world and expects things to be done his or her way
   C. Intellectual: No longer interested in magical world, but now thinks concretely—how things are and how they work
   D. Social
      1. Experiments with ways to interact successfully with teachers and peers
      2. Prefers associating with own sex
      3. Cultural and ethnic patterns of others difficult to understand
III. **Risk factors**
   A. Poor school adjustment or inappropriate school
   B. Frequent illness or using illness as a way to escape new developmental tasks
   C. No primary caregiver to listen to him or her
IV. **See guidelines for specific factors to be noted in physical examination.**

| INJURY PREVENTION

I. **Review safety protocol.**
   A. Many new challenges face children from 6–9 years of age as they reach a wider environment and have less surveillance of their activities. First-aid courses and injury-prevention classes need to be available for children.
II. **Accident frequency**
   A. Accidents most common in this age group
      1. Bicycles, particularly riding without proper helmet
      2. Skateboards and in-line skates, without proper equipment
      3. Contact sports—equipment and supervision needed
      4. Swimming accidents

    5. Guns—where ammunition not locked away

III. Societal health problems

  A. Problems they are soon to be faced with are drugs, sexual abuse, eating disorders, alcohol, and smoking.

    1. Special attention and education needed

    2. Learn how to handle advances made by strangers

  B. Peer group pressure needs to be countered by a caring adult.

    1. Home-alone children must have strict regulations and emergency planning.

CHILD ABUSE

I. **Age-specific factors**

  A. Children should now be able to verbalize any unwanted physical touching or attacks.

    1. May be better able to talk away from parents—for instance, during privacy of physical examination

II. **Areas to investigate**

  A. Sexual abuse, corporal punishment, overreaction to pain, confronting sexual harassment and harassers

III. **At-risk child**

  A. Continued health problems

  B. Unhappy, depressed versus aggressive, arrogant

  C. Verbal and psychological abuse

  D. No caring adult with whom to relate

NOTES

6-YEAR WELL CHILD VISIT

The attitudes of competence, self-worth, and initiative that the 6-year-old has developed provide the impetus to separate more completely from family and home. Both the child and family enjoy their increasing independence. Attending school and associating with teachers and peers provide the child with new challenges to develop his or her own capabilities and self-confidence within the enlarging world.

I. **Developmental process**
   A. Parents
      1. Understand the importance of change from home- and family-centered child to teacher- and peer group-centered child
      2. Have consistent expectations of appropriate behavior
      3. Continue to provide safe, supportive environment
      4. Child abuse identified
   B. Child
      1. Maintains appropriate behavior, accepting cultural values of family
      2. Busy and happy with projects at school and with friends
      3. Continues to turn to family for support

II. **Family status**
   A. Parental concerns and problems: Ability to identify problems and to cope
   B. Illnesses in family since last visit
   C. Parental assessment of child's development
   D. Family interaction and support for each other
      1. Organization of responsibilities for each member
      2. Review and updating of emergency planning
      3. Meetings for group decisions, problem solving, and sharing of experiences
      4. Sibling rivalry problems; referrals as needed
   E. Fear of violence or abuse identified

III. **Health habits**
   A. Nutrition and diet history
      1. Adequate diet offered
      2. Intake of food during school hours; snacks
      3. Child learning basics of nutrition
      4. Ethnic eating patterns evaluated
      5. Continued involvement in shopping and preparation of foods
   B. Sleep
      1. Restful 10 hours with fewer disturbances from nightmares
      2. Falls asleep easily unless overtired or overstimulated
      3. Beginning to realize when he or she needs rest and sleep
   C. Elimination
      1. Managing independently
      2. Family routine allows regular time of bowel movements.
      3. Problems or discomforts discussed with caregiver

4. Enuresis: See Enuresis in Part II.
5. Encopresis: Refer to physician.

IV. **Growth and development**

A. Physical

1. Growth follows established pattern.

a. Participates in activities to develop endurance and large muscles, such as climbing, swimming, running

b. Develops muscle coordination with games of rhythm, music, and using large balls

c. Baseball requires slowly developing eye–hand coordination.

d. Activity program needed that is designed to develop individual skills.

e. Family emphasis on importance of physical fitness

f. Careful supervision to de-emphasize competitive games until child is physically and emotionally ready

2. Teeth

a. Loses teeth in the same order as eruption

b. Child takes responsibility of daily care.

c. Dental care available

B. Speech development

1. Articulates all sounds by 6–7 years

2. Correctly uses verb tenses, plurals, pronouns

3. Vocabulary increases, and most words used appropriately

C. Emotional development—Erikson: Initiative versus guilt. Child demonstrates that he or she feels competent to manage daily routine, can make friends, and can accept and return affection of primary caregivers.

1. Enthusiastic about daily happenings but cautious about routine changes and new experiences

2. Enjoys companionship of peers but continues to want to do things his or her way

3. Instigates and carries through new projects

4. Continues to turn to caregivers for affection and approval

5. If these attitudes are not present, further assessment is needed.

D. Intellectual development—Piaget: From intuitive learning to concrete thinking. Child continues through sufficient experiences to distinguish fact from fantasy. His or her world of reality is established through increased memory and ability to symbolize experiences.

1. Learning

a. Enjoys school, learning of facts; rather than "What does that do?" child asks, "How does it work?"

b. Turns to stories of actual adventures; no longer interested in fairy tales

c. Can define ways to solve a problem and understand its consequences

2. Language

a. Enjoys words, riddles, puns

b. Experiments with sounds—chants, songs, poems

c. Exchanges factual information, but has trouble expressing ideas and feelings

    E. Social development: Continuing task is to learn to interact successfully with those in child's enlarging world of school and community.

       1. Inconsistent behavior in trying to find successful interactive patterns

       2. Frequent changes in friendships

       3. Depends on own rules for expected ways of acting for self and playmates

       4. Turns to adults as guides to cultural and moral behavior; internalizes behavioral patterns of culture

    F. Risk factors

       1. Family

          a. Needs not being met

          b. Inappropriate and inconsistent expectations of child

          c. Abuse of any family member

       2. Child

          a. Inappropriate behavior patterns

            (1) Lack of behavior control

            (2) Not showing guilt when doing wrong

            (3) No appropriate role models

          b. Developmental lags (specifically neurologic and speech)

          c. Inability to relate appropriately to siblings, peers, and adults

          d. Poor adjustment to school

V. Physical examination

    A. Appearance

       1. Body proportion

       2. Muscle development

    B. Behavior

       1. Makes eye contact

       2. Cooperative

       3. Interested in visit

       4. Able to contribute to history taking

    C. Growth

       1. Continues on established pattern

       2. Investigate if more than two standard deviations in height or weight

    D. Specific factors to note during routine physical examination

       1. Skin: Excessive bruises, burns

       2. Eyes: Equal tracking

       3. Ears: Mobility of tympanic membrane

       4. Teeth: Losing teeth in order of appearance; occlusion; cavities

       5. Throat: Tonsils—size, color, pitting

       6. Heart: Sinus arrhythmia

       7. Abdomen: Muscle tone, hernia

       8. Genitalia: Irritation, discharge, phimosis

       9. Musculoskeletal: Muscle development, strength, tone; scoliosis

      10. Neurologic: Coordination—gait, skip, hop; fine motor—draws triangle horizontal, vertical

    E. Parent–child interaction
        1. Parent—pride and affection evident
        2. Child—responds to parent in positive manner
    F. Assessment
    G. Plan

NOTES

OVERVIEW

ANTICIPATORY GUIDANCE FOR THE PERIOD OF 6–9 YEARS

I. **Parents**

   A. Appreciate role of establishing family standards and cultural values

   B. Discuss expectations with child and devise plans toward cooperation in maintaining them

   C. Plan sufficient time with child to listen and talk about experiences

   D. Provide opportunities for successful experiences at school and with friends

II. **Child**

   A. Physical

      1. Slower growth pattern for both sexes but agility and coordination improving

      2. Early-maturing girls can begin hormonal changes by age 9; evident by developing chubbiness

      3. Diet: Learning to take responsibility for eating balanced diet

      4. Elimination: Boys have more evidence of encopresis and enuresis; important to elicit this information and refer to physician

      5. Safety: Accident-prone behavior needs evaluation.

   B. Emotional

      1. Successful experiences are important to continue child's growth toward self-esteem and self-confidence. Without these, a feeling of inferiority can take over child's attitude toward self and his or her ability.

      2. See guidelines for characteristics of temperament.

   C. Intellectual

      1. Developing ability to think realistically helps child manage self and affairs effectively.

      2. See guidelines for school and learning expectations for each age group.

   D. Social

      1. Child turns from needing only a few friends to expecting to become a member of a group or gang. Community activities such as scouts, church, and sports can provide appropriate groups.

      2. See guidelines for age-appropriate expectations.

III. **Risk factors**

   A. Poor school adjustment, not working up to capacity

   B. Using aggressive behavior to gain attention

   C. Accident-prone or frequent illnesses

   D. Depending on TV or computer games for entertainment rather than enjoying companionship of others

IV. **Safety and accident prevention**

   A. See guidelines for accident prevention.

V. **Watch for:**

   A. Development of a positive or negative attitude toward self and world

      1. Positive role model; authority figure who demonstrates gentleness, fairness, affection, respect, and cooperation

2. Adult who listens carefully to child's ideas and helps him or her express ideas and feelings
3. Self-fulfilling prophecy "I'm OK"
4. Family, school, and community taking responsibility to help child develop positive behavioral pattern

B. Now is the time to identify children without a supportive adult and to make appropriate referrals and follow-up.

NOTES

ANTICIPATORY GUIDANCE FOR THE PERIOD OF 6–9 YEARS

Like the other age periods, the years 6–9 are not a single unit. Contrasting a 6-year-old and a 9-year-old shows what a big step this is. The 6-year-old retains many characteristics of earlier periods, including struggling to find a way to establish him- or herself with peers and turning back to the family for overt shows of affection. In contrast, the 9-year-old is a firm member of the gang, accepting its rituals and rules and taking disappointments and hurts stoically. This period, the first that can be recalled chronologically, includes years of freedom, fun, and fond memories.

I. **Expectations of this period**
   A. By 9 years, the child:
   1. Is separating from the family and making independent decisions
   2. Can relate successfully to peers and adults other than parents
   3. Enjoys school and is eager to learn
   4. Instigates projects; has perseverance and derives pleasure from completing tasks
   5. Turns to family for support and approval
   6. Is guided in behavior by rules of family and peers and understands consequences of behavior

II. **Family status**
   A. Basic needs being met; self-direction in coping with problems
   B. Parents
   1. Take pride in and enjoy child
   2. Foster independence and new experiences
   3. Take time for listening, discussions, and support
   4. Give responsibility as child demonstrates he or she can accept it
   5. Act as a moral guide and role model of love and affection
   6. Spend time to see that family rules are adhered to
   7. Report abuse of any family member
   C. Child
   1. Moves away from a close association with family to own peer group
   2. Accepts household responsibilities and schedules
   3. Returns to family for support and belonging
   4. Begins challenging family values with the values of peers and school; moral judgment limited by inability to appreciate views of others
   5. Learns to accept consequences of actions

III. **Health patterns**
   A. Nutrition
   1. Learns nutritional standards such as basic four food groups; knows nutritious foods versus junk foods
   2. Participates in meal planning and shopping
   3. Keeps chart for adequate calories and nutrition as needed
   B. Elimination
   1. Responsibility for regular schedule

2. Boys have more frequent problems with constipation and soiling than girls—refer to physician if a continuing problem.
   3. Enuresis: See Enuresis in Part II
C. Sleep
   1. Individual pattern (8–10 hours)
   2. Older child can stay up later than younger child; this gives parents time with each child and gives the children a feeling of individuality.
   3. Can awaken on time in the morning and has sufficient energy for day's activities
D. Exercise
   1. High energy level and muscular development require adequate opportunity for exercise.
   2. Supervised sports program in and after school for both boys and girls
   3. Free play periods—safe environment, necessary limits
   4. TV watching limited
E. Responsibility for own health
   1. Adequate role models
   2. Realizes pleasure and advantage of good health and disadvantage of illness
      a. Knowledge and willingness to obtain health care
      b. Social and emotional problems identified—parents or school personnel used as resource
F. Safety
   1. Realistic thinking promotes more cautiousness.
   2. Accident-prone children: Investigate causes.
   a. Awkwardness
   b. Daredevil behavior to get attention from peers
   c. Unstable environment causing inattention and high level of frustration
IV. **Growth and development**
A. Physical
   1. Growth continues at a slow pace for both sexes.
      a. Chubbiness at 8–9 years does not mean future obesity; after puberty there is usually a return to the previous pattern.
      b. Muscle growth equal for both sexes; amount of exercise now determines muscle strength.
   2. Teeth—"age of the loose tooth"
      a. Teeth replaced in same order as eruption of deciduous teeth
      b. Dental care: Discuss fluoride treatments with dentist if no fluoride in drinking water
   3. Eyes: By 7 years, visual acuity of 20/20–20/30
   4. Speech
      a. Articulation: Refer to speech therapist if problems with enunciation, slurring, or fluency continue.
      b. More complex sentences used (5–7 words).
      c. Rapid increase in vocabulary
      d. Careless enunciation can be improved by whistling, repeating jingles

and tongue twisters, and singing; listening to tape of own voice also
is helpful.

5. Development of secondary sex characteristics: Organ enlargement begins
   2–4 years before puberty.

   a. Girls: Growth spurt at 9–14 years; breast enlargement at 8–13 years;
      menses at 10–16 years

   b. Boys: Growth spurt at 10.5–13.5 years; enlarged testes at 9.5–13.5 years

6. Childrearing practices

   a. School athletic program: Title IX specifies equal time and money for
      girls and boys.

   b. 6–7 years

      (1) Child learns to interact and to play according to rules but finds
          it difficult to be a loser.

      (2) Physical coordination allows simple games such as kickball; eye–
          hand coordination and depth perception are insufficient for much
          success at more skilled games.

      (3) Muscle strength and development progress rapidly; equipment is
          needed to enhance this.

      (4) Endurance is greatly improved, but signs of fatigue need to be iden-
          tified.

   c. 8–9 years

      (1) Sportsmanship a gang standard

      (2) Child can interact well enough to enjoy team sports.

      (3) Girls need sufficient opportunities to develop muscle strength and
          have team participation.

B. Emotional development—Erikson: Industry versus inferiority. Building on
   previously developed attitudes of self-confidence, competence, and independence, the child attempts new projects. Completing these projects fosters
   pleasure and satisfaction in doing and succeeding. These same skills apply to
   participating in school and making new friends successfully. Without opportunities for these successes, feelings of inferiority develop.

   1. Temperament

      a. Egocentric thinking continues until age 7–8, when child can include
         peer group in his or her world.

      b. Affection: Turns from family to teacher and peer group for affection
         and approval

      c. Spontaneous and enthusiastic; enjoys new outside world

      d. Assertive: Attempts to persuade others to do things his or her way;
         demands own share, own turn, and own belongings

      e. Self-concept: Sees self as different from others and begins to perceive
         own abilities

      f. Self-identity: Moves away from family; becomes dependent on
         gang's assessment

      g. Self-esteem: Approval or disapproval of those important to him or
         her reflects view of self.

      h. Sexual identity: Interacts best with own sex (both adults and peers);
         takes on society's role expectations; by age 8–9, curiosity; needs facts
         and proper vocabulary

    i. Frustration: Learns to cope with disappointments; learns to have more realistic expectations

2. Risk factors

    a. Attitudes of defiance, rebellion, aggression, and overpassivity need careful, intense workup.

    b. Treatment now is more likely to be successful than in the future.

3. Childrearing practices

    a. Independence of parents and child; important to have specific times together for planning, companionship, support

    b. Carefully watch child's success and failure in school and with friends; promote open communication so that understanding of problems is possible.

    c. Provide opportunities for successful experiences.

        (1) Appropriate school experience for child's ability

        (2) Playmates available of same size, age, and interests; playing with older or younger child causes child to be bossed or to do the bossing with no possibility of reciprocal interaction.

    d. Affection and approval

        (1) Child keen enough to know when approval is undeserved; demands and gives honest opinions

        (2) Child needs help expressing affection and love; compassionate role model needed

    e. Seek help if:

        (1) Child continues to be unsuccessful in school or in making friends

        (2) Child cannot control acting out or is predominantly passive in behavior

        (3) Communication between parents and child is poor

C. Intellectual development—Piaget. During this period, child progresses from learning through intuition to learning through concrete experiences. Difference between fantasy and reality is being sorted out and replaced by facts and order, systematic thinking, organizing, and classifying. Problems need to be tested in actuality; hypotheses are not yet comprehended.

1. Expectations

    a. 6–7 years

        (1) Still learning intuitively, but with good memory and building up of experiences will soon become a realist

        (2) Ready for learning

        (3) Can still be unrealistic in explanations of events

        (4) Can remember letters and numbers

        (5) Expends much energy in learning to manage away from home and to interact with teacher and peers—can cause learning difficulties if this becomes an overriding concern

    b. 7–8 years

        (1) Learning concretely; logical reasoning improving

        (2) Can sit still longer

        (3) Lengthening attention span and improving listening skills

    c. 8–9 years

        (1) Looks for cause and effect (scientist)

        (2) Comprehends reading material more easily

        (3) Time and place: past becomes important; interest in far-off places

        (4) Basic writing, spelling, reading skills accomplished

    d. Identify intellectual behavior by:

        (1) Successfully adapts to new situations

        (2) Changes thinking to new requirements

        (3) Manages self and affairs effectively

        (4) Has acute sense of humor

        (5) Is goal-directed

    e. Risk factors

        (1) Difficult and unhappy adjustment away from home

        (2) Inappropriate schooling for child's abilities

    f. Childrearing practices

        (1) Sincere, consistent interest in child's schoolwork

        (2) Participation in school organizations by parents

        (3) Defined, realistic expectations of child, following teacher conference and own judgment

        (4) Consistent insistence on child's appropriate behaviors

        (5) "What's the hurry?": If social or academic problems arise, this is the best time to give the child a chance to catch up.

            (a) Boys: One of the youngest and smallest in the class

            (b) Girls: One of the youngest in the class, with a maternal history of late pubertal maturation; by sixth or seventh grade, still a little girl while classmates are becoming young ladies; socially a misfit at a crucial time of development

2. Language

    a. Vocabulary development important for expression of increasing range of feelings and experiences

    b. Expresses ideas and feelings; used as a coping and problem-solving mechanism

    c. Childrearing practices

        (1) Vocabulary development

            (a) Encourage word games, crossword puzzles, word tests of synonyms and antonyms, dictionary use.

            (b) Provide new experiences and find specific new words from these experiences.

            (c) Encourage reading: Read to child until reading skills are sufficient for child to take over; visit library.

            (d) TV: learning from pictures and voices; can cause difficulty in shifting to letters

        (2) Help in developing communication skills

            (a) Expressing feelings; finding precise vocabulary

            (b) Stating problems; defining problem areas

(c) Developing "think tank" solutions

(d) Predicting outcome of each solution

(e) Appropriate listener available

(3) Bilingual home

   (a) Most children handle bilingualism successfully.

   (b) If problems, child should develop proficiency in one language, then return to the second.

(4) Listening skills

   (a) For awareness of speech, encourage memorizing and reciting, repeating digit lists (backward and forward), learning nonsense verse.

   (b) Music: Have child learn to play an instrument and read music.

   (c) Encourage child to repeat statements of others before giving an answer.

   (d) Constant high background noise discourages efforts to listen.

   (e) Approving adult with whom to talk

(5) Writing skills

   (a) By 6 years: Has muscle control for printing large letters

   (b) By 7–8 years: Writes simple, short sentences; one idea or fact, few adjectives or adverbs

   (c) By 9 years: Can write compositions of 200 words

   (d) Spelling: Connecting sound to written form demands attention to detail, a difficult task for a child with other concerns.

D. Social development

1. Expectations

  a. 6–7 years

    (1) Successfully managing a whole day at school; taking the bus; eating away from home, bathroom independence; now able to sit still, listen, answer questions, and, most particularly, be aware of what others are doing

    (2) Interaction with teacher established

    (3) Still controls behavior for attention and approval

    (4) Makes friends with a few classmates

  b. 7–8 years

    (1) Enjoys school; eager to learn

    (2) Reliable, accepts behavioral expectations

    (3) Makes friends but changes affections frequently

    (4) Groups have loose ties and easily change members.

    (5) Rules not absolute, change to serve own purpose

  c. 8–9 years

    (1) Exceptional period of good health, good academic skills, good friends, and few concerns

    (2) Peer groups: Behavioral phenomenon that appears to develop in all societies

      (a) Rules and rituals are rigid and form boundaries of behavior.

(b)   Leadership by those who are largest (in boys' group) and the best talkers (in girls' groups) and who can understand feelings of other gang members

(c)   Satisfies need for companionship and approval

(d)   Needs opportunity to compare gang values with standards of family

(e)   Perpetuates segregation; continued sex discrimination, even beyond this age group (fraternities, lodges, service clubs); usually part of a neighborhood group, which perpetuates ethnic affiliations

(f)   Organized peer groups such as scouts, church groups continue society's cultural patterns.

2. Risk factors

   a. Inability to form and maintain friendships

   (1)   Becomes a loner or makes extra demands on teacher for approval by being especially helpful (teacher's pet)

   (2)   Uses pets as center of affection (most common in girls who have difficulty maintaining friendships)

   (3)   Uses unacceptable behavior to get attention from peers—class clown, daredevil, thief

   (4)   Label received from gang can continue throughout school years— fatty, clown, teacher's pet.

   b. Peer group with unacceptable behavioral standards

   (1)   Appreciate that peers are necessary to child for approval and affection; criticism and maligning of friends demand that child defend those on whom he or she depends for self-esteem.

   (2)   Open discussion important

   (3)   Maintenance of family behavioral standards

   (4)   Referrals as needed

   c. Overwhelmed by pressure of school and peers; acting out or passive behavior

   d. Divorce particularly shattering

   (1)   Awareness of others and their feelings

   (2)   Fear of abandonment

3. Childrearing practices

   a. Expectation that family values and standards will be upheld

   b. Review developmental tasks accomplished and identify those unmet

   c. Provide loving, approving adult with time to talk with and listen to child

   d. Provide child advocate for developing a plan to remove unattainable pressure on child, and find a way to have child operate in an environment in which he or she can succeed.

   e. Environmental and family inadequacies necessitate referral of family to social service agencies or parent education classes.

4. Sexual identity

   a. 6–7 years: Begins to prefer playmates of own sex

   b. 7–8 years

(1) Prefers company of own sex, to whom child relates more easily

(2) Boys aspire to maleness, girls to femininity; affected by mass media

(3) Parents and teachers of child's sex used as role models

   c. 8-9 years

      (1) Curiosity and interest in other sex

         (a) Secretive whisperings about sex; off-color stories; experimenting and inspection of each other; searching in dictionary for words

         (b) Appropriate time for information and vocabulary to be supplied before emotions become mixed with facts

      (2) Sex roles more clearly defined and adhered to

         (a) Boys more aggressive and set higher vocational goals than girls

         (b) Girls less aggressive and less motivated for success than boys; new role of women is slow to change these deep cultural patterns; role models helpful

      (3) Parents' attitudes and actions are models for love and affection.

E. Safety

   1. Statistics—frequency and type of accidents (age 5-14 years)

Mortality Rates	Boys (per 100,000)	Girls (per 100,000)
Motor vehicles	13.3%	7.8%
Pedestrian	5.2%	3.3%
Drowning	5.6%	1.3%
Fires and flames	1.9%	1.5%
Falls	0.5%	0.2%

   2. Education

      a. Responsibilities given as child proves reliable

      b. Awareness of incidence of accidents

      c. Discussions and prevention planning

      d. Emergency plans established and rehearsed

   3. Accident-prone children

      a. Accidents follow stressful events

      b. Accidents more frequent when aggressive behavior is reactive pattern

      c. Accidents used as means of getting attention

V. **Suggested reading**

   A. Levant R. *Between Father and Child*. New York: Penguin 1991.

   B. Langdon MJ. *Back Off—How to Confront and Stop Sexual Harassment and Harassers*. New York: Simon & Schuster, 1993.

   C. Silverstein O. *The Courage to Raise Good Men*. West Haven, CT: National Education Association, The Academic Building, 1994.

OVERVIEW

9- TO 11-YEAR WELL CHILD VISIT

I. **Individualized guidelines**

    A. Chronological age does not determine the preadolescent's physical and psychological stage of development, so information in these guidelines must be individualized for each child.

    B. See guidelines for overall picture of these years.

II. **Family**

    A. Onset of this transitional period depends on child's genetic, physical, and environmental history. Parents' and child's understanding of child's individual growth pattern can make this a successful and happy period.

    B. Because children of the same age may be at different developmental levels, peers and gangs will find they are shifting their interests and loyalties.

III. **Parents**

    A. Maintain family and moral standards

    B. Provide opportunity for health care and counseling as needed

    C. Provide appropriate schooling, recreational, and community activities

    D. Give child opportunities to make independent decisions as he or she demonstrates ability to be responsible and accept the consequences of activities

    E. Provide consistent and caring listener

    F. Abuse of any family member identified

IV. **Child**

    A. Understanding and accepting individual pattern of development

    B. Physical

        1. See guidelines for physical changes and development of secondary sex characteristics.

        2. Takes responsibility for good health habits

        3. Use guidelines for parameters of physical changes.

        4. Safety: Aware of incidence of accidents and prevention planned

    C. Emotional

        1. Period of confusion and indecision. Through trial and error, child is working toward developing confidence and self-esteem to become an independent, reliable member of society. This can make for a very self-conscious, indecisive, stubborn, argumentative preadolescent.

        2. Continues to need family to provide acceptance and feeling of self-worth

    D. Intellectual

        1. Transitional period from concrete thinking to abstract thinking, giving child ability to express ideas and feelings better and to begin to accept ideas of others. However, because child does not have the experience to realize practical limitations, he or she can have impractical expectations of others and be critical of those around him or her.

    E. Social

        1. Peers, teachers, and other adults outside family give child opportunity to observe other cultures and values. Behavior is still directed by need to be accepted by those important to him or her. An understanding adult is important for child to turn to for support to maintain expected behavior.

V.   Risk factors
   A. Not using language to express feelings; resorting to aggressive behavior
   B. Inappropriate environment of school and peers
   C. Frequent illnesses or accidents
   D. Presence of drugs in peer group
VI.   See guidelines for specific factors to be noted in physical examination.

INJURY PREVENTION

I.   Review safety protocol.
   A. Injury is the main cause of death and disability in adolescents. Confusing drive toward establishing independence and self-esteem can lead to "trying out" and "showing off."
   B. Parents and community need to provide safety education, counseling, and a safe environment.
   C. Accident-prone adolescents need referrals and follow-up.
II.   Main concerns
   A. Traffic accidents: Cars, bicycles, pedestrian
   B. Water safety: Boating, diving, swimming alone
   C. Sports: appropriate conditioning, proper equipment, good supervision
   D. Firearms: Unloaded gun and ammunition kept in separate locked cabinets
   E. Increased danger if drugs, alcohol, or smoking present
   F. Unsafe environment at home and for play
   G. Most accidents occur 3–6 p.m.

CHILD ABUSE

I.   Physical abuse
   A. Adolescent should be willing to express how injuries and abuse occurred; if reticent, referral and follow-up important
   B. Sexual abuse for both boys and girls needs to be discussed.
II.   At-risk child
   A. Physically handicapped, mentally retarded
   B. Frequent illnesses and continuing health problems
   C. Accident-prone and underachievers
III.   At-risk caregivers
   A. No caring adult

NOTES

NOTES

9- TO 11-YEAR WELL CHILD VISIT

The third cycle of growth comprises the physical and psychosocial steps from childhood to adulthood. It is divided into two periods: a transitional stage of preadolescence (roughly ages 9–11) and adolescence (ages 12–17). Children enter and exit these stages according to their genetic, environmental, and physical status. The preadolescent period has been defined as one of mismatch: the child's peers are the same chronological age but their physical development, interests, and abilities can be at different stages.

I.   **Developmental process**
  A. Parents
      1. Understand this natural process of growth and change
      2. Establish and maintain home, school, and social guidelines and standards
      3. Provide a safe, supportive environment
      4. Abuse of any family member identified
  B. Child
      1. Appreciates importance of this growing process
      2. Maintains school and family responsibilities and standards
      3. Develops ability to assess peer group values relative to own values
II. **Family status**
  A. Parental concerns and problems: Ability to identify problems and to cope; single parents, divorce, remarriage, step-parents, step-siblings
  B. Parents' and child's assessment of development
  C. Family interaction and support for each other
  D. Review and updating of emergency planning
III. **Health habits (as maintained by child)**
  A. Nutrition
      1. Understands basic nutritional requirements during this rapid growth period
      2. Takes responsibility for and obtains adequate diet
      3. Participates in food shopping and preparation
  B. Sleep
      1. Maintains adequate schedule of sleep and rest to meet needs
      2. Can discuss sleep disturbances if present
  C. Hygiene
      1. Takes pride in good grooming
      2. Understands and copes with body changes—increased perspiration, menstruation, acne, weight increase
      3. Can discuss problems and concerns
IV. **Growth and development**
  A. Physical
      1. Parameters of second period of rapid growth, lasting 2–4 years
          a. Onset: Girls, 9–13 years; boys, 11–14 years
          b. Height: Girls, 3 ½ in/yr; boys, 4 ½ in/yr

      c. Weight: Girls, 10 lb/yr; boys, 12 lb/yr

  2. Body changes

      a. Extremities grow faster than trunk and head.

      b. Facial proportions change; nose and chin enlarge first.

      c. Figure changes: Girl's pelvis enlarges; boy's shoulders enlarge.

      d. Subcutaneous fat increases.

      e. Skin: Increased function of sweat glands and increased activity of sebaceous glands

  3. Secondary sex characteristics

      a. Girls

          (1) Breast enlargement: 8–13 years

          (2) Axillary hair: 11–13 years

          (3) Pubic hair: 10–12 years

          (4) Menarche: 10–16 years

      b. Boys

          (1) Genitalia enlargement: 9–13 years

          (2) Axillary hair: 12–14 years

          (3) Facial hair: 11–14 years

          (4) Pubic hair: 12–15 years

B. Emotional development—Erikson. Task of pubescence (prepuberty) is to begin developing an identity independent of family and peers. First steps in this process are:

  1. Increased self-awareness, self-consciousness, self-appraisal

  2. Preoccupation with how one measures up to peers

  3. No longer accepts only parental evaluation, but beginning to use values of peers as criteria by which to judge own values

  4. Continues to need family for acceptance and feeling of self-worth

C. Intellectual development—Piaget. This stage marks the progression from concrete thinking to formal operation, the ability to conceptualize and hypothesize, and the beginning of abstract thinking.

  1. Excitement of thinking through possibilities leads to argumentativeness.

  2. Joy of putting across ideas and listening to ideas (of peers) leads to a constant need for gabfests, long telephone conversations, and writing of songs and verse.

  3. Learning is rapid and efficient if school provides a challenging program.

D. Social development

  1. School: Wide range of physical, emotional, and intellectual growth of students makes age grouping unsatisfactory; individual programming of classes and extracurricular activities is essential.

  2. Community activities (scouts, church, sports, volunteer work)

      a. Provides contact with a wider group than child's own clique

      b. Provides projects that help child reach beyond self-interests

  3. Sexual maturity

      a. Boys are becoming more masculine, girls more feminine.

      b. Interest in each other continues to increase.

    c. New self-consciousness makes physical appearance to the opposite sex an overriding concern.

    d. Behavioral patterns are less established than in the past because society's expectations and adult role models have been changing.

    e. Facts are needed on reproduction, female body, male body, terminology, birth control, venereal disease.

  4. Antisocial behavior

    a. Drugs: Knowledge of classification and street names, availability, effects, physical and emotional problems with use needed; group discussion classes helpful

    b. Sexual experimentation

      (1) Dependence on peer group for acceptance and attention

      (2) Role models from television, movies, friends, relatives

      (3) Ability to conceptualize consequences of behavior

    c. Need for consistent, caring adult to help adolescent evaluate behavior

    d. Destructive acts toward society

      (1) Impulsive behavior

      (2) Inability to delay gratification

      (3) Inability to give and accept affection

      (4) Lack of consistent, caring adult

  5. Developing sense of community

    a. Cooperation with others—family, school, peers

    b. Leadership qualities and self-actualizing activities

    c. Willing to participate in volunteer projects

E. Risk factors

  1. Family

    a. Poorly defined parental roles

    b. Lack of clear and consistent expectations for child's behavior

    c. Inability to allow preadolescent to participate in decision-making process

  2. Child

    a. Abnormal eating habits

    b. Inability to gain peer acceptance

    c. Socially unacceptable behavior

    d. No caring adult for support and open communication

V. **Physical examination**

A. Growth: Continuing on established pattern; deviations reflected by growth spurt (see Appendix B, Physical Growth NCHS Percentiles)

B. Appearance and behavior

  1. Overall hygiene, appropriateness of dress

  2. Posture

  3. Coordination

  4. Self-assurance

  5. Communication skills

      6. Interest in health care

      7. Eye contact

  C. Specific factors to note during routine physical examination

      1. Skin

         a. Enlargement of pores

         b. Bruises and burns

      2. Hair: Becoming oily

      3. Dental occlusion; need for orthodontia

      4. Decrease in lymph tissue (dependent on maturational level)

      5. Heart: Heart rate slower, particularly in athletes; normal blood pressure slowly rises

      6. Breasts: Breast budding; gynecomastia in males

      7. Genitalia

         a. Boys

            (1) Pubic hair at first sparse and straight

            (2) Enlargement of testes

         b. Girls

            (1) Pubic hair sparse and straight along labial border

            (2) Labia enlarged

            (3) Vaginal discharge

      8. Musculoskeletal: Increased muscle mass, strength, tone; scoliosis; leg length discrepancy

  D. Parent–child interaction

      1. Parent

         a. Allows child to have health maintenance visit alone, but is made aware of any problems and care plans

         b. Expresses health care concerns with provider and child

         c. Discusses emerging sexual development openly with child

      2. Child

         a. Discusses concerns with parent and provider regarding sexual abuse, fear of violence, dealing with strangers

         b. Open communication with parent—trusting, supportive relationship

         c. Peer pressure about sexual activity, experimenting with drugs or alcohol

VI. Assessment

  A. Physical

  B. Developmental

  C. Emotional

  D. Environmental

VII. Plan

  A. Immunizations: Complete schedule as needed.

  B. Screening: Hematocrit, urinalysis, blood-pressure check, hearing and eye tests

  C. Problem list (devised with child); SOAP for each

  D. Appropriate timing for office, home, or telephone visits; continue individual scheduling.

| OVERVIEW

ANTICIPATORY GUIDANCE FOR THE PERIOD OF 9–11 YEARS

I. **Expectations for this period**

    A. Family, school, and community provide opportunities for child to continue on path to maturity.

    B. Adolescent understands and accepts own pattern of growth.

II. **Health**

    A. Adolescent takes responsibility for maintaining good health habits and coping with physical changes.

    B. Sports activities appropriate to developmental stage

    C. Health care available

III. **Emotional**

    A. Moving toward having sufficient self-esteem to make appropriate decisions

    B. Can predict and accept consequences of decisions

IV. **Intellectual**

    A. Continuing to move forward from concrete thinking to hypothesize or think abstractly, leading to indecision and being impractical and critical of others

    B. Language an important tool in this development

    C. Lack of language skills can lead to continued use of aggressive acts.

V. **Social**

    A. Family and school behavioral standards needed

    B. Sexual identify established; appropriate time for sex education

    C. Peer group: See guidelines.

VI. **Safety**

    A. Accident prevention important

    B. Accident proneness needs further evaluation.

VII. **Watch for:**

    A. Unhappy child

    B. Failure to live up to potential in school

    C. Lack of significant, appropriate adult role model

    D. Now is the time when home, school, and community need to identify these boys and girls and provide them with the care, respect, and help they need to become self-actualizing and positive members of society.

NOTES

NOTES

ANTICIPATORY GUIDANCE FOR THE PERIOD OF 9–11 YEARS

Review the previous anticipatory guidelines to help identify accomplished or unaccomplished developmental tasks. This is a transitional period and a time of new challenge. The strengths and weaknesses brought to these preadolescent years will influence the success of the passage from childhood to adulthood. Especially important during preadolescence are the understanding and guidance of the family, school, and community organizations to ensure the optimal opportunities for each child to continue his or her path to maturity.

I. **Expectations of this period**

    A. Knowledge of sequence of physical changes of preadolescence, to predict individual pattern of growth

    B. Understanding of the development from concrete to abstract thinking, to assess the preadolescent's ability to assume responsibilities and independent activities, to think through planned activities, and to predict outcomes

    C. Opportunities for the preadolescent to have successful accomplishments, thereby understanding own capabilities and continuing to develop self-esteem and self-worth

    D. Consistent, caring adult to insist that standards of behavior be upheld and to act as appropriate role model, source of encouragement, and patient listener

II. **Family status**

    A. Basic needs being met; referrals as needed

    B. Parents

        1. Understand use of communication skills and problem-solving techniques

        2. Appreciate changing family dynamics and need for developing opportunities for independent decision-making by child

    C. Child

        1. Able to establish close relationships outside family

        2. Maintains school and home responsibilities and behavioral standards

        3. Keen interest in outside activities such as sports, church, or community groups

        4. Continues to return to family for support

    D. Identify sexual abuse to or by any family member.

III. **Health patterns**

    A. Nutrition: Status of growth cycle and level of activity determine nutritional requirements.

        1. Period of most rapid growth is the year before puberty; chubbiness before and during this year may lead to extreme dieting, which may interfere with optimal growth.

        2. Child assumes responsibility for nutritional standards, adequate intake, and appropriate eating habits.

    B. Health maintenance

        1. Knowledge about appropriate care of skin, hair, body odor, menses

        2. Respect extreme self-consciousness; appropriate fitness and grooming classes available

3. Exercise: Team sports and competition favor those who mature early; individual sports activities are needed for late maturers so that they also may continue to develop and appreciate their capabilities.
4. Health supervision and counseling available
5. Sickness treated and evaluated; attitude toward illness assessed
6. Health care available
7. Proneness to accidents evaluated for underlying causes and referrals made as needed

IV. **Growth and development**

A. Physical
1. Growth pattern evaluated: See growth and development of well child visit.
2. Awkwardness expected because of large muscle growth before refinement of fine motor muscles
3. Teeth: Dental care available; orthodontia as needed
4. Speech
   a. Enjoyment of and interest in words, rhymes, puzzles
   b. Increasing vocabulary to handle expanding knowledge and expression of ideas and emotions
   c. Problems in speech, articulation, or syntax need referrals.

B. Emotional development—Erikson: Identity versus role confusion. First task is to move from security of family and friends and develop positive self-identity. Another task is to develop ability to make independent decisions and to understand and assume their consequences. Thus, development of child's self-esteem and integrity continues.
1. The first steps of these tasks need careful attention so that the taking on of independent activities can be geared to both the physical and intellectual stages of development.
2. Risk factors
   a. Regressive patterns of overdependence on family, shyness, passivity, or aggression
   b. Use of illness as a means of avoiding new challenges
   c. Use of food, either too much or not enough, as a means of gaining attention and satisfaction
   d. Lack of opportunities for taking on new responsibilities
   e. Inability to make and maintain friends; becoming a loner

C. Intellectual development—Piaget: Period of transition from concrete thinking to formal (abstract) thinking. Horizons are broadened to include such learning as calculus and appreciation of the images in poetry. However, because preadolescents do not have the experience to realize the practical limitations of life, they can be indecisive, accept impractical ideas, and lack understanding of others.
1. Opportunities provided for taking on new responsibilities with careful supervision
2. Reading and experiences broaden the understanding of others.
3. Academic programs stimulate independent work.
4. Discussion groups help child formulate and express ideas and listen to and counter ideas of others.

5. Risk factors
   a. Unsuccessful in maintaining scholastic expectations
   b. Inappropriate school for developmental stage and ability
   c. Assuming responsibilities beyond ability to understand and assume consequences of these actions
6. Language becomes the most important tool in understanding and accepting the new experiences of this transitional period.
   a. Aggressive acts replaced by use of communication skills and problem-solving techniques.
   b. Peer groups and "best friend" used to try out new ideas
   c. Broad reading programs introduce cultural heritages.
   d. Consistent, caring adult who listens to problems and new ideas and provides alternative approaches
   e. Risk factors
      (1) Too much time watching TV and computer play inhibits discussions with peers and family and limits vocabulary development.
      (2) Failure to use language to express feelings and ideas; still resorting to aggression to take control
      (3) Lack of consistent listener to provide a sounding board for feelings and ideas

D. Social development: It is important for the preadolescent to turn to peers, school, and community groups to observe the cultures, mores, and values of others. Evaluating these in relation to family patterns and establishing one's own standards take an extended period of trial and error, with reinforcement of appropriate behavior by a significant adult.
   1. Guidelines established by family for behavioral standards, curfews, and extracurricular activities
   2. Guidelines indicate parents' interest and concern and provide the security of behavioral limits.
   3. Sexual identity
      a. Depends on stage of growth and development with respect to awareness of and interest in opposite sex
      b. Girls' maturing earlier than boys makes chronological age activities difficult, as in sports, clubs, discussion groups, social events.
      c. Now is the time to provide information and vocabulary about sex, before emotions become mixed with facts.
   4. Peer group
      a. Positive developmental process
         (1) Facilitates learning about interpersonal relationships
         (2) Source of support, guidance, and esteem
         (3) Role model for appearance and behavior
         (4) Leads to awareness of social class, prestige, and power of belonging to "right" group
         (5) Pressure to perform provides opportunity for testing out own values and evaluating them against values of others.

    b. Parental role

      (1) Continue expecting conformance to family behavioral limits, values, and standards

      (2) Understand importance of peer group to preadolescent

      (3) Reserve evaluation of peer group until concrete evidence available

      (4) Remember that preadolescent considers criticism of group a personal attack

      (5) When intervention is necessary, explain parental responsibility to protect child. Genuine concern can be appreciated by preadolescent and used as a means of extracting him- or herself from an unhappy situation.

  5. Risk factors

    a. Antisocial behavior

    b. Poor school performance

  6. Childrearing practices

    a. Time to investigate and evaluate carefully forces that are causing preadolescent to reject this next step toward becoming a responsible member of society

    b. Appropriate intervention and referrals

E. Safety

  1. Statistics: Frequency and type of accidents (age 5–14 years)

Mortality Rates	Boys (per 100,000)	Girls (per 100,000)
Motor vehicles	13.3%	7.8%
Pedestrian	5.2%	3.3%
Drowning	5.6%	1.3%
Fires and flames	1.0%	1.5%
Falls	0.5%	0.2%

  2. Education

    a. Responsibilities given as child proves reliable

    b. Awareness of incidence of accidents

    c. Discussions and prevention planning

    d. Emergency plans established and rehearsed

  3. Accident-prone children

    a. Accidents follow stressful events.

    b. Accidents more frequent when aggressive behavior is reactive pattern.

    c. Accidents used as means of getting attention

V. **Suggested reading**

A. Benedict H. *Safe, Strong, and Streetwise.* Boston: Little, Brown & Co., 1987.

B. *Female Juvenile Prostitution: Problems and Responses.* Arlington, VA: National Center for Missing and Exploited Children, 1992.

C. Greenberg KE. *Runaways.* Minneapolis: Lerner Publishing Co., 1995.

D. Johnson L, Rosenfeld G. *Divorced Kids.* New York: Fawcett Crest, 1990.

E. Kraizer S. *The Safe Child Book: A Commonsense Approach to Protecting Children and Teaching Children to Protect Themselves.* New York: Dell Publishing Co., 1985.

F. Start E. *Everything You Need to Know About Sexual Abuse.* New York: The Razen Publishing Group, 1993.

G. "Where the Lies Take You" (video). Minneapolis: WHISPER (Women Harmed in Systems of Prostitution Engaged in Revolt), 1995.

NOTES

| OVERVIEW

12- TO 17-YEAR WELL CHILD VISIT

I. **Guidelines**
   A. During these years, increasing stability of physical and psychological development can be expected. These guidelines can be used to identify the essential parameters of this development.
      1. Family
         a. Assessment of child's growth toward maturity, with successes and concerns identified; problem-solving session planned and referrals made as needed
         b. Identify any abuse of family members
      2. Adolescent
         a. Physical
            (1) Changes can be predicted and a more realistic thought process can help the adolescent understand and appreciate uniqueness.
            (2) Concerns and problems identified and referrals made as needed
            (3) Accepts responsibility for good health habits and safety practices for self and others
            (4) Physical abuse identified
         b. Emotional
            (1) Develops a more self-directed and assured behavior pattern
            (2) Establishes confidence to rely on self-esteem and competence
            (3) Becomes more discriminating in making friends and group involvement
         c. Intellectual
            (1) Can think more realistically about own capabilities and values
            (2) Becomes more tolerant of others
            (3) Feels comfortable in society and takes on role of a responsible member of society
         d. Social
            (1) Less dependent on peer group for self-confidence
            (2) Establishes own standards of behavior and values
            (3) Accepts own values and self-awareness of sexual role
            (4) Awareness of violence and abuse

II. **Risk factors**
   A. Substance abuse
      1. Changes in behavioral habits
      2. Changes in emotional stability
      3. Withdrawal from friends and family activities
   B. Risk of suicide: Talking about this is a serious call for help; careful evaluation and intervention are indicated.
   C. Adults who may be guilty of sexual harassment or abuse

III. **See guidelines for specific factors to be noted in physical examination.**
   A. Aggressive and abusive pattern of behavior of adolescent and peer group

| INJURY PREVENTION

I. **Review safety protocol.**

A. As adolescent matures towards self-confidence and taking the responsibility for own actions, he or she is more capable of preventing injury to self and others.

B. Careful supervision and definite regulations needed until these stages of maturity are reached

II. **Safety concerns**

A. Main concern continues to be automobile accidents, including drinking and driving.

B. Added to this is the attitude of infallibility ("that won't happen to me"). The reality of these life-threatening situations can be made clear by injury prevention planning and experiences of working with the police, visits to the emergency room, and talking with accident victims. This is serious business and needs to be taken seriously.

| CHILD ABUSE

I. **Age-specific factors**

A. Children of this age are well aware of the possibility of abuse to them.

1. Fear of violence is one of their main concerns.

2. Sexual harassment and actual sexual abuse also of great concern

3. Presence of drugs, alcohol, smoking, etc. is a great threat.

4. Strangers, neighbors, relatives can be perpetrators of abuse.

5. Adolescents can abuse each other with their irresponsible acts; therefore, families, schools, and community need to work together to help provide a safe environment.

6. Each adolescent needs a responsible, caring adult to help keep him or her safe from harm.

NOTES

| **12- TO 17-YEAR WELL CHILD VISIT**

The adolescent is now settling into a more stable growth and behavioral pattern. The individuality of this process can be identified and strengths and problems assessed. Physical changes can be predicted, and the emergence of a more realistic thought process helps the adolescent understand and appreciate his or her uniqueness.

I. **Developmental process**
   A. Parents
       1. Provide opportunities for adolescent to make independent decisions
       2. Assess with adolescent appropriateness of these decisions
       3. Allow increased independence when teenager can make appropriate and realistic decisions and bear the consequences of his or her activities
   B. Adolescent
       1. Understands physical changes and takes responsibility for health maintenance
       2. Successful accomplishments at home, at school, and in extracurricular activities
       3. Accepts sexuality and establishes own standards for sexual behavior
       4. Sexual abuse to or by adolescent discussed

II. **Family status**
   A. Basic needs being met; referrals as needed
   B. Parents
       1. Assessment of adolescent's development
       2. Concerns identified
       3. Family communication skills and problem-solving techniques assessed
       4. Problem-solving session including parent and adolescent planned; referrals as needed
   C. Adolescent
       1. Understands and accepts individuality of development
       2. Accepts consequences of behavior
       3. Concerns and problems identified
       4. Able to relate to and cooperate with parents or another significant adult
       5. Problem-solving sessions planned; referrals as needed

III. **Health habits**
   A. Health maintenance
       1. Attitude toward and appreciation of health maintenance
       2. Knowledge of requirements for good health
       3. Availability of health supervision and crisis care
       4. Accident prevention:
           a. Driver education
           b. Swimming and lifesaving proficiency
           c. Knowledge of sports injuries; appropriate equipment, supervision, physical fitness needed for particular activity

      d. First-aid course and emergency planning available

      e. Proneness to accidents evaluated for underlying causes

   5. Prevention of infectious diseases

      a. Knowledge of communicability, symptoms, course of disease, complications, sequelae

      b. Most common infectious diseases of adolescents: Mononucleosis, upper respiratory infections, herpes, hepatitis, gonorrhea

   6. Information for sexually active adolescents

      a. Knowledge of endocrine and reproductive systems

      b. Birth-control information

      c. Symptoms of physical problems and infections

      d. Pregnancy testing and abortion counseling

B. Nutrition

   1. Knowledge of nutritional requirements

   2. Nutritional assessment for poor weight gain, slow muscle tissue growth, obesity, intense physical activity

      a. 24-hour recall or diary of food intake

      b. Eating habits: More than three meals per day to spread metabolic load for better absorption

      c. Evaluate intake of protein, milk products, fruits, vegetables, grains.

         (1) Protein: Two servings/day; high percentage of fish, poultry, dried beans, peas, nuts

         (2) Milk products: Two servings/day, including cheese and ice cream

         (3) Fruits and vegetables: Four servings/day, including potatoes

         (4) Cereal and grains: Four servings/day

         (5) Fluids: Increase intake to compensate for increase of sweat glands; avoid caffeine and soda.

      d. Athletes and those who need to gain weight: Increase the size of servings of high-value foods (whole-grain bread, cereal, potatoes, cheese, nuts)

      e. Eating disorders (both boys and girls); referrals and follow-up

   3. Refer to nutritionist as needed.

C. Sleep

   1. Established pattern of work and sleep

   2. Sufficient sleep to maintain daily schedule

   3. Willing to discuss problems

D. Elimination

   1. Established schedule

   2. Understanding and knowledge to cope with problems

   3. Symptoms of urinary tract infections known

   4. Willing to ask for help as needed

E. Menstruation

   1. Regular periods

   2. Premenstrual symptoms

   3. Menstrual discomforts

    4. Able to maintain daily schedule

    5. Willing to ask for information and help

  F. Nocturnal emission

    1. Understanding of normal physical development

    2. Willing to ask for information and help

  G. Masturbation

    1. Infrequent experimenting is normal.

    2. If a frequent and obsessive practice, intervention and referral needed

IV. Growth and development

  A. Physical

    1. Slower rate of growth in height and weight; return to percentiles of preadolescent pattern

    2. Facial features and adult stature by 18 years for females and 20 years for males

    3. Muscle strength and size influenced by sex hormones as well as by nutrition and exercise

    4. Endurance depends on lung capacity, heart size, and muscle strength, as well as on sex hormones and physical fitness.

    5. Speech

      a. Voice changes in resonance and strength in both sexes but more pronounced in males

      b. Problems in articulation, pitch, and rhythm need investigation.

    6. Sexual maturity

      a. Adjusting to body changes and functions

      b. Accepting societal standards for sexual identity

      c. Developing own values for and self-awareness of sexual role

  B. Emotional development—Erikson: Self-identity versus role confusion. These years see the development of a more self-directed and assured behavioral pattern. As in all steps to maturity, optimal growth is more easily reached when opportunities are available to try out and experiment with new roles in an understanding and safe environment.

    1. More even-tempered and cooperative

    2. Self-directed in planning educational and vocational goals

    3. More discriminating in making friends and group involvement

  C. Intellectual development—Piaget: Concrete thinking to formal operation; ability to conceptualize and hypothesize

    1. Continues to be excited about presenting ideas and countering ideas of others; debating and discussion groups help organize and define ideas and force him or her to listen to ideas of others.

    2. Can think realistically about vocational goals

    3. Accepts own capabilities and appreciates own values

  D. Social development

    1. Continues to establish own standards of behavior and values

    2. Becomes less dependent on peer groups for social stature and behavior pattern

    3. Increased tolerance and appreciation of others

   4. Antisocial behavior less evident
      a. Developing better judgment toward and control of drug use, smoking, alcohol, and sexual behavior
      b. Can respond to school and community counseling groups
   5. Destructive acts toward society
      a. Impulsive behavior
      b. Need to gain attention from peer group
      c. Inability to delay gratification
      d. Inability to give and accept affection
      e. No consistent, caring adult with whom to relate
   6. Developing sense of community
      a. Cooperation with others—family, school, peers
      b. Leadership qualities and self-actualizing activities
E. Risk factors
   1. Family, school, community
      a. Not providing an understanding and safe environment
      b. Punitive measures of behavior control attempted in place of open communication, problem-solving techniques, and defined behavioral standards
      c. Unrealistic expectations of adolescent's ability to control and take responsibility for actions
   2. Adolescent
      a. Physical problems not under medical supervision
      b. Failure to accept physical appearance and capabilities
      c. Failure to take on role of a self-directed, caring individual
   3. Indication of substance abuse and risk of suicide
      a. Changes in patterns of sleep, eating, friendship, and school performance
      b. Changes in personality: Boredom, agitation, bursts of anger, apathy, evasiveness, carelessness
      c. Increasing attitude of discouragement and disgust with world
      d. Difficulty accepting disappointment and failure
      e. Lack of supportive companion to share and evaluate new perceptions of role for self and obligations to society
      f. Suicidal calls for help
        (1) Talking about ways of committing suicide
        (2) Giving away prized possessions
        (3) Previous attempts
        (4) Withdrawal from friends and family
V. Physical examination
A. Growth: Height and weight percentiles return to preadolescent pattern.
B. Appearance and behavior
   1. Grooming and hygiene
   2. Posture

3. Coordination
4. Self-assurance
5. Communication
6. Interest in health care
7. Eye contact

C. Specific factors to note during routine physical examination
1. Hair: Oily; body hair appears on chest and face in males, axilla in both sexes
2. Skin: Acne on face, back, chest; large pores; presence of bruises, burns, bites evaluated
3. Lymph: Decreased lymph tissue
4. Teeth: Caries; dental hygiene; need for orthodontia
5. Heart: Decreased heart rate; increased blood pressure
6. Lungs: Decreased respiratory rate
7. Breasts: Breasts developing; gynecomastia in males
8. Genitalia

   a. Males
      (1) Pubic hair: Increase in amount to adult distribution; becomes coarse and curly
      (2) Penile enlargement continuing
      (3) Enlargement of testes

   b. Females
      (1) Pubic hair: Increase in amount to adult distribution; becomes coarse and curly
      (2) Labia mature
      (3) Vaginal discharge

9. Musculoskeletal: Increased muscle mass, strength, and tone; scoliosis; leg length discrepancy

D. Parent–adolescent interaction
1. Parent
   a. Expects adolescent to take responsibility for health care
   b. Made aware of health problems and care plan
   c. Follow-up visits and financial responsibility planned
2. Adolescent
   a. Turns to parents for support and comfort
   b. Discusses health care plans with parents and health professionals

VI. Assessment
A. Physical
B. Developmental
C. Emotional
D. Environmental

VII. Plan
A. Immunizations: Complete schedule as needed.
B. Screening: Hematocrit; urinalysis; blood pressure; hearing and eye tests
C. Problem list (devised with adolescent); SOAP for each

   D. Appropriate timing for office, home, or telephone visits; continue individual scheduling.

NOTES

| **OVERVIEW**

ANTICIPATORY GUIDANCE FOR THE PERIOD OF 12–17 YEARS

I. **Expectations**

    A. Parents and adolescents appreciate the strengths needed to become an independent, responsible, and caring member of society.

    B. Family, school, and community provide opportunities for development of these strengths.

    C. Adolescent develops pride in own capabilities and accepts responsibility for his or her actions.

    D. Adolescent is better able to accept changes in family structure (divorce, remarriage, step-siblings).

II. **Adolescent**

    A. Health

        1. Period of rapid growth, so adequate nutrition essential

        2. Accepts responsibility for health maintenance

    B. Emotional

        1. Can evaluate positive attitudes toward self and others

        2. Negative attitudes: May need referrals

    C. Intellectual: Continuing ability to think abstractly leads to more accurate and tolerant assessment of self and others.

    D. Social: At home, in school, and in community, now a responsible, caring member

III. **Watch for:**

    A. Many positive experiences at home, at school, and in the community

    B. Expresses feelings, hopes, and concerns

    C. Caring, responsible adult to listen and to respect ideas, and to help keep him or her safe from harm

NOTES

|ANTICIPATORY GUIDANCE FOR THE ADOLESCENT YEARS

In these fascinating and challenging years, both the parents and the adolescent come to understand and appreciate the strengths and individuality needed to become an independent, responsible member of society.

I. **Adolescent**
   A. Accepts and develops pride in capabilities
   B. Works toward vocational goals
   C. Establishes independent values that provide a framework to assess appropriate behavior
   D. Has role models of caring, responsible members of society

II. **Family status**
   A. Basic needs being met; self-direction in coping with problems
   B. Parents
      1. Have positive attitudes toward changing emotional ties between selves and adolescent
      2. Provide time to listen (not argue) and encourage adolescent to verbalize new ideas and feelings
      3. Provide role models for maintaining family mores and cultural values
      4. Identify sexual abuse to or by any family member
   C. Step-parents
      1. Shift in family relationship demands that parents be role models of mature, caring people.
      2. Understand and appreciate adolescent's individuality
      3. Poor adjustment can lead to behavioral and school problems for the adolescent and jealousy and abuse by the parent; make referrals as needed.
   D. Adolescent
      1. Single-parent home
         a. Has extra responsibility
         b. Feels left out of some activities
         c. Misses attention of other parent
         d. Can be embarrassed by having only one parent
      2. Divorce
         a. Better able to understand the problems
         b. Relieved by cessation of family discord
         c. Can feel despair and abandonment
      3. Remarriage
         a. Can appreciate and be happy for parent
         b. Glad to be relieved of some of the responsibility he or she has been carrying
         c. Jealousy and resentment possible if parent has been dependent on adolescent for emotional satisfaction
   E. Step-siblings
      1. Each child must be seen as an individual.

    2. Parents establish a caring relationship with each child.

    3. Parents provide opportunities for open communication.

    4. Children given opportunity to take part in and develop outside interests

  F. Siblings

    1. Different developmental stages cause different needs and expectations.

    2. Important to provide privacy and respect for each person's possessions

    3. Expect a united front if one sibling is hurt or maligned.

III. Health patterns

  A. Nutrition: Period of rapid physical growth, so attention to adequate nutrition essential

    1. Considerations: Ethnic food habits, past growth pattern, nutritional history, familial diseases such as high blood pressure, heart attacks, diabetes, obesity

    2. Nutritional requirements

      a. Boys: 45 kcal/kg, or 25 cal/lb

      b. Girls: 38 kcal/kg, or 20 cal/lb

    3. Problems to be evaluated

      a. Inadequate food

      b. Obesity

      c. Anorexia nervosa or bulimia

      d. Poor eating habits

  B. Health maintenance—responsibility assumed by adolescent

    1. Established patterns of grooming, elimination, sleep

    2. Physical fitness and pride in maintaining good health

    3. Accepts responsibility of sexual behavior

    4. Seeks help when problems arise

  C. Exercise

    1. Variability of growth pattern makes individualized program necessary.

    2. Endurance and muscle strength improving, but type of activity geared to stage of development

    3. Girls: Equal opportunities and equal money allotted for their activities (Title IX); school programs evaluated

    4. Evaluate growth progress by frequent measurement of height, weight, muscle mass, and energy level.

  D. Safety and accident prevention

    1. Can accept reality that accidents can happen to him or her

    2. Impulsive and aggressive behavior can be a reactive pattern to stressful events.

    3. Able to identify and assume responsibility for own actions

    4. Can control activities for benefit of others

IV. Growth and development

  A. Physical

    1. Individual growth expectation recognized

    2. Information on the order of expected body changes provided

3. Self-consciousness and rapid body changes can cause overconcern with health problems.

   a. Parents and health professionals appreciate reality of the problem to the adolescent.

   b. Care plan devised with parent, adolescent, and professional

   c. Identify use of illness as a way of avoiding emotional or social concerns; plan intervention and referrals.

B. Emotional development—Erikson: The preadolescent developmental task of beginning to establish an identity as an independent, self-sufficient, caring person continues during the next years.

   1. Positive developmental process

      a. Shows confidence in own judgment and accepts consequences of actions

      b. Appraises own abilities and works toward vocational goals

      c. Decreased self-concern, increased understanding of others

   2. Negative developmental process

      a. Lack of self-esteem and confidence in potential abilities

      b. Frequent illnesses, accidents, and periods of depression

      c. Continued use of self-destructive behavioral patterns, such as drugs, promiscuity, cheating, stealing

C. Intellectual development—Piaget: Development from concrete thinking to formal operation continues at an individual pace.

   1. First steps identified by ability to think abstractly

      a. Conceptualizes and theorizes about ideas that include several variables; seen by parents as having difficulty making decisions and being slow to start projects

      b. Theorizes from own perspective and cannot incorporate ideas of others; seen by parents as stubborn, uncooperative, argumentative

      c. Idealistic in problem solving because expectations are unrealistic; seen as disgust with stupidity of adult world

   2. Final steps toward formal operation

      a. Makes decisions on basis of more accurate appraisal of options, so can become independent of societal and peer pressure

      b. Incorporates ideas of others, so can become more tolerant of both peers and adults

      c. Experience leads to less idealism about the ease of solving problems.

      d. Feels comfortable in society and takes on role of responsible member of society

D. Social

   1. Beyond their academic purpose, schools are a safe environment that can be used as a common meeting ground.

      a. In the school environment, adolescents intellectually and emotionally can:

         (1) Appreciate other cultures and mores

         (2) Observe a wide range of socioeconomic strata, with their respective privileges and inequalities

        (3) React to the importance placed on academic performance and the pressures of testing and scoring

        (4) Try out and develop interpersonal skills

    b. School provides opportunities for adolescent to develop abilities, find pride in accomplishments, and obtain leadership skills.

    c. Adolescent needs teachers and administrators who will maintain standards by which actions and abilities can be fairly judged.

  2. Community

    a. Provides adolescent with opportunity to observe and take part in projects that serve other segments of society

    b. Maintains sufficient recreational activities to provide wholesome outlets for adolescents' energy and need to be together

    c. Demonstrates interest, concern, and pride in its adolescent population

  3. Family continues its important role.

    a. Provides safe, wholesome environment

    b. Offers help and encouragement when problems occur

    c. Respects adolescent's ideas and opinions

    d. Gives open, honest answers and suggestions when asked

    e. Demonstrates roles of caring, responsible citizens

V. Suggested reading

  A. Coles R. *The Moral Life of Children.* Boston: Houghton Mifflin, 1986.

  B. Giggans P, et al. *What Parents Need to Know About Dating Violence.* Seattle: Seal Press, 1995.

  C. Goodman L. *Is Your Child Dying to Be Thin?* Pittsburgh: Dorrance Publishing, 1992.

  D. Pipher M. *Reviving Ophelia—Saving the Selves of Adolescent Girls.* New York: Ballantine Books, 1994.

NOTES

| COMMON CHILDREARING CONCERNS: TEMPER TANTRUMS

Temper tantrums are a developmental stage in learning to cope with frustration and gain self-control. In *The Process of Human Development* (see Suggested Reading below), five sequential stages in the development of self-control are identified:

1. Passive acceptance: Bewilderment and noncompliance
2. Physical aggression: Biting, hitting, throwing objects, running, stamping feet
3. Verbal aggression: Using "no," name calling, making demands, using expletives
4. Socially acceptable behavior: Bargaining, accepting alternative means or goals
5. Cooperation: Compromising own wishes and maintaining self-control

These stages may overlap, but they "resolve quickly in normally developing children."

I. **Manifestations of frustration**

A. Infant

1. Uncontrolled crying can be caused by baby's inability to stop once he or she has started.
2. Requires quiet soothing and rocking to let baby know there is comfort
3. If such crying spells occur frequently, physical and environmental factors need investigation.

B. Toddler

1. Still completely ego-centered; own needs and wishes come first
2. Does not tolerate well fatigue, hunger, pain, overstimulation
3. Schedule, physical condition, nutrition, and family patterns of behavior should be investigated.
4. Best to head off temper tantrums by carefully noting precipitating events and trying to avoid them
5. Having to make choices can be frustrating to a toddler. A definite schedule and decisive tone of voice ("Now it is time to eat," "Now it is time for bed") can help toddler accept rules and standards of world.

C. Preschool child

1. Verbal aggression best ignored
2. Adults are excellent role models. Parents should express frustration in positive ways, such as by singing, laughing, reciting poetry, and stating clearly why they are upset.
3. A 4-year-old realizes he or she can get attention by using forbidden words.
   a. If child is getting enough attention and having success in daily routine, this language will soon pass.
   b. Playing word games with child and listening to his or her stories seem to be the best ways to handle this problem.
4. Preschoolers are learning socially acceptable ways of handling frustration.
   a. Language skills should now be sufficient for child to state wishes and needs.

      b. Child is becoming expert in bargaining.

    5. A 4-year-old is usually still working on these skills and may still occasionally lose control and have a temper tantrum. Adult should help him develop positive ways of handling frustration.

    6. By age 5, the child has become an expert in bargaining. Girls learn this skill earlier than boys; boys need more supervision and male role models to help them control their behavior through words rather than aggression.

    7. Learning self-control enhances self-esteem; punishment control only lessens child's feeling of being able to control self.

  D. School-age child

    1. If uncontrolled outbursts of frustrations persist at this age, referral to appropriate professionals is imperative.

    2. School, family, and environmental pressures must be evaluated before new skills in behavior control can be established.

    3. Frequent outbursts at this age may be a precursor of delinquency.

    4. Child's ability to control own behavior is seen in success with peers and teachers, in school, and at home.

    5. School-age child has come a long way since toddlerhood; with caregivers providing good examples and guidance, child has learned to stand up for what he or she thinks is right and yet is willing to cooperate and bargain when appropriate.

II. Caregivers' responsibilities

  A. Appreciate that they are role models with respect to behavior patterns for coping with anger and frustration.

  B. Demonstrate processes of bargaining, accommodation, compromise, and cooperation.

  C. Review the successes or problems the child is encountering with each developmental task.

  D. Understand the child's individual temperament and let a fiery-tempered child know that he or she must work harder than others to build behavior control.

  E. Respect the child's need to protect own self-esteem and growing need for independence.

  F. Identify precipitating events that lead to loss of self-control, and head them off.

  G. Create a family environment in which all members are expected to respect and help one another.

  H. Help the child develop positive ways of expressing anger and frustration to experience the satisfaction of learning to control behavior.

    1. Set up "time-out" periods or a "thinking bench" to be used when child's behavior is unreasonable.

    2. Watch for and praise successful attempts at self-control.

    3. Help child develop a vocabulary to express feelings, and talk about one's own feelings so that the child will learn how adults handle their frustrations.

    4. Learn songs and poems to use to relieve anger and frustration.

    5. Provide child with plenty of opportunity for physical exercise.

    6. Make available a caring adult with whom the child can share concerns.

    7. Understand that parents' own emotional states may be reflected in child's behavior.

III. **Tips for handling temper tantrums**
   A. Infant: Hold closely, rock, play music, sing.
   B. Toddler
      1. Pick up, hold under caregiver's arm (child may be frightened by loss of control), keep calm, sing.
      2. Do not reason or explain.
   C. Preschooler
      1. Do not allow child to hurt self or others; hold under caregiver's arm if necessary.
      2. Walk out of room if possible.
      3. Do not try to reason or explain.
      4. Do not take the episode too seriously; respond with a casual statement, such as, "Oops, see if you can't hold on to your temper" or "Now that you are 4, you don't need to do that anymore; tell me why you are angry."
      5. Praise child for getting behavior under control.
      6. Do not use threats or punishments.
   D. In public
      1. Remove child from scene; walk with child outside until he or she calms down.
      2. Take child home if possible.
      3. Help child practice how to act in public and set limits he or she knows about before going out.
      4. Carefully study child's world to make sure such episodes are not his or her only way of getting attention.
   E. Refer to limit-setting protocol.

IV. **Risk factors**
   A. Children who are too quiet, too good, and too shy; their behavior may be controlled by low self-esteem or fear of punishment.
   B. Sudden burst of destructive acts toward self or others may occur, as child has not learned a positive way to cope with frustrations.
   C. Early identification and family interaction need further investigation or referral for these destructive behaviors.

V. **Suggested Reading**
   A. Schuster C, Ashburn S. *The Process of Human Development*, 3d edition. Philadelphia: JB Lippincott, 1992.

COMMON CHILDREARING CONCERNS: TOILET TRAINING

Toilet training is a developmental task of toddlerhood. Success will help the toddler continue to develop awareness of his or her own ability for self-control and self-esteem. There appears to be a critical period at about 18 to 24 months of age when the child becomes aware of body functions; attempts at training too early or too late may influence long-range behavior.

I. **Indications of readiness**

   A. Maturation of muscles and nerves to allow voluntary sphincter control

   B. Myelination occurs in a cephalocaudal direction, so the ability to walk well indicates that myelination has occurred in the trunk of the body and that sphincter control is possible.

   C. Body awareness: Toddler shows discomfort in soiled diapers, can locate pain, and is developing some coordination.

   D. Toddler can follow simple directions and use language to make wishes known.

   E. Toddler·can anticipate and postpone events in daily schedule.

   F. Toddler is not under any new stresses.

   G. Toddler has primary caregivers to look to for approval and attention.

II. **Technique**

   A. Pretraining when the above indicators are present

      1. Have child observe others using bathroom.

      2. Talk about it as an expected accomplishment; comment with appropriate word when child is observed having bowel movement (BM) so that he or she becomes aware that this will get attention.

      3. Have potty chair or insert ring for toilet seat available.

      4. Use training pants occasionally.

      5. Toddler shows awareness of plan by bringing to caregiver's attention that he is having a BM; this is the beginning of gaining the child's cooperation and may take more time and effort than seems necessary.

      6. This is only one of the many tasks the toddler is attempting to master at this age, so frequent lapses may occur.

   B. Bowel control

      1. First make sure toddler is becoming aware of the connection between the potty chair and the BM.

      2. If child's bowel movements are regular, use the potty chair at those times.

      3. If no regularity is apparent, watch for signal from child and then take him or her to the bathroom. This is where patience and perseverance by the caregivers are rewarded.

      4. Leave child on potty chair for only a short time; long sitting sessions may lead him or her to rebel. Child may be afraid of the toilet seat.

      5. Do not distract child with books or toys; he or she is there for one reason.

      6. Treat success as a normal expectation. Overenthusiasm may cause child to use toileting as a way to get attention; positive feedback should be reserved for other daily activities.

      7. If training is unsuccessful, re-evaluate maturation indicators and repeat pretraining techniques. It seems to take more time and effort to train boys than girls, particularly if they are larger than average.

C. Daytime bladder control
1. Follows BM control, as voiding signal is less intense
2. Small bladder size makes control more difficult.
3. Watch for increasingly long periods of dryness, as this signifies an increase in bladder size.
4. Put child on potty chair before and after meals, naps, and playtime; treat as usual part of daily schedule.
5. Dress child in clothing that is easy to remove.
6. Boys may prefer to sit backward on toilet seat.
7. Treat success casually.

D. Nighttime bladder control
1. Follows daytime control; may not be accomplished until after age 3 years
2. Bladder must have capacity of 8 oz before child will be dry all night.
3. Getting child up at night may be helpful in the short term but is not a good long-term solution to nighttime voiding.
4. Put child on toilet or potty chair as soon as awake, whether dry or not, to develop routine.
5. Outside pressure makes child feel inadequate and discouraged with ability to please those important to him or her.
6. In a happy, healthy child, bladder control is a natural process.

E. Success
1. Depends on toddler's physical maturation
2. Depends on parents' positive attitudes and patience in following through and helping child

F. Problems: See Enuresis in Part II.

NOTES

COMMON CHILDREARING CONCERNS: LIMIT SETTING*

Discipline can best be defined as training that helps a child develop self-concept and character. Parents are often hesitant to set firm and consistent limits on their children because they are afraid of damaging their psyche or fear that their children won't love them or feel loved by them if they are stern. On the contrary: Being allowed to act in a way the child knows should not be tolerated causes him or her anxiety and insecurity. Children feel their parents do not love them if parents fail to make an effort to help them develop inner controls.

The ultimate goal for any child is parental approval; children will do their best to live up to parental expectations. For example, if a mother conveys the impression that she does not expect her toddler to go to bed without a struggle, a struggle will surely ensue. If parents expect their son only to get by in school, he probably will; if the same parents were to expect A's, the child would probably strive to achieve them. Parental disapproval helps children develop a conscience; they know that, after committing a naughty deed, they have not measured up.

Health care providers involved in routine physical concerns must not neglect the issue of discipline, especially as the child develops initiative and autonomy. The following points can be discussed with parents, and it is generally helpful to raise the issue before the need arises and to reinforce significant areas when the parents have a specific concern.

I. **Principles of limit setting**
   A. United front
      1. Parents must be in accord.
      2. Parents must agree on what limits will be.
      3. Parents must agree on penalties for infractions.
   B. Consistency
      1. Rules must be consistently enforced.
      2. Expectations must be consistent.
      3. Child should not be allowed to perform unacceptable behaviors at some times and be punished for similar behaviors other times.
   C. Limits clearly delineated
      1. Parental expectations must be defined.
      2. Rules and regulations must be clear.
   D. Behavioral expectations in relation to child's developmental and intellectual level
      1. A 12-month-old cannot be relied on not to touch something because mom or dad said "no."
      2. A 2-year-old does not understand what can happen if he or she goes in the street or gets into a car with a stranger.
      3. A school-aged child can be expected to understand that he or she must go home after school before playing with friends.
      4. If expectations are made clear to the child, he or she will strive to achieve them.

---

*This section written by Elizabeth Dunn.

E. "Bumping point": Every parent has a point up to which he or she can be pushed. Children quickly learn this point and use it to their own advantage.

F. Unemotional approach

   1. Children repeat behaviors that they know get a parental response, whether positive or negative.

   2. A toddler learning to walk takes another step when parents laugh and applaud.

   3. The perfect entertainment for a school-aged child on a boring rainy day is to tease a sibling and watch Mom hop.

   4. Overreacting under stress and in anger leads to irrational threats and perhaps violence.

G. Stress that the deed is bad, not the child.

   1. Attack the deed, not the child; this preserves the child's respect for self and parent.

   2. "Breaking windows (throwing stones, etc.) is a naughty thing to do."

   3. Children need to know, however, that they are responsible for their actions.

H. Immediacy of action

   1. For most effective learning, especially with a toddler or preschool child, the consequences of inappropriate behavior should not be delayed.

   2. With older children and adolescents, a conference with parents may be more appropriate; in this case, the consequence is delayed.

   3. Do not say, "Wait 'til your father gets home!" This threat can cause an enormous amount of anxiety for a child and makes it appear not only that Dad is the bad guy but also that Mom does not care enough to set limits. Alternatively, for a child whose father comes home from work and then usually spends his time in front of the TV, a secondary gain may be involved in the form of attention (albeit negative attention).

I. Punishment must fit the crime.

   1. There should be a logical connection between the two; banning after-school play for 2 weeks for an infraction unrelated to such activity is usually not only inappropriate but also unhealthy.

   2. Punishment should not exceed the child's tolerance.

   3. Punishment should not negate educational aims.

   4. Coming in half an hour after curfew does not warrant restricting an adolescent for 1 or 2 months; instead, make the curfew half an hour earlier next time and give the child one of the parent's tasks the next day because "Dad is so tired from waiting and worrying."

   5. As the child gets older, parental disapproval is often the only punishment needed; guilt at letting parents down is often punishment enough.

J. Punishment should educate.

   1. Punishment is done for and with children, not to them.

   2. Spanking

      a. Produces an external rather than an internal motive for controlling the impulse and therefore does not help develop child's conscience

      b. Cancels the crime

      c. Relieves sense of guilt too readily

      d. Parental anger often escalates with spanking, resulting in injury

   3. Isolation
      a. Appropriate length of time ("until you can act like a young lady") is preferable to isolating for a specified length of time once child is old enough to understand what behaviors are expected.
   4. Sit on chair: Tell child timer is set for 3 minutes; do not say, "Sit there until I tell you you can get up."
   5. Restrictions on privileges
      a. For bike rule infraction, take bike away.
      b. TV restrictions work well for most children.
      c. Best not to restrict learning experiences such as a scout camping trip
      d. Withhold positive rewards such as social or verbal approval.
      e. Never offer a reward that cannot be fulfilled.
K. Treat children with respect.
   1. This teaches them to respect in turn.
   2. Allow them to share in decision-making process.
   3. Children model behaviors they see in parents; be the kind of person you expect your child to be.
   4. Earliest approach to limit setting is based on baby's ability to learn.
L. Threats are useless.
   1. Any self-respecting child will try to see whether parents will follow through; threats are an invitation for unwanted behaviors.
   2. Threats are often made in a moment of anger and may be unreasonable.
M. An ounce of prevention is worth a pound of cure and is certainly easier on parents.
   1. Clearly define limits.
   2. Remove temptation.
   3. Do not pick on insignificant things.
   4. Do not threaten with punishment that you cannot or are unwilling to carry out.
   5. Distract child if it looks as though he or she is getting in trouble.
   6. When child is losing control, pick up and remove him or her.
   7. If you know the child has misbehaved, do not ask whether he or she has done the misdeed. Confront child with it and thereby avoid tempting him or her to lie.

COMMON CHILDREARING CONCERNS: SIBLING RIVALRY*

Sibling rivalry occurs when children feel displaced, frustrated, angry, and unloved. It is normal for an older child to feel jealous at the arrival of a new baby. Competition and feelings of envy can also occur among older siblings; fighting between brothers and sisters is common. However, if such behavior is allowed to continue, it can persist into adolescence and even adulthood.

Often the arrival of a second child occurs when the first child is at the developmentally stressed age of 2 years. All children show signs of regression after the birth of a sibling, and it is best to allow this regression to occur without interference. If the parents continue to reinforce positive behavior, the older child will gradually begin to feel as important and loved as the younger sibling, and the relationship between the two will become stronger and more supportive.

Parents are responsible for establishing a positive, supportive environment in which competition among siblings is reduced and replaced by a caring, concerned, affectionate relationship. This takes place over a long period of time. Parents must be fair and consistent in teaching children both by example and by good management of negative behavior.

One successful method used to change negative behavior is "time out." This is a proven method in which the fighting children are separated and sent to separate rooms. All the combatants are treated equally, with no favoritism. Parents must praise and encourage positive play, rewarding good behavior and discouraging name calling, baiting, and arguments.

Feelings of jealousy naturally occur at the birth of siblings. If this event does not interfere with the time spent with the older child or affect the love and affection shown, these feelings eventually dissipate.

The age of the child is an important factor in sibling rivalry. The younger the older child, the greater will be the degree of rivalry. Children age 5 years or older are fairly secure and therefore less intensely jealous of a new baby. Anticipatory guidance is advisable; parents should set the stage well in advance of the birth. A few simple practices may help decrease the jealousy between the first child and the new baby.

1. Take the older child to the prenatal exam to hear the baby's heartbeat.
2. Allow the child to feel the baby move in Mom's tummy.
3. When talking about the new baby, use terms such as "our baby" and describe what babies do (wear diapers, coo, smile, etc.).
4. Borrow a small baby or visit a friend with a newborn to acquaint the child with babies.
5. Have a special time each day, called "our time," to be spent reading or playing with just the older child.
6. Read books together (many are available at the library) about arrival of new baby.
7. Supply the older child with a doll, a baby of his or her own.
8. Establish the older child in a new bed or room long before the baby is due.

After the baby arrives:

1. Allow the child to visit you in the hospital each day.
2. Phone the child daily from the hospital.

---

*This section written by Rose Boynton.

3. Bring a special gift to the child when you come home with the baby.
4. Allow the child to assist in baby care by bringing you diapers and so forth.
5. Spend some time each day exclusively with each child.

   Parents must be fair about the attention they give each child. If a child matures in a loving, sharing, charitable environment, he or she will have the self-esteem needed to grow into a well-rounded, strong adult who likes and enjoys his or her siblings.

I. **Sibling interaction**

   A. Siblings interact independently of other family relationships; relationships with parents and extended family members may be more or less intense, or more or less caring.

   B. Birth order influences development of the sibling bond. Because all children in the family both initiate behaviors and react to others' behaviors, this development continues into and through adulthood.

   C. Families provide a social arena in which children learn to explore language, observe behavior (both negative and positive), and learn to assess their influence on other people. Therefore, children's personalities outside the family and their ability to deal socially with others are first established with family members.

   1. Children without siblings are more critical of themselves and often find peer relationships more uncomfortable and difficult to sustain than do children with siblings. Single children relate to older people and adults much more successfully than to children their own age. Single children are perfectionists, expecting perfect behavior from others as well as from themselves. As Leman states in *The Birth Order Book*, "Only children often quietly wish they could move in, take over, and 'do it right.' "(see Suggested Reading).

   2. First-born children are often confident, conscientious, organized children who grow up to be hard-driving, successful adults. A lot of pressure is exerted on the oldest child, who receives more attention and more discipline and has more expectations made on him or her. He or she is the pathfinder and the one all the other children in the family look up to.

   3. Middle children learn social skills early in life. They learn how to negotiate and that it is futile to compare themselves constantly with others. They are forced to form their own identities, usually by adolescence, and grow up to be people-oriented adults.

   4. Last-born children are often pleasant, cheerful, outgoing, and uncomplicated. They can be impatient, spoiled, and clownish. Last-borns live in the shadow of their older siblings. They are often criticized and not taken seriously. Often they get attention by clowning, making jokes, or behaving badly in school, but they secretly wish to be very successful.

   D. Gender influences the interaction between siblings. Rivalry is likely to be most intense in a family with two boys; however, if such brothers are born close together, there is less chance for the older one to establish clear superiority. In a family with two girls, rivalry is likely to be much less serious; the father is usually the key family figure, and the girls compete for his attention. In a family with a girl and a boy, rivalry is much less serious, the difference in expectations of the two sexes having been made clear since birth.

    E. Sibling rivalry is an important consideration in the age spacing of children in families. The children closest in age often share experiences and friends and therefore form a stronger bond than do siblings born 8 or 9 years apart. Siblings born close together become more reciprocal in their relationship and are more intimate and intensely involved with each other than are siblings born years apart.

II. Parents can influence sibling rivalry

    A. Set a good example; be supportive of all the children in the family, and reinforce positive behavior within the family.

    B. Teach the children to be loyal to each other regardless of the anger they feel toward each other; allow competition between them to be verbalized and to be resolved openly and swiftly.

    C. Verbalize the frustration the angry child is feeling; always show concern and compassion for the child.

    D. Try to teach the children constructive ways of expressing feelings of rivalry rather than punishing them for negative rivalrous behaviors.

    E. Expect the children to be accountable for their words and actions, and thereby teach them coping skills.

    F. Be consistent; the punishment should fit the crime.

    G. Separate the children for a period of time if they are constantly fighting ("time out").

    H. Treat the children with respect, and show confidence in their ability to get along.

III. Sibling rivalry in step-families

    A. Difficult problem: Family system is complex due to the large number of persons involved, and often parents are preoccupied with their own new marriage.

    B. Special attention should be focused on cementing a bond between step-parent and step-child. Allow time to build a caring relationship.

    C. Children in step-families are often angry and sad at the loss of their original families.

    D. Children should be taught that sharing is a key component to success, and the advantages of sharing within the family should be pointed out to them.

    E. Step-families must clearly and consciously work out the rules of the family; children should be included in this process.

    F. Adolescents find the new family structure in step-families difficult; often they withdraw from both parents and become closer to their siblings.

IV. Siblings of handicapped children

    A. Sibling relationships between handicapped and nonhandicapped children are more complex; special problems arise due to the intense nature of the relationship.

        1. Siblings of a handicapped child

            a. Resent the attention and time given to the handicapped child

            b. Fear catching the condition

            c. Feel anger toward the disabled child because they feel ignored and unappreciated by parents

            d. Feel upset by the unfairness of the family situation; long for a normal family

    e. Feel embarrassed by the handicapped sibling

    f. Feel guilty about their hostility toward their sibling

    g. Feel confused about their role in caring for the sibling

    h. Fear that outsiders won't accept the handicapped child

2. Parents of a handicapped child

    a. Communicate with the handicapped child; be truthful about the degree of the handicap and open about the problems of working with him or her.

    b. Treat all the children individually, reinforcing their positive characteristics.

    c. Schedule quality time to be spent with the nondisabled children.

    d. Strive to attain a normal home life by providing a comfortable home environment that welcomes the participation of other children in family activities.

    e. Establish or join a support group in which each family member obtains a balanced perspective on his or her role in the family and can compare his or her experiences with those of others.

NOTES

CHILD ABUSE*

By definition, child abuse is divided into four groups: physical abuse, emotional or physical neglect, emotional abuse, and sexual abuse.

Physical abuse may be present in a child with evidence of bruises, lacerations, head trauma, human bites, burns, hematomas, fractures or dislocations, or injury to the abdomen (evidenced by a ruptured liver or spleen or fractured ribs), all seen on the physical examination.

Emotional and physical neglect are more difficult to identify, more subtle in their presentation, and more likely to have been going on for some time. Such neglect implies that the caregiver cannot care for the child or protect the child from danger. Examples are the child who is emotionally distraught or the child with failure to thrive, who often has an inadequate diet, shows signs of poor growth, is depressed and developmentally delayed, and occasionally (but not always) is dirty and unkempt.

Emotional abuse is exemplified by the child who seems unable to relate to others and is apathetic, lacking any emotion because he or she is constantly berated, beaten, rejected, or ignored. Infants as well as older children can be emotionally abused.

Sexual abuse, the sexual exploitation of infants or children by an adult, may include exhibitionism, fondling or digital manipulation, masturbation, or vaginal or anal intercourse. The sexual abuser may be a stranger but more often is someone known to the family or even a member of the family. Father–daughter incest accounts for 75% of all cases of incest.

Child abuse is most often identified in the pediatric office; the nurse practitioner or pediatrician must be able to recognize the signs and symptoms of such abuse.

I. **Physical abuse**

   A. Physical signs

      1. Bruises: Explained or, often, unexplained welts or abrasions on the face, body, back, thighs; may also be several surface areas in different stages of healing, often recurring and suggesting the shape of the article used to inflict them (belt, whip)

      2. Evidence of human bites

      3. Ocular insult

      4. Fractures or dislocations in various stages of healing

      5. Unexplained rupture of spleen, liver, or pancreas

      6. Neurologic findings

      7. Signs of poisoning

      8. Unexplained burns: May appear on soles, palms, back, buttocks, or genitalia, often in pattern of cigarette, cigar, electric burner, or iron; rope burns around neck, body, or extremities

   B. Behavioral signs

      1. Excessively aggressive or withdrawn

      2. Suspicious of adults

      3. Speaks in dull voice

---

*This section written by Rose Boynton.

4. Often feels he or she deserves the battering
5. Lies very quietly during examination with vacant stare
6. May not report injury inflicted by parent
7. Seeks affection inappropriately
8. Has poor self-esteem

II. **Physical neglect**
   A. Physical signs
      1. Failure to thrive (poor growth pattern, developmental delay, malnourishment)
      2. Inappropriate dress
      3. Poor hygiene
      4. Lack of supervision in dangerous activities, or abandonment
      5. Absence of medical care; unattended physical problems
   B. Behavioral signs
      1. Excessive crying
      2. In infants, ruminating behavior
      3. Begging for food
      4. Poor school attendance, delinquency, falling asleep in school, stealing
      5. Alcohol or drug abuse
      6. States that "no one cares"

III. **Emotional neglect**
   A. Physical signs
      1. Failure to thrive
      2. Hyperactivity
      3. Speech disorder
   B. Behavioral signs
      1. Developmental delays
      2. Habitual sucking, rocking, ruminating, head banging, or destructive or antisocial behavior
      3. Sleep disorders, repeated nightmares, constant waking to see whether parents are there
      4. Phobias
      5. Difficulty in learning, poor school performance
      6. Inability to play for any length of time
      7. Inappropriate adult behavior; not childlike
      8. Wounding of self or attempted suicide

IV. **Sexual abuse**
   A. Physical signs
      1. Genital, urethral, vaginal, or anal bruising or bleeding
      2. Swollen, red vulva or perineum
      3. Positive culture for sexually transmitted disease (gonococcus, venereal warts)
      4. Recurrent urinary tract infections

     5. Recurrent streptococcal pharyngitis

     6. Recurrent abdominal pain

     7. Enuresis

     8. Encopresis

     9. Pregnancy

     10. Foreign body in genital area

  B. Behavioral signs

     1. Child knows and uses sexual terms.

     2. Excessive sexual play

     3. Sleep disturbances (nightmares)

     4. Appetite disturbances

     5. Avoidance behavior or excessive aggressive behavior

     6. Temper tantrums

     7. Poor school attendance, performance

     8. Excessive masturbation

     9. Running away

     10. Suicide attempts

V. Role of medical provider

  A. Identify and make diagnosis of child abuse.

  B. Openly and candidly discuss abuse with parent.

  C. Treat for medical injuries or neglect.

  D. Report to department of welfare or child protection unit, again notifying parent.

     1. To protect child

     2. Initiate steps to ensure that abuse will not recur.

     3. Failure to report child abuse is a class A misdemeanor.

  E. Request referral or consultation to medical or surgical staff, social worker, or other specialists as appropriate.

VI. Predisposing factors

  A. Most abusive parents were themselves abused children and show little ability to cope with adult life. Although they resent their own upbringing, they look for approval from other adults by repeating the abusive pattern.

  B. Many abusive caregivers are impulsive, immature persons who cannot solve their own problems. They have trouble establishing meaningful relationships and feel alone, stressed, and overwhelmed. They are mistrustful of others and therefore unwilling to ask for help in caring for their children.

  C. Other factors that predispose a caregiver to child abuse: Mental illness, inability to control temper, unrealistic expectations of a child at a specific age, and particularly inability to handle parental stress or stress caused by poverty, unemployment, or chronic illness of the child.

  D. The caregiver may not have bonded with the child at birth and therefore feels insecure about his or her parenting abilities.

  E. Abuse can be seen in all social and economic backgrounds.

  F. In many cases, one parent is the active abuser and the other parent condones this behavior; therefore it continues.

VII. Management

A. Complete medical history must be outlined in the chart. Review the former medical record, especially noting dates and occurrences of unexplained trauma, burns, or broken bones.

B. Thorough physical examination must be performed and appropriate laboratory work and x-ray studies requested.

C. Any positive physical findings should be photographed and a collaborating physician called in to verify the findings

D. A social worker provides the necessary psychological workup, helping with the plan of care and contacting local agencies.

E. Always notify the parents and explain to them that you are reporting the diagnosis.

F. Severity of the abuse determines the need for follow-up care. The primary concern in working with families involved in child abuse is to protect the child. The health care team determines the need for hospital care or the need to separate the child from the family.

G. After making the diagnosis and plan of care, report the findings to the appropriate agencies within 24–48 hours.

NOTES

BIBLIOGRAPHY

American Academy of Pediatrics. *TIPP—The Injury Prevention Program: A Guide to Safety Counseling in Office Practice.* Department of Publications, Elk Grove Village, IL, 1994.

American Academy of Pediatrics. *Caring for Your Baby and Young Child.* New York: Bantam Books, 1991.

American Academy of Pediatrics. *Child Abuse: A Guide to References and Resources in Child Abuse and Neglect.*

Brazelton T. *Infants and Mothers: Differences in Development.* New York: Dell, 1986.

Erikson E. *Childhood in Society.* New York: WW Norton, 1991.

Fraiberg SH. *The Magic Years.* New York: WW Norton, 1991.

Kagan J, Coles R. *The Twelve to Sixteen Year Old.* New York: WW Norton, 1972.

Pillitteri A. *Maternal and Child Health Nursing,* 2d ed. Philadelphia: JB Lippincott, 1995.

Schowalter JE, Anyan WR. *The Family Handbook of Adolescence.* New York: Knopf, 1981.

Schuster C, Ashburn S. *The Process of Human Development,* 3d ed. Philadelphia: JB Lippincott, 1992.

Singer D, Revenson I. *How a Child Thinks: A Piaget Primer.* New York: New American Library, 1978.

Stone LJ, Church J. *Childhood and Adolescence,* 3d ed. New York: Random House, 1984.

Valadian I, Porter D. *Physical Growth and Development from Conception to Maturity.* Boston: Little, Brown, 1977.

II

Management of Common Pediatric Problems

Elizabeth S. Dunn

Part II covers common pediatric health problems within the scope of practice for a nurse practitioner and others responsible for the delivery of primary health care. It is developed according to the SOAP format, an outline form that includes subjective data, objective data, assessment, and plan.

The subjective data include the information with which the child or parent presents or the provider expects to elicit in a history of the presenting illness.

The objective data include the information that would be obtained from the physical examination as well as from laboratory tests.

In the assessment, the differential diagnoses for each management problem are listed and include relevant information to help the provider make an accurate diagnosis.

The plan consists of various treatment modalities used in managing the case. Specific pharmaceutical treatment as well as symptomatic treatment comprise the plan.

Additionally, for each protocol there is an extensive education section that includes pertinent information for parents. It incorporates physical care, psychosocial issues, medication information, and general information about the presenting problem.

The etiology, incidence, communicability, and incubation period have been included for each protocol where applicable. Similarly, indications for follow-up, complications, and indications for consultation or referral are part of every protocol.

Before initiating a treatment plan for any management problem, several factors must be recognized and assessed. First, a high anxiety level may interfere with the parent's or child's ability to hear and remember the recommended plan; the provider should recognize this anxiety and deal with it. Second, the ability to follow through with recommendations should be assessed; for example, a parent already stressed by the daily care of several small children may find the additional tasks involved in coping with a sick child overwhelming. Third, given that compliance is enhanced by knowledge, it is essential to evaluate the parent's or child's understanding of the disease and treatment. The provider must be aware of potential barriers to compliance, such as ethnic or religious customs or restrictions, and address them as necessary. Fourth, with regard to pharmaceuticals, it is necessary to ascertain whether the family can afford the prescribed medication, how they intend to measure the dosage, whether they understand the route of administration, whether they can give it at proper intervals, and whether they know the importance of continuing the medication for the duration prescribed.

Protocols are included for some of the most common childhood problems. Space has been left at the end of each protocol for changes and additions, as specific practices and geographic locations may necessitate minor revisions. For most effective use, each protocol should be carefully reviewed by the health care team and amended, if necessary, for their particular health center. Once reviewed and amended by the nurse practitioner and collaborating physician, they can be used as guidelines for practice as required for nurses practicing in an expanded role.

Indications for use and dosages for drugs are from current literature. However, because medicine is a constantly changing science, recommendations for management and standards for use of drugs are subject to frequent change. For that reason, current recommendations should be reviewed on a regular basis.

Anorexia and bulimia have been included in this section. Although they are not necessarily problems that should be managed solely in the primary health care setting, the health care provider is responsible for the diagnosis, referral, and coordination of care of these contemporary issues. They are presented with pertinent background information, presenting signs and symptoms, indicators for diagnosis, broad guidelines for management, and referral sources. Space has been left for the health care provider to list local resources at the end of each of these protocols.

AIDS is included as an informational source; it is not a protocol for management. In addition, suicide prevention is discussed in a section written by Rose Boynton. It contains pertinent background information, indicators for diagnosis, and management techniques.

ACNE

An inflammatory eruption involving the pilosebaceous follicles characterized by comedones (open and closed), pustules, or cysts

I. **Etiology**

    A. Pilosebaceous follicle activity is stimulated by increased androgen levels during puberty. Desquamation of the follicular wall occurs, creating a number of cells that, combined with sebum, result in a plug obstructing the lumen of the follicle. *Corynebacterium acnes* enzymes hydrolyze these trapped sebaceous lipids, causing distention and rupture of the sebaceous ducts.

    B. An inflammatory reaction occurs in the dermis with the release of the keratin, bacteria, and sebum.

II. **Incidence**

    A. Affects 30%–85% of adolescents

    B. Generally disappears by the early 20s in males, somewhat later in females

    C. Severe disease affects males 10 times more frequently than females.

III. **Subjective data**

    A. Vary according to degree of severity; complaints include:

        1. "Bumps," blackheads, whiteheads, pimples, cysts, scarring

        2. Pain on application of pressure

        3. Premenstrual flare

    B. Location: Face, chest, back, buttocks

    C. Pertinent subjective data

        1. Does patient see acne as a problem and want treatment for it?

        2. Does acne flare with stress or emotional upheaval?

        3. Does acne flare premenstrually?

        4. Do seasonal changes affect acne (improve in summer or worsen with high humidity)?

        5. Is acne worse in response to certain foods? What are they?

        6. What treatment has been used in the past?

        7. What was the response to previous treatment?

        8. Has female patient been on birth-control pills?

        9. Are there any associated endocrine factors?

            a. Are menses regular?

            b. Does patient complain of hirsutism?

      10. Does patient use cosmetics or creams on skin?

            a. Determine type—oil- or water-based.

      11. Is patient exposed to heavy grease and oil?

    D. *Note:* Often patient will not complain of symptoms because of embarrassment. It is the responsibility of the nurse practitioner to raise the issue.

IV. **Objective data**

    A. Inspect the entire body. Lesions may be found on the face, earlobes, scalp, chest, back, buttocks; they generally recur in the same areas.

B. Lesions

   1. Mild acne

      a. Closed comedones (whiteheads)

      b. Open comedones (blackheads)

      c. Occasional pustules

   2. Moderate acne

      a. Comedones, open and closed

      b. Papules

      c. Pustules

   3. Severe acne

      a. Comedones, open and closed

      b. Erythematous papules

      c. Pustules

      d. Cysts

C. Scarring may be present in any stage.

D. Hair is often very oily.

V. Assessment

A. Diagnosis easily made by appearance of different lesions on skin

B. Assess degree of involvement, both physical and emotional, to determine the best therapeutic plan.

VI. Plan

A. Mild acne

   1. Exposure to sunlight. Start with brief periods (15–20 minutes), extending the time daily by 5 minutes. Too much sun exposure can exacerbate acne.

   2. Topical agents

      a. Benzoyl peroxide—a potent antimicrobial agent as well as an exfoliant, a sebostatic, and comedolytic agent. Water-based agents are less irritating than alcohol-based ones.

         (1) Use one of the following:

            (a) Desquam-X (clear aqueous gel)

            (b) Benzagel (clear alcohol gel)

            (c) PanOxyl (clear alcohol gel)

            (d) Persa-Gel (clear acetone gel)

         (2) Begin with 5% used once daily. (With fair or sensitive skin, use every other day and increase frequency accordingly.)

         (3) Follow-up telephone call in 2 weeks. If no sensitivity, gradually increase application to twice daily.

      b. Tretinoin (Retin-A) 0.025% cream—a comedolytic agent

         (1) Initially, use on a small area every other day and increase use to once daily if no irritation develops.

      c. Local antimicrobials

         (1) T-Stat pads (antimicrobial agent). Use once daily.

         (2) Cleocin T lotion, gel, or solution. Use once daily.

3. Recheck in the office in 1 month. Continue regimen if condition responds to treatment. If there is no response to treatment and no sensitivity to the medication:

   a. Increase strength of benzoyl peroxide preparations to 10% used once daily. Increase frequency to twice daily after 2 weeks if no sensitivity.

   b. Increase strength of Retin-A to 0.05% cream or 0.025% gel used once daily. Increase frequency to twice daily after 2 weeks if no sensitivity.

   c. During early treatment, increase in inflammatory lesions is common. Improvement may take as long as 2 months.

4. Further follow-up individualized according to patient's needs and degree of response to therapy

B. Moderate acne

1. Benzoyl peroxide gel (types and dosages as above)

2. Retin-A cream 0.05%

3. Hot soaks to pustules five or six times a day

4. Tetracycline 250 mg qid or 500 mg bid

5. Recheck in 4 weeks.

   a. With no improvement and no local irritation:

      (1) Increase tetracycline to 1.5 g/day for 2 weeks, then 2 g/day for 2 weeks.

      (2) Increase strength of keratolytic gel to 10% or increase Retin-A to 0.1% cream or change to 0.025% gel.

   b. With marked improvement, decrease tetracycline to 250 mg bid.

6. Recheck again in 4 weeks.

   a. With no improvement:

      (1) Continue tetracycline at 2 g/day.

      (2) Use keratolytic gel at bedtime, Retin-A in the morning.

   b. With improvement:

      (1) Decrease tetracycline to 250 mg qid, or discontinue if already decreased to bid.

      (2) Continue with topical medication.

7. Continue individualized follow-up

   a. Every 4–8 weeks while on tetracycline

   b. Every 3–6 months while on topical medication

8. *Note:* If patient is an adolescent female, either on the birth-control pill or seeking oral contraception, order Ortho Tri-Cyclen #28.

   a. Has minimal intrinsic androgenicity

   b. Studies have shown clinically significant improvement in total acne lesions and inflammatory lesions.

C. Severe or inflammatory acne

1. Topical medication as above

2. Hot soaks to inflamed lesions five or six times a day

3. Tetracycline 250 mg qid

4. Recheck in 4 weeks. With no improvement, increase tetracycline as above.

5. Refer to dermatologist if no improvement.

D. Notes:

1. Limit refills on tetracycline to ensure follow-up visits.

2. Sulfur can be comedogenic.

3. Keratolytic gels penetrate better than creams or solutions.

4. When discussing acne, do not hesitate to touch the area so patient does not feel he or she is "dirty." Tell patient blackheads are not dirt, but oxidized melanin.

5. Psychological scarring may occur.

6. Appropriate therapy should be instituted if patient perceives acne as a problem.

7. "Prom pills"—emergency clearing of inflammatory acne for a prom, wedding, or other major event: Prednisone 20 mg every morning for 7 days

VII. Education

A. Acne is chronic. It cannot be cured, but it can be controlled. Acne flare-ups occur in cycles, both hormonal and seasonal.

B. Explain etiology (for psychological support).

C. When local treatment is instituted, acne may appear worse before it improves.

D. For mild and moderate acne, aim is to dry and desquamate the skin. Expect some dryness, peeling, and faint erythema of the skin.

E. Topical medication

1. If marked erythema and pruritus develop in response to topical medication, discontinue use temporarily and then resume with less frequent application.

2. Apply 20–30 minutes after gentle washing.

3. Apply lightly to affected area. Do not rub in vigorously.

4. Expect a feeling of warmth and slight stinging with application.

F. Hygiene

1. Avoid abrasive agents (over-the-counter scrubs).

2. Shampoo frequently; no special shampoo is necessary.

3. Change pillowcase daily.

4. Do not pick or squeeze lesions. This retards healing and causes scarring.

5. Use face cloth and hot water for soaks. Try to soak for 10–20 minutes five or six times a day.

6. Wash face gently three times daily with mild soap; excess scrubbing can exacerbate acne.

7. Facials may exacerbate acne.

8. Use only water-based cosmetics.

    a. "Oil-free" is not necessarily water-based.

    b. Use loose powder and blush.

9. Acne medications can be applied under cosmetics and sunscreens.

10. Avoid oily sunscreens. Sundown and PreSun are generally acceptable.

G. Avoid foods that seem to make acne worse.

H. Overexposure to sunlight can have adverse effects, alone or in combination with Retin-A and tetracycline. It may be necessary to discontinue these medications in the summer.

I. High humidity and heavy sweating exacerbate acne, as does exposure to heavy oils and grease.

J. Tetracycline

1. While on medication, restrict exposure to sunlight.

2. Do not take if there is any chance of pregnancy.

3. Take 1 hour before or 2 hours after a meal.

4. If unable to take four times a day because of schedule, take 500 mg every 12 hours. Nurse practitioner should acknowledge that it may be a problem for an adolescent to have an empty stomach four times a day.

5. Patient must take the full dose for at least 1 month for effective treatment.

6. Moniliasis may occur in females.

K. Discuss use of over-the-counter preparations. Explain to adolescent (and parent, if applicable) that it is more cost-effective to follow the treatment regimen than to try all the latest acne products for the dramatic cures that advertisements promise.

L. Birth-control pill may need to be changed to one that does not contain norgestrel, norethindrone, or norethindrone acetate.

M. T-Stat should be applied with the disposable applicator pads. Drying and peeling can be controlled by reducing the frequency of application.

VIII. Follow-up

A. Acne is chronic. Treatment should be continued until the process subsides spontaneously.

B. Return visits need to be individualized according to severity of acne and emotional needs of patient. Once control has been achieved, however, frequency of follow-up can be decreased. Patient may need to remain on a 250–500mg daily maintenance dose of tetracycline for several months, in which case 6–12-week return visits should continue. If patient is on topical medications alone, after acne is controlled the frequency of application can be adjusted by patient, and telephone follow-up may be sufficient.

IX. Complications

A. Psychological problems

B. Secondary bacterial infection

C. Scarring

X. Consultation/Referral

A. Moderate acne: Consult for treatment. If no improvement noted after treatment with tetracycline for 2 months, consult before continuing treatment plan.

B. Severe or inflammatory acne: Consult for treatment. Refer if no improvement noted after treatment with tetracycline for 1 month. May require more aggressive therapy, such as treatment with isotretinoin (Accutane).

C. Severe or resistant acne in a woman if accompanied by hirsutism, irregular menses, or other signs of virilism

NOTES

NOTES

AIDS (ACQUIRED IMMUNE DEFICIENCY SYNDROME)

A severe, debilitating disease that destroys the immune system. It is characterized by increased vulnerability to bacterial, protozoan, fungal, and other
viral infections as well as by malignancies. These opportunistic infections
eventually cause death.

I. **Etiology**

A. RNA cytopathic human retrovirus, human immunodeficiency virus, type 1
(HIV-1) causes virtually all AIDS cases outside West Africa and southern
Europe. HIV can be isolated from everyone with AIDS or its clinical prodrome.
At least two thirds of HIV-infected individuals develop AIDS.

B. Virus infects the CD4+ lymphocyte. When stimulated by an antigen, the
infected CD4 cell replicates the HIV instead of itself. The new HIV then
infects other T cells. With its CD4+ lymphocytes depleted, the immune
system is impaired by severely diminished antibody production. Overwhelming infections then occur when organisms, some of which do not generally
cause disease, invade the body.

II. **Communicability**

A. HIV is a low-contagion virus and is not spread by casual contact.

B. No documented instances of transmission to family members other than by
sexual contact

C. Not transmitted by fomites, by hugging, social kissing, or shaking hands, or
through swimming pools or hot tubs

D. No known cases of AIDS transmission by insects

E. HIV is transmitted by blood, blood products, semen, transplacental infection,
vaginal secretions, and possibly breast milk.

F. Higher incidence of transmission from infected men to women than from
infected women to men.

G. In anal intercourse, transmission is twice as likely to occur to the receptive
partner as to the insertive partner.

H. Humans are the only known reservoir of HIV.

I. HIV cannot reproduce outside a living cell.

III. **Exposure categories**

A. Homosexuality. About 58% of AIDS victims are homosexual or bisexual.

B. Bisexuality

C. Heterosexual contact with person with high-risk behaviors. Risk increases in
relation to the number of sexual encounters. Accounts for 8% of adults and
adolescents with AIDS.

D. Prostitution

E. Intravenous drug use. About 25% of AIDS patients use IV drugs, most commonly heroin and cocaine.

F. Receipt of blood transfusion, blood components, or tissue

G. Hemophilia (1%)

H. Individuals of Haitian ethnic background comprise 3.6% of those infected
in the United States. Most of these individuals are not involved in high-
risk behaviors.

    I. Infants or children of high-risk individuals. 91% of pediatric patients with AIDS younger than 13 years have mothers with, or at risk for, HIV infection.

IV. **Incubation period**

    A. Six months to 5 years or more

    B. Antibodies develop in 2 weeks–4 months (average, 6 weeks). If an exposed person shows no antibodies after 4 months, he or she has not been infected.

    C. AIDS symptoms appear an average of 18 months after infection. (Dormant periods have been estimated to be 1.9 years for children up to age 4 at time of infection to 8.23 years for people aged 5–59 years at time of infection.)

V. **Incidence**

    A. AIDS

        1. First reported in United States in mid-1981

        2. 20,000 cases had been reported in the United States by spring 1986.

        3. By August 1987, 40,532 cases reported

        4. By 1991, over 160,000 cases reported

        5. On Jan. 1, 1993, total cases reported were 242,146.

        6. As of June 1996, total cases reported were 548,102.

            a. Adults and adolescents

                (1) Males: 462,152

                (2) Females: 78,654

            b. Children younger than 13 years: 7,296

        7. 1% of patients with AIDS are adolescents.

        8. 18% of patients with AIDS are 20–29 years old, representing infection as teens.

    B. Incidence by exposure category

        1. Pediatric (younger than age 13)

            a. Hemophilia: 3%

            b. Mother with or at risk for HIV: 90%

            c. Receipt of blood transfusion, blood components or tissue: 5%

            d. Unidentified risk: 2%

        2. Males age 13–19

            a. Men who have sex with men: 33%

            b. Intravenous drug use: 7%

            c. Men who have sex with men and inject drugs: 5%

            d. Hemophilia or coagulation disorder: 41%

            e. Heterosexual contact: 3%

            f. Receipt of blood transfusion, blood components, or tissue: 4%

            g. Unidentified risk: 7%

        3. Females age 13–19

            a. Intravenous drug use: 15%

            b. Hemophilia or coagulation disorder: 1%

            c. Heterosexual contact with individuals with high-risk behaviors: 55%

            d. Receipt of blood transfusion, blood components, or tissue: 7%

            e. Unidentified risk: 22%

C. Age at time of diagnosis (totals as of June 1996)
1. Under 5 years: 2,899 males, 2,888 females
2. 5–12 years: 853 males, 656 females
3. 13–19 years: 1,647 males, 927 females
4. 20–24 years: 15,061 males, 4,936 females
5. 25–29 years: 64,715 males, 13,316 females
6. 30 and older: 380,729 males, 59,475 females
D. Infection by AIDS virus
1. Data not truly representative of all people estimated to be infected by HIV. Cumulative totals reported in United States are:
   a. Adults and adolescents: 71,888
   b. Children younger than 13: 1,329
2. Current worldwide cumulative counts of infected individuals
   a. 10–12 million adults
   b. One million children
3. People infected with HIV
   a. Have no visible signs of illness
   b. May not be aware that they harbor the virus
   c. Can transmit the virus throughout their lifetime
   d. Will not necessarily get AIDS
   e. May get AIDS-related complex, with symptoms taking as long as 9 years to appear
E. Less than 2% of individuals with AIDS in United States are children.
1. 1982: 16 cases
2. 1983: 35 cases
3. 1984: 48 cases
4. 1985: 132 cases
5. 1986: 410 cases
6. 1993: 4,051 cases
7. June 1996: 7,298
F. Health care workers (6.8 million in United States)
1. Documented cases of occupational transmission through September 1992: 32; as of June 1996: 51
2. Cases with possible occupational transmission through September 1992: 69; as of June 1995: 108
VI. **Mortality (Statistics may be inaccurate due to underreporting or underdiagnosis)**
A. 63% of those with a diagnosis of AIDS have died.
B. All infected individuals are expected to die from AIDS or opportunistic infections.
C. Centers for Disease Control and Prevention statistics indicate that as of June 1996, 338,831 adults and 7,296 children younger than age 13 have died from AIDS.
D. 70% of those with AIDS die within 2 years of diagnosis.
E. 80% of children with AIDS have died within the first 2 years of diagnosis.

    F. In 1987, AIDS was the 15th leading cause of death in United States.

    G. In 1989, AIDS was the second leading cause of death in males age 25–44.

    H. In 1991, AIDS was estimated to be the fifth leading cause of death in females age 25–44.

VII. Diagnostic indicators

    A. AIDS

        1. Positive history of exposure to risk factors

        2. Low birth weight

        3. Failure to thrive or poor growth rate; unexplained weight loss of greater than 10 lb

        4. Hepatosplenomegaly

        5. Diffuse lymphadenopathy

        6. Recurring fever and/or night sweats

        7. Recurrent severe viral or fungal infections

        8. Episodic or chronic diarrhea

        9. Persistent cough; shortness of breath

      10. Persistence of an infection despite appropriate treatment

      11. Infections in diffuse sites rather than a single site

      12. Candidiasis

      13. Chronic interstitial pneumonitis

      14. Increased bruising; unexplained bleeding

      15. Giardia or other opportunistic infections

      16. *Pneumocystis carinii* pneumonia

      17. Kaposi's sarcoma (most common cancer seen with AIDS); pink or purple blotches on or under skin and inside mouth, nose, eyelids, or rectum

      18. Positive HIV antibody test

    B. Congenital AIDS

        1. Pediatric AIDS is predominantly perinatally acquired (91% of cases).

        2. Fetal transmission both transplacentally and during delivery is 25% to 30% in United States. If infected during pregnancy, risk of transmission to fetus is 27%, as opposed to a 16% risk if infected before pregnancy.

        3. Positive history of risk factors in mother

        4. Prematurity

        5. Low birth weight (small for gestational age)

        6. Failure to thrive

        7. Respiratory infections

        8. Dysmorphic features

            a. Microcephaly

            b. Hypertelorism

            c. Prominent forehead

            d. Flat nasal bridge

        9. Positive HIV antibody test after 4 months of age

VIII. Differential diagnosis

    A. Congenital immunodeficiency disorders

1. X-linked agammaglobulinemia: B-cell deficiency characterized by recurrent bacterial sinopulmonary infections, diarrhea, otitis media
2. Wiskott-Aldrich syndrome (chronic granulomatous disease): T-cell deficiency characterized by severe eczema, thrombocytopenia with platelets of reduced size and function, recurrent infection with encapsulated bacteria
3. Ataxia-telangiectasia: T-cell deficiency characterized by telangiectasias, ataxia, recurrent sinopulmonary infection, malignancy, dysarthric speech
4. DiGeorge anomolad: T-cell deficiency characterized by hypertelorism and ear anomalies; abnormalities of aortic arch and neonatal tetany candidiasis are common.
5. Severe combined immunodeficiency: T- and B-cell deficiency characterized by low immunoglobulin levels and by absent antibody responses with recurrent or chronic bacterial, fungal, viral, and protozoan infections

IX. Plan

A. Order blood test for HIV after appropriate counseling and signing of informed consent. Schedule return visit to inform patient of results of HIV testing.
B. Blood test should include complete blood count, differential, platelets, liver function tests, BUN, TP albumin, serology for syphilis, hepatitis B screen.
C. Chest x-ray
D. Urinalysis
E. Tuberculosis test
F. Pap test, vaginal cultures, endocervical tests for GC, chlamydia
G. Urethral test for GC, chlamydia
H. Referrals
   1. Local AIDS service groups
   2. Social workers (for physical and financial assistance)
   3. Mental health personnel
I. List local referral sources here.

J. There is no known cure for AIDS. Opportunistic infections can be treated with appropriate therapy, although they may not respond. Over 200 investigational drugs have been tried, but none has effectively halted or reversed the immunodeficiency.
K. There are ongoing pharmacologic advances in HIV research. The solution for the HIV pandemic, however, lies in the development of an effective

vaccine. Trials are in progress to study the efficacy of vaccines in preventing HIV infection.

1. Antiretroviral drugs—improve overall health and reduce HIV levels in blood

2. Nucleoside analogs—inhibit activity of reverse transcriptase and prevent spread of HIV into new cells but do not stop viral replication in infected cells

    a. Zidovudine (AZT): Prolongs quality and duration of life by delaying progression of immunodeficiency and onset of symptoms

    b. Zalcitabine (Hivid): Approved for use in combination with AZT for adults with advanced infection

    c. Didanosine (ddI): Used for treatment of adults and children who cannot tolerate zidovudine or in whom AZT treatment has failed

3. Protease inhibitors—act against an enzyme, HIV protease. When protease is inhibited in infected cells, a noninfectious virus results.

    a. Invirase

    b. Crixivan

    c. Norvir

L. Routine monitoring of clinical status: Growth, nutrition, development, associated infections

M. Prophylaxis for *P carinii* pneumonia as indicated (trimethoprim–sulfamethoxazole)

N. Aggressive treatment of HIV-associated infections

X. **Education**

A. General public

1. Education best method of controlling spread of AIDS. Prevention requires both education and behavior change.

2. Intravenous drug abuse is the most important factor in maternal spread.

3. Sexual promiscuity increases chances of contracting AIDS; sexual partners should be chosen with care.

4. Couples who have had a mutually monogamous relationship for at least 6 years will not contract AIDS through sexual intercourse unless one or both partners has illicitly used intravenous drugs.

5. Use latex condoms for sexual intercourse (vaginal or rectal); they afford some protection, as does nonoxynol-9, either on a condom or intravaginally.

6. Do not have sex with prostitutes or intravenous drug abusers.

7. Avoid sexual activities that could cause tears in the vaginal or rectal lining or injury to the penis.

8. Avoid oral contact with vagina, penis, or rectum.

9. Rectal intercourse is particularly dangerous, as the rectal mucosa tears easily and provides direct access to the circulatory system by HIV.

10. Genital ulcers (herpes) facilitate transmission of the virus.

11. Transmission occurs less easily from women to men than from men to women.

12. A pregnant woman infected with HIV is more apt to develop AIDS than a nonpregnant woman with the virus. An infected pregnant woman can also transmit the virus to the fetus.

13. Because a number of reports have implicated breast-feeding as a mode of transmission, HIV-infected mothers should avoid breast-feeding.

14. Do not share syringes, needles, or other implements used for injecting drugs.

15. Do not donate blood if you have a history of homosexual activity or illicit drug use.

16. Donating blood poses no threat to the donor.

17. Do not get a tattoo.

18. Virus can be transmitted by acupuncture if instruments are not properly sterilized.

19. Ear piercing should be done only under aseptic conditions in a physician's office.

20. Do not share toothbrushes, razors, or any other personal effects that can be contaminated by body fluids.

B. Health care workers

1. Intact skin is an effective barrier against HIV; health care workers with exudative dermatitis or lesions should not provide direct patient care.

2. Hands should be washed carefully and thoroughly before and after patient contact and after any contact with body fluids.

3. Gloves should be used for any contact with body fluids (blood, vomitus, feces, urine); gloves should be discarded and hands washed after contact.

4. Gloves should be worn by all dental personnel.

5. Body spills should be disinfected with bleach (1 part bleach to 10 parts water); this solution should be prepared daily.

6. Use chlorine bleach in laundry for items soiled with blood, urine, feces, or vomitus.

7. Avoid accidental puncture by lancets, needles, and other sharp objects.

8. All used needles, lancets, and other sharp objects should be disposed of in puncture-proof containers.

9. Disposable diapers, dressings, syringes, gloves, and so forth should be placed in plastic bags, which should be tied securely.

10. Disposable Ambu-bags should be used for mouth-to-mouth resuscitation.

11. Use masks for direct, sustained contact with patients who are coughing.

12. Protective eye wear (goggles) should be worn if splattering of body fluids is anticipated.

13. Gowns are necessary only if soiling of clothing with body fluids is anticipated.

14. Continuing education programs concerning infection control procedures should be ongoing in every health care facility.

C. Children

1. Children with AIDS and members of their families should not receive live virus vaccines.

2. Children with AIDS who have cutaneous eruptions or draining lesions that cannot be covered should not attend school or day care.

3. Children with AIDS who have bloody diarrhea or inappropriate behaviors, such as biting of an unusual frequency that would result in transfer of blood from the biter, should not attend school or day care.

4. Children with AIDS should not attend school or day care during outbreaks of chicken pox or other communicable diseases. Advise home tutoring when child with AIDS is at risk of getting infections from other children.

5. For all children, a comprehensive sex education curriculum should be instituted at the earliest age possible.

D. Adolescents

1. The high incidence of AIDS in 20–29-year-olds (20% of cases of AIDS) clearly indicates infection in the adolescent years. Behavioral intervention programs such as comprehensive substance abuse and HIV prevention education must be provided to adolescents by parents, schools, and health care providers.

2. 20% of all people with AIDS (adults ages 20–29) were probably infected in their teenage years.

3. As of January 1, 1993, there were 912 cases of AIDS in teenagers.

4. 51.5% of adolescent females report having intercourse between ages 15–19.

5. 25.6% of 15-year-old females have had intercourse.

6. Adolescents who have intercourse at younger ages are more likely to have multiple partners.

7. Adolescents are less apt to use condoms after drinking or using drugs.

8. Use of crack cocaine is associated with high levels of risk-taking and sexual activity.

9. By age 21, 25% of teens have been infected with a sexually transmitted disease.

10. Homelessness, poverty, and abuse increase exposure to HIV.

NOTES

| **ALLERGIC RESPONSE TO HYMENOPTERA**

A local or systemic reaction to the sting of an insect, generally a bee, wasp, or hornet

I. **Etiology**
   A. Hypersensitivity is an IgE-mediated response. Generally an initial exposure is followed by re-exposure, and the rechallenge elicits the reaction.
   B. Hymenoptera
      1. Bee family: Bees, honey bees
      2. Wasp family: Yellow jackets, wasps, hornets
   C. Ant family: Fire ants of southeastern United States (attack en masse)

II. **Incidence**
   A. 90% of children experience a normal reaction of less than 2″ in diameter and less than 24 hours in duration.
   B. 10% of children have a large local reaction greater than 2″ in diameter and lasting up to 7 days.
   C. Anaphylaxis occurs in 0.4%–0.8% of the general population.
   D. About 50 deaths from stings occur in United States every year.

III. **Subjective data**
   A. History of bite or sting
   B. Local reaction
      1. Swelling and redness at site of sting
      2. Intense local pain
   C. Systemic reaction. May be a combination of the following:
      1. Anxiety initially
      2. Nausea
      3. Itching
      4. Sneezing, coughing
      5. Hives or frank angioedema, with various parts of skin swollen
      6. Swelling of lips and throat
      7. Difficulty swallowing
      8. Difficulty breathing
      9. Stridor
      10. Respiratory compromise with ultimate collapse
      11. Vertigo

IV. **Objective data**
   A. Local reaction
      1. Local wheal and flare reaction with central punctum
      2. Edema around sting site
      3. Normal reaction
         a. Swelling less than 2″ in diameter
         b. Duration less than 24 hours

    4. Large local reaction
        a. Swelling greater than 2″ in diameter
        b. Duration 1–7 days
  B. Systemic reaction—signs of anaphylaxis; generally occur within 30 minutes
    1. Anxiety
    2. Urticaria
    3. Dysphagia
    4. Laryngeal edema
    5. Bronchospasm
    6. Dyspnea
    7. Cyanosis
    8. Drop in blood pressure and pulse

V. Assessment
  A. Hymenoptera sting by history (honey bee if stinger left intact)
  B. Differential diagnosis of anaphylaxis
    1. Vasopressor syncope—self-limited. No pulmonary involvement, rarely occurs when child is prone, blood pressure and pulse do not drop, child rouses after breathing amyl nitrite.
    2. Cardiac failure
    3. Anxiety attack
    4. Penicillin allergy
    5. Obstruction in laryngotracheobronchial tree
    6. Aspiration of foreign body

VI. Plan
  A. Normal local reaction
    1. Remove stinger.
    2. Topical application of ice
    3. Diphenhydramine (Benadryl), 5 mg/kg/day in four divided doses (less than 10 kg, 12.5—25 mg tid or qid)
    4. Calamine lotion
  B. Large local reaction or multiple stings
    1. Local measures as above
    2. Prednisone, 1 mg/kg/day for 5 days, may be helpful.
  C. Systemic reaction
    1. Apply tourniquet proximal to sting.
    2. Remove stinger; shave off stinger of honey bee (has reverse serrations).
    3. Administer epinephrine 1:1,000, 0.01 ml/kg SC (maximum 0.3 ml); rub injection site to speed absorption. Repeat in 15–30 minutes.

Kilos	Pounds	Dosage (ml)
10	22	0.1
15	33	0.15
20	44	0.2
25	55	0.25
30 & over	66	0.3

4. Transport patient immediately to emergency room.

5. Refer patient to allergist for testing and possible immunotherapy.

6. Order EpiPen and instruct patient or parent in its use.

VII. Education

A. Do not wear perfumes, hair spray, aftershave, etc. when outside.

B. Wear neutral colors; flowery prints are apt to attract bees.

C. Do not walk barefoot outside. Yellow jackets, the most aggressive hymenoptera, nest in the ground.

D. Avoid flower beds, playgrounds, picnic areas, and trash or garbage disposal areas.

E. Do not run or engage in physical activity after a sting.

F. The honey bee stinger has reverse serrations and leaves its stinger in the skin, with the venom sac attached to it. The venom sac continues to eject venom and will empty completely if compressed. Do not squeeze it; instead, shave the stinger off.

G. 70% of deaths due to hymenoptera are caused by airway edema or respiratory compromise.

H. 85% of children who go into anaphylactic shock do so within the first 15–30 minutes of exposure.

I. Anaphylaxis has occurred as late as 6 hours after exposure, but this is highly unusual.

J. Steroids do not help against the initial insult but will help against a delayed recurrence after initial treatment.

K. Skin testing for allergy may yield a false-negative result if done too soon after treatment for a sting; wait 3–4 weeks after a sting before doing such testing.

L. Immunotherapy reduces the risk of life-threatening complications from 60% to less than 5%.

M. EpiPen spring-loaded syringes contain epinephrine in a premeasured dose. EpiPen delivers 0.30 mg, EpiPen Jr. 0.15 mg.

N. Parents should notify school, day care, camp, and other caregivers of reaction and have EpiPen available for child at all times.

O. Child should wear a Medic Alert bracelet.

VIII. Follow-up

A. Make contact after discharge from hospital to ensure that parent or child has made appointment with allergist for testing.

IX. Complications

A. Anaphylaxis after rechallenge

B. Delayed systemic reaction

X. Consultation/Referral

A. Refer any patient who has had an immediate systemic reaction to allergist.

B. Consult with allergist on any patient who has had a large local reaction.

NOTES

NOTES

ALLERGIC RHINITIS AND CONJUNCTIVITIS

An allergic response characterized by chronic, thin, watery nasal discharge with or without concurrent conjunctival discharge, inflammation, and pruritus

I. **Etiology**

A. IgE-mediated immunologic reaction to common inhaled allergens (pollens, molds, dust, animal dander)

B. Seasonal allergic rhinitis generally caused by nonflowering, wind-pollinated plants

C. Allergens vary seasonally and by geographic distribution and commonly include tree pollens in the early spring, grasses in late spring and early summer, and weeds primarily in the fall. However, in many areas, various weeds pollinate from spring through fall.

D. Perennial allergic rhinitis caused by animal dander, dust, and molds

E. The mediators cause increased permeability of the mucosa and produce vasodilation, mucosal edema, mucous secretions, stimulation of the itch receptors, and a reduction in the sneezing threshold.

F. Foods not a common cause of allergic rhinitis

II. **Incidence**

A. Allergic rhinitis is the most common atopic disease.

B. Usually seen after 3–4 years of age

C. Affects about 10% of the population

III. **Subjective data**

A. Nasal stuffiness—varies from mild to chronic obstruction

B. Rhinorrhea—bilateral, thin, watery discharge

C. Paroxysms of sneezing

D. Itching of nose, eyes, palate, pharynx

E. Conjunctival discharge and inflammation

F. Mouth breathing

G. Snoring

H. Fatigue, irritability, anorexia may be present during season of offending allergen.

I. "Allergic salute"—rubbing tip of nose upward with palm of hand

J. Recurrent nose bleeds

K. Pertinent subjective data to obtain

1. History of associated allergic symptoms—asthma, urticaria, contact dermatitis, eczema, food or drug allergies

2. Family history of allergy

3. Does child always seem to have a cold, or does it occur at specific times of the year (perennial versus seasonal)?

4. Are symptoms worse in any particular season?

5. Do parents or child notice that symptoms are worse after exposure to specific allergens, such as animals, wool, feathers, going into attic or cellar, etc.?

6. Are symptoms worse when child is indoors or outside?
7. What do parents or child think causes symptoms?
8. Can child clear nose by blowing?
9. What makes child feel better?
10. How much do symptoms bother child and family?

IV. Objective data

A. Allergic shiners—bluish cast under eyes
B. Allergic crease—transverse nasal crease at junction of lower and middle thirds of nose
C. Clear mucoid nasal discharge
D. Pale edematous nasal mucosa
E. Nasal turbinates swollen, may appear bluish
F. Nasal phonation
G. Mouth breathing
H. Conjunctivae may be inflamed. "Cobblestoning" of upper lids may be present.
I. Tearing
J. Edema of lids
K. Laboratory test: Nasal smear positive for eosinophilia

V. Assessment

A. Diagnosis. Differentiate between the following:
1. Seasonal allergic rhinitis occurs seasonally as a result of exposure to airborne pollens, generally tree pollens in late winter and early spring, grass pollens in spring and early summer, and weeds in late summer and early fall.
2. Perennial allergic rhinitis occurs all year but is usually worse in winter due to increased exposure to house dusts from heating systems, pets, wool clothing, and other allergens.

B. Differential diagnosis
1. Infectious rhinitis or recurrent colds: By detailed history
2. Foreign body: Unilateral purulent nasal discharge with foul odor
3. Vasomotor rhinitis: Symptoms precipitated by exposure to temperature changes or specific irritants (smoke, air pollutants, strong perfume, chemicals). Symptoms appear and disappear suddenly.
4. Rhinitis medicamentosus: By history of chronic use of nose drops
5. Acute or chronic sinusitis: Nasal mucosa usually inflamed and edematous, discharge generally mucopurulent; possible low-grade fever
6. Cystic fibrosis: Consult if nasal polyps are present.

VI. Plan

A. Involve child in treatment plan as much as developmental level allows.
B. Pharmacologic therapy
1. Antihistamines relieve rhinorrhea, sneezing, and itching.
2. Decongestants improve nasal congestion.
3. Nasal cromolyn and steroids suppress the entire inflammatory process in the nose but do little to relieve ocular symptoms or systemic manifestations.

4. Optimal results obtained with a combination of nasal cromolyn or steroids and an antihistamine or decongestant

5. Antihistamines for seasonal rhinitis

   a. Ages 6–12 years

      (1) Diphenhydramine, 5 mg/kg/day (more than 10 kg, 12.5—25 mg tid or qid)

      (2) Clemastine (Tavist) syrup, 0.5 mg/5 ml–1 tsp every 12 hours

      (3) Cetirizine (Zyrtec) syrup, 5 mg/5 ml—1 to 2 tsp orally daily, depending on severity of symptoms

   b. Ages 12 and over

      (1) Clemastine and phenylpropanolamine (Tavist-D), one tablet every 12 hours

      (2) Cetirizine (Zyrtec) 5 to 10 mg once daily, depending on severity of symptoms

      (3) Astemizole (Hismanal), one 10-mg tablet every 12 hours

6. Decongestant—antihistamine combination

   a. Actifed, Sudafed

   b. Dimetapp

7. Cromolyn sodium nasal solution: Nasalcrom, one spray in each nostril three or four times a day (children over 6 years), or Nasacort AQ, two sprays in each nostril once daily (children over 12 years)

8. 0.5% ketorolac tromethamine (Acular) ophthalmic solution

   a. One or two drops in each eye four to six times a day

   b. For maximum effect, use at regular intervals as directed.

C. Avoidance

   1. Identify and avoid offending allergens (see Environmental Control for the Atopic Child, p. 290).

   2. Seasonal allergic rhinitis: Ragweed, trees, grasses, molds

   3. Perennial: House dust, feathers, animal dander, wool clothing or rugs, mold

D. Desensitization. Referral indicated if:

   1. Symptoms are severe and cannot be controlled with symptomatic therapy.

   2. Recurrent serous otitis occurs with resultant hearing loss.

   3. Symptoms become progressively worse or asthma develops.

   4. Allergen avoidance is impossible.

VII. Education

A. Advise parents that this is a chronic problem, although symptoms sometimes decrease with age and then disappear.

B. Exacerbation of symptoms may occur, particularly as child approaches puberty.

C. Discuss indications for hyposensitization

   1. Inability to suppress symptoms with conservative treatment

   2. Inability to avoid allergens

   3. Severe symptoms affecting child's normal lifestyle—school, sleep, play

   4. 30% to 50% of children with allergic rhinitis who are not treated develop asthma.

   5. Desensitization is a lifelong process.
D. Discuss specific allergen control (see Environmental Control for the Atopic Child).
E. Advise child and parents of possible hearing loss due to serous otitis.
F. Notify school of child with hearing loss.
G. Side effects of antihistamines
   1. Sedation—often resolves with continued use; nightmares
   2. Excitation, nervousness, tachycardia, palpitations, irritability
   3. Dryness of mouth
   4. Constipation
H. Antihistamines relieve nasal congestion, itching, sneezing, rhinorrhea. Continuous therapy is more efficacious than sporadic use.
I. Astemizole (Hismanal)
J. Cromolyn nasal solution
   1. Inhibits release of histamines
   2. Generally takes 2–4 weeks for full effect
   3. Antihistamines and decongestants can be used concomitantly during initial phase of treatment and can be discontinued once cromolyn becomes effective in controlling symptoms.
   4. Treatment with Nasalcrom should be started before expected exposure to allergens and, in seasonal allergic rhinitis, continued until pollen season is over.
K. Nasacort AQ
   1. Reduces nasal stuffiness, discharge, sneezing
   2. Maximum benefit achieved in 1 week
L. Child should not wear soft contact lenses when using Acular.
M. Acular may cause transient stinging or burning.
N. Child with allergic rhinitis is more prone to upper respiratory and ear infections.
O. Child cannot clear nose by blowing it.
P. Child may not be able to chew with mouth closed.
Q. Epistaxis may be a problem because of nose picking and rubbing. Control nose bleed by compressing lower third of nose (external pressure over Kiesselbach's triangle) between fingers for 10 minutes.

VIII. Follow-up
A. Return visit or telephone follow-up in 2 weeks for re-evaluation. Contact sooner if adverse reaction to medication occurs.
B. If no response to medication, increase dosage to control symptoms. Re-evaluate in 2 weeks. Change type of antihistamine if indicated.
C. If symptoms under control, continue medication until suspected allergen no longer a threat. Medication may then be used as needed to control symptoms.
D. Return visit whenever child or parent feels symptoms are worse or medication has ceased to control symptoms.

IX. Complications
A. Bacterial infection
B. Recurrent serous otitis media

    C. Malocclusion

    D. Psychosocial problems

X. **Consultation/Referral**

    A. Symptoms have not abated after a trial period of 4 weeks on antihistamines.

    B. Parent or child sees symptoms as a major problem and requests skin testing.

    C. Recurrent serous otitis affects hearing or school progress.

NOTES

ANOREXIA NERVOSA

A symptom complex of nonorganic cause resulting in extreme weight loss in the preadolescent or adolescent

I. **Etiology**

A. Generally hypothesized to be due to reactivation at puberty of the separation–individuation issue, as the adolescent attempts to maintain or initiate a sense of autonomy and separateness from the mother.

B. Starvation gives the adolescent a sense of identity and control over what is happening to her body.

II. **Incidence**

A. Affects about 3% to 4% of adolescents

B. 90% to 95% of anorexics are female; onset between ages 13 and 20 in 75%

C. Most patients are from middle to upper socioeconomic families, but they can be of any race, gender, age, or social stratum seen commonly among members of the same family.

D. Generally seen in perfectionists or "model children" with poor self-images. They are high achievers academically and often engage in strenuous physical activity such as varsity sports or vigorous exercise programs. Parents are often overprotective, controlling, and demanding. Children feel unable to live up to parental expectations despite strict adherence to these expectations.

E. 80% of anorexics respond to therapy in terms of body weight, although other psychosocial problems may be prolonged. Amenorrhea persists in 13%–50% even after weight returns to normal or is stabilized at 85%–90% of ideal weight.

F. Mortality from physiologic complications or suicide is 5%–18%. Most common cause of death in anorexia is suicide, not medical complications.

III. **Subjective data**

A. Weight loss

B. Amenorrhea—absence of three consecutive menstrual periods

C. Constipation

D. Abdominal pain

E. Cold intolerance

F. Fatigue

G. Insomnia

H. Depression, loneliness

I. Dry skin and hair

J. Headaches (hunger headaches)

K. Fainting or dizziness

L. Anorexia

M. Pertinent subjective data to obtain

1. Preoccupation with food and dieting

a. History of dieting

b. Denial of hunger

c. Patient finds food revolting but may spend time preparing gourmet meals for others

        d. History of food rituals

    2. Morbid fear of gaining weight

    3. Weight history—highest and lowest weights achieved

    4. Vomiting after meals

    5. Low self-esteem, poor body image; patient complains of being fat, when in reality she is not.

    6. Excessive exercising

    7. Use of laxatives, diuretics, or other medications to control weight

    8. Recent family or social stress

    9. History of unpleasant sexual encounter; patient may be using starvation to try to halt development of secondary sex characteristics.

    10. History of sexual activity; condition may be unconscious attempt to abort a pregnancy.

  N. *Note:* Anorexia may be identified in its early stages by a conscientious health care provider eliciting a history during a routine health maintenance visit. Any combination of the above should create a high index of suspicion. (See Appendix J, Are You Dying to be Thin?)

IV. Objective data

  A. Weight loss of 20% or more of body weight or, in prepubertal patients, failure to gain height and weight

  B. Emaciation: Patient appears gaunt, skeletal.

  C. Bradycardia

  D. Hypotension

  E. Hypothermia

  F. Skin: Dry and flaky, lanugo hair, loss of subcutaneous fat, yellow

  G. Hair loss: Scalp and pubic

  H. Extremities: Edema, cyanosis, mottling, cold; slow capillary refill in hands and feet

  I. Compulsive mannerisms (eg, hand washing)

  J. Apathy, listlessness

  K. Loss of muscle mass

  L. Occasionally, scratches on palate from self-induced vomiting

  M. Laboratory findings

    1. Usually normal until later stages of malnutrition

    2. With malnutrition

        a. Leukopenia—characteristic of starvation

        b. Lymphocytosis

        c. Low sedimentation rate

        d. Low fibrinogen levels

        e. Low serum lactic dehydrogenase estrogens

        f. Low T3

        g. Electrolyte imbalance if vomiting

        h. BUN--high with dehydration, low with low protein intake

        i. Cholesterol levels often dramatically elevated in starvation states

  j. Liver function tests may be mildly elevated.

  k. Blood glucose low or low normal

  3. Cranial MRI to rule out hypothalamic tumor if neurologic symptoms present and in all males (cerebral atrophy often seen)

V. Assessment

  A. Diagnosis is made by evaluation of the subjective and objective data. Primary among these are the adolescent's intense or morbid fear of being fat, a poor or distorted body image, and a loss of 20% or more of body weight (patient weighs less than 75% of mean weight for age). See Appendix K, DSM-IV Diagnostic Criteria for Eating Disorders.

  B. Differential diagnosis

  1. Inflammatory bowel disease

  2. Endocrine disorder

  3. Psychiatric illness (eg, schizophrenia, depressive disorder)

  4. Pregnancy (starving to abort pregnancy)

VI. Plan

  A. Outpatient treatment

  1. Refer to psychotherapist.

  2. Refer to nutritionist.

  3. Weekly visit to check weight and urine (water loading detected by specific gravity)

  4. Refer family for counseling and/or parents' group.

  5. Restrict physical activity. This helps maintain weight by decreasing energy expenditure and also can motivate sports-minded teen to eat properly in order to resume activity.

  6. Daily structure should include three meals a day.

  7. Clearly identify parameters for admission

  a. Weight less than 75% of ideal body weight or less than a preset minimum weight

  b. Dehydration

  c. Electrolyte imbalance

  d. EKG abnormalities

  e. Severe bradycardia, hypotension, hypothermia, orthostatic changes

  f. Failure to make progress as an outpatient in 4 weeks (weight gain of less than 1 lb/week)

  g. Refusal to eat

  h. Suicidal ideation

  i. Severe depression

  B. Hospitalization indicated with severe malnutrition or for failure to make progress as an outpatient over a 4-week trial. Treatment includes:

  1. Family therapy

  2. Behavior modification

  a. Operant conditioning with positive reinforcers

  b. Negative reinforcers

    3. Pharmacotherapy

       a. Amitriptyline

       b. Cyproheptadine

VII. Education

A. This is a chronic condition and may require medical management and counseling for as long as 2–3 years.

B. A consistent approach by all caregivers and family members is necessary.

C. Aversion to food decreases as self-image improves.

D. Emphasis should be on weight gain, not eating.

E. Recommended weight gain is about 3 lb/week. Too rapid weight gain may cause adolescent to begin dieting again, as it reinforces perceptions of being ineffective, powerless, and worthless.

F. Weekly weights preferable to daily weights

G. Adolescent may drink copious amounts of water or conceal weights on body before weigh-in.

H. Bathroom use may need to be monitored for prevention of self-induced vomiting after meals.

I. Laxative use may continue if not closely monitored.

J. Anorexics who are cured generally stabilize at 85%–90% of normal weight.

K. Television use should be monitored. Cultural influences such as television promote a preoccupation with food. In addition, television and fashion magazines are dedicated to a "thin is in" image, an ideal figure that few can hope to achieve.

L. Hospitalization should not be perceived as a punishment but rather as an adjunct or intensification of treatment.

M. It is increasingly difficult with some insurance plans to secure inpatient hospitalization for treatment of anorexia. Despite established and accepted criteria developed for each patient, in many instances patients are not accepted for intensified treatment unless overtly suicidal (and that does not include the not-so-subtle signs of laxative and appetite suppressant abuse).

N. Acknowledge the fact that the adolescent feels fat. Avoid telling her she looks thin, as that can be perceived as a compliment.

O. Clearly identify threats to health; cold hands and feet, amenorrhea, syncope represent a physiologic reaction to starvation, much like an animal in hibernation.

P. Explain that unless the anorexic is dehydrated, most laboratory values (except for cholesterol, which is almost always elevated) will be within normal limits.

VIII. Follow-up

A. Schedule on an individualized basis. Many patients need to be seen on a weekly basis, sometimes biweekly until stabilized. It is an ongoing problem, and the child may need to be followed for years.

B. Contact patient or family after all referrals to ascertain that appointments have been made and kept, as well as to provide support.

IX. Resources

A. National Association of Anorexia Nervosa and Associated Disorders, Inc. (ANAD), Box 7, Highland Park, IL 60035; (708) 831-3438

B. Massachusetts Eating Disorder Association, 1162 Beacon St., Brookline, MA 02146; (617) 738-6332

    C. National Anorexic Aid Society, 1925 E. Dublin-Granville Rd., Columbus, Ohio 43229; (614) 436-1112

    D. American Anorexia/Bulimia Association, Inc., 418 E. 76th St., New York, NY 10021; (212) 734-1114

    E. Center for the Study of Anorexia and Bulimia, 1 W. 91st St., New York, NY 10024; (212) 595-3449

X. **List local referral sources.**

NOTES

APHTHOUS STOMATITIS

Recurrent small, painful ulcers on the oral mucosa, commonly known as canker sores

I. **Etiology**
   A. Cause unknown
   B. Emotional and physical factors often precede eruptions and have been implicated in the etiology, but no definite proof is available.
   C. Certain foods, especially chocolate, nuts, and fruits, can precipitate lesions, as can trauma from biting or dental procedures.
   D. Herpes simplex is not the cause.

II. **Incidence**
   A. Most common between ages 10 and 40
   B. Estimated prevalence: About 20% of the general population

III. **Subjective data**
   A. History of tingling or burning sensation preceding eruption for up to 24 hours
   B. Complaint of canker sores or recurrent painful oral lesions
   C. Pertinent subjective data to obtain. Do lesions occur after a specific triggering factor such as:
      1. Trauma
      2. Ingestion of certain foods—chocolate, tomatoes, nuts
      3. Ingestion of drugs
      4. Stress, emotional or physical
      5. Premenstrually

IV. **Objective data**
   A. Lesions
      1. Single or multiple
      2. Small: 1–10 mm
      3. Oval, shallow
      4. Light yellow or gray
      5. Erythematous border
   B. Distribution: Buccal or labial mucosa, lateral tongue, pharynx
   C. Rarely any systemic symptoms or adenopathy

V. **Assessment**
   A. Diagnosis is made by the characteristic appearance of the lesion, its recurrent nature, and the absence of systemic symptoms.
   B. Differential diagnosis
      1. Herpes simplex: Lesions are on the skin, most commonly at the mucocutaneous junction.
      2. Herpangina: Elevated temperature, sore throat, vesicular eruptions on an erythematous base on the anterior pillars; no lesions on gingival or buccal mucosa

VI. **Plan**
   A. Triamcinolone (Kenalog in Orabase) applied to lesion three times daily

B. Topical anesthetics for pain: Chloraseptic mouthwash every 2 hours (for children over 6 years of age) or Xylocaine Viscous Solution: Over 12 years of age: 1 tbsp (15 ml or 300 mg) swished around mouth every 4 hours (dosage is 4.5 mg/kg). For children 5–12: 0.75–1 tsp every 4 hours.

C. Tetracycline mouth rinse (250 mg/5 ml) four times a day for children over 8 years of age. Keep in mouth for 2 minutes, then swallow. Tetracycline compresses four to six times a day for 5–7 days can also be used for children over 8 years of age.

D. Toothpaste swish: Brush teeth and swish the toothpaste around the mouth after meals and at bedtime.

E. Oral hygiene: Rinse mouth gently with warm water.

VII. Education

A. With recurrent lesions, use Kenalog in Orabase as soon as tingling or burning is felt. This may be useful in aborting aphthae or shortening duration of ulcers.

B. Topical anesthetics

1. Dry lesion before using topical anesthetic.

2. Apply to lesion only; do not use on surrounding skin.

3. Topical anesthetics provide pain relief for about 1 hour; do not overuse. Do not eat within 1 hour after using.

4. Do not use more than 120 ml (about 8 tbsp of Xylocaine Viscous) in 24 hours for children over 12. Maximum 40 ml for children ages 5–12.

C. Tetracycline compresses abort lesions, shorten healing, and prevent secondary infection.

1. Dissolve 250 mg tetracycline in 30 ml water. Apply for 20–30 minutes.

2. Do not eat or drink for a half-hour after treatment.

D. Identify trigger factor if possible; avoid specific foods or drugs thought to be precipitating factors.

E. Use soft toothbrush if trauma seems to precipitate lesions.

F. Encourage liquids.

G. Bland diet is helpful; avoid salty or acidic foods.

H. Recurrences are common.

I. Lesions heal in 1–2 weeks.

J. Lesions are not the same as cold sores.

VIII. Follow-up

A. Telephone follow-up in 24 hours if child is not taking liquids well.

B. Routine follow-up visit not indicated

IX. Complications

A. Dehydration in a small child with several lesions (see Appendix D, Clinical Signs of Dehydration).

X. Consultation/Referral

A. Infants

B. Signs or symptoms of dehydration

C. Child with very large or many lesions, or with concurrent skin, ocular, or genital lesions

NOTES

ASTHMA

A disease of the lungs characterized by reversible or partially reversible airway obstruction, airway inflammation, and airway hyperresponsiveness. The usual manifestations are wheezing, cough, and dyspnea, although any of the three can be the sole presenting complaint. It is the most common chronic disease and the most serious atopic disease in children.

I. **Etiology**
    A. Hyperreactivity of the tracheobronchial tree to chemical mediators
    B. Allergens
        1. Environmental inhalants such as dust, molds, animal dander, pollens
        2. Food allergens such as nuts, fish, cow's milk, egg whites, and chocolate provoke asthma in about 10% of children.
        3. Anaphylactic reaction
    C. Upper and lower viral respiratory tract infections
        1. Viral infections are more common in younger children, particularly those in day care, who may easily have more than 12 infections a year.
        2. In the younger age group, viral infections are the primary cause of asthma attacks.
    D. Exertion—exercise-induced asthma
    E. Rapid temperature changes—cold air, humidity
    F. Air pollutants: Smog, smoke, paint fumes, aerosols
    G. Emotional upsets: Fear, anxiety, anger
    H. Gastroesophageal reflux

II. **Incidence**
    A. Prevalence of asthma has been increasing. An estimated 5.2% of children under 18 years of age are affected.
    B. Before puberty, twice as many males are affected as females. At puberty, the incidence becomes about equal.

III. **Subjective data**
    A. Onset may be abrupt or insidious.
    B. Generally preceded by several days of nasal symptoms (sneezing, rhinorrhea)
    C. "Allergic salute"—rubbing tip of nose upward with palm of hand
    D. Dry, hacking cough
    E. Tightness of chest
    F. Wheezing
    G. Dyspnea
    H. Anxiety, restlessness
    I. Rapid heart rate
    J. Pertinent subjective data to obtain
        1. History of upper respiratory tract infections, particularly in infants
        2. History of allergic rhinitis or atopic dermatitis
        3. Family history of atopic disease (eg, allergic rhinitis, bronchial asthma)
        4. History of inciting factors that may have initiated current attack

     5. Review of environment (eg, pets, heating system)

     6. History of bronchospasm occurring after vigorous exercise

     7. History of recurrent pneumonia or bronchitis

K. Clues to diagnosis in nonacute phase

   1. Symptoms

     a. Cough. Exercise-induced asthma may be manifested as a cough with no wheezing.

     b. Wheezing—episodic. Acute wheezing may indicate aspiration of a foreign body.

     c. Shortness of breath

     d. Tightness of chest

     e. Excessive mucous production

   2. Pattern of seemingly isolated symptoms

     a. Episodic or continuous with acute exacerbations

     b. Seasonal, perennial, or perennial with seasonal exacerbations

     c. Frequency of symptoms

     d. Timing—after exercise, consider exercise-induced asthma; during night, consider gastroesophageal reflux.

   3. Factors precipitating symptoms

     a. Exposure to common triggers—allergens, viral infections, exertion, pollutants, emotional upheavals, cold air

L. History negative for symptoms that would indicate other chronic diseases (eg, cystic fibrosis, cardiac disease)

   1. Wheezing associated with feeding

   2. Failure to thrive

   3. Sudden onset of cough or choking

   4. Digital clubbing

IV. Objective data

A. Rales; sibilant or sonorous throughout lung fields

B. High-pitched rhonchi

C. Prolonged expiratory phase; exhales with difficulty

D. Bilateral inspiratory wheezing. Sometimes expiratory wheezing as well, which reflects exacerbation of the process. Patient with severe respiratory distress may not have enough air exchange to generate wheezing.

E. In infants, inspiratory and expiratory wheezing with tracheal rales

F. Hyperresonance to percussion

G. Tachypnea

H. Evidence of hyperinflation; child sits upright with shoulders hunched forward to use accessory muscles of respiration

I. Fever, if concurrent infection

J. History or signs of atopic disease; rhinitis, flexural eczema

K. In infants, intercostal and suprasternal retractions

L. Flaring of alae nasi

M. Altered mental status; indicates impaired gas exchange

N. Examination may be negative in a child with mild or moderate asthma who presents between episodes, except for signs of allergic rhinitis.

O. Examination negative for clinical features suggests other diseases: Failure to thrive, digital clubbing, cardiac murmur, unilateral signs.

P. Laboratory findings and diagnostic procedures

1. In mild or moderate acute attacks, laboratory studies are not generally indicated; diagnosis is generally clinical, depending on history and physical examination.

2. X-ray studies are not generally indicated except to rule out a foreign body or infectious process.

3. For recurrent episodes or mild asthma, skin testing and cytology provide the most valuable data.

4. Pulmonary function tests (PFTs)

   a. Spirometry. A 10% improvement in the forced expiratory volume in 1 second or a 25% increase in the mean forced expiratory flow at 25%–75% of vital capacity after inhaling a bronchodilator indicates reversible airway obstruction. Simple spirometry can be done in the primary care physician's office.

   b. Bronchial challenge tests. Refer to pulmonologist for testing and evaluation.

5. A complete blood count is generally not indicated for diagnosis, but if it is done, eosinophilia would indicate allergies. Blood gases should be analyzed with a severe episode.

V. Assessment

A. Acute asthma attack—diagnosis clinical, dependent on history and physical examination

B. Asthma

1. Diagnosis is generally made by history of symptoms and pattern of occurrence, physical examination, and if indicated PFTs.

2. Severity can then be classified clinically or with PFTs.

   a. Mild asthma

   (1) Fewer than two attacks a week

   (2) Few symptoms between attacks

   (3) No significant lifestyle disruptions

   (4) Peak expiratory flow rate (PEFR) greater than 80% of normal

   b. Moderate asthma

   (1) More than two attacks a week

   (2) Exacerbations may last several days.

   (3) Symptoms between attacks

   (4) May have nocturnal symptoms two or three times a week

   (5) Disruption of lifestyle

   (6) Exercise tolerance decreased

   (7) PEFR 60%–80% of normal

   c. Severe asthma

   (1) Daily wheezing with frequent, often severe exacerbations

   (2) Low-grade coughing and wheezing almost constantly

    (3) Poor exercise tolerance

    (4) Nocturnal symptoms almost nightly

    (5) School or work attendance affected

    (6) PEFR less than 60% of normal

C. Differential diagnosis

  1. Infectious bronchitis: Elevated temperature, poor response to epinephrine, negative family or patient history of atopy

  2. Foreign body in trachea or bronchi: Especially common in young children with negative history of atopy and unilateral wheezing. Confirm with bronchoscopy if history, physical examination, and x-ray studies are inconclusive.

  3. Bronchiolitis: Most common in infants under 6 months, although it can occur in children up to 2 years of age. Temperature is variable; infant presents with paroxysmal cough, dyspnea, tachypnea, shallow respirations, marked hyperresonance, and markedly diminished breath sounds. A challenge with epinephrine usually does not cause improvement. Strongly suspect asthma if child has a second episode of bronchiolitis.

  4. Pertussis: Rule out by history of exposure; nasopharyngeal cultures in children under 11 years or within 2 weeks of onset of symptoms or serology in patients over 11 years with an illness of greater than 2 weeks' duration

  5. Cystic fibrosis: Rule out by previous history and, if indicated by history and physical examination, sweat test.

  6. Laryngotracheobronchitis: Usually seen in children under 3 years; characterized by insidious onset, with history of upper respiratory tract infection; harsh, barking cough with severe inspiratory stridor; slightly elevated temperature

  7. Bronchopneumonia: Dyspnea, tachypnea; rales may be present; expiratory wheezes generally not present; in advanced, consolidative phase, decreased breath sounds

VI. Plan

A. Acute severe attack

  1. Immediate treatment

    a. Albuterol (nebulized) 5 mg/ml

      (1) Dosage: 0.10–0.15 mg/kg (up to 2.5 mg)

      (2) Frequency: Every 20 minutes, up to three doses

      (3) Observe at least 1 hour.

      (4) Refer stat if no response.

    b. Oxygen as needed

    c. Poor response: Refer to emergency room.

    d. Stable with good response after 1 hour of observation, normal respiratory rate, PEFR greater than 70%–90% baseline with no retractions or dyspnea

      (1) Discharge home.

      (2) Continue albuterol every 3 to 4 hours for 24 hours.

      (3) Continue routine medications.

      (4) Call stat if symptoms recur.

  e. Incomplete response after first nebulizer treatment
    (1) Consult physician.
    (2) Repeat nebulized albuterol.
    (3) Monitor heart and respiratory rate.
  f. If improved after repeat nebulizer treatment, may go home with medications after 1 hour of observation
    (1) Prednisone 1–2 mg/kg/day in three divided doses for 3 days
    (2) Reassess after 3 days.
    (3) Dose need not be tapered.
    (4) Recheck in 48–72 hours.
    (5) Initiate inhaled corticosteroids at that time.
  g. If diminished consciousness or unable to generate PEFR
    (1) Administer epinephrine hydrochloride 1:1,000 SC, 0.01 mg/kg (up to 0.3 mg), every 15–20 minutes, for up to three doses.
    (2) Auscultate chest and heart after each dose. Do not repeat if pulse is over 180/minute.
    (3) Refer stat to emergency room for probable status asthmaticus.

B. Long-term treatment
  1. Goal of treatment is to control chronic symptoms, maintain normal activity levels, maintain normal or near-normal pulmonary function, and prevent acute episodes.
  2. Frequency of exacerbations can be diminished by continuous therapy.
  3. Side effects of prescribed drugs diminish with long-term administration.
  4. Mild or episodic asthma
    a. Inhaled beta-agonist as needed for wheezing
    b. Re-evaluate if a $beta_2$-agonist is needed on a daily basis. This usually indicates need for additional therapy.
  5. Moderate asthma
    a. Inhaled $beta_2$-agonist three or four times a day
    b. Inhaled cromolyn sodium, two inhalations two to four times a day, or inhaled corticosteroids, two inhalations two or three times a day. If control not achieved, increase inhaled corticosteroid or add
    c. Oral beta-agonist or
    d. Theophylline (particularly if nocturnal asthma)
  6. Severe asthma: Refer to asthma specialist.
    a. Inhaled beta-agonist as needed
    b. Inhaled corticosteroid
    c. Long-acting bronchodilator (oral $beta_2$-agonist or theophylline)
    d. Oral corticosteroid
  7. Exercise-induced asthma
    a. Inhaled beta-agonist, two puffs before exercise. Repeat in 2 hours as needed if exercise sustained.
    b. Alternative: Inhaled cromolyn sodium, two inhalations before exercise

   c. If control not achieved, use inhaled beta$_2$-agonist, two inhalations, and inhaled cromolyn sodium, two inhalations 5–10 minutes after albuterol inhalation.

  8. Peak flow monitoring program with moderate or severe asthma

  9. Environmental control

VII. Medications

  A. Beta-agonists: Albuterol (Proventil, Ventolin), metaproterenol (Alupent)

    1. Metered-dose inhaler: Two inhalations every 4–6 hours (one inhalation every 4–6 hours if under age 12)

    2. Powder inhaler: One capsule every 4–6 hours

    3. Nebulizer solution

      a. Albuterol: 0.10–0.15 mg/kg every 4–6 hours, up to 2.5 mg

      b. Metaproterenol: 0.3–0.5 mg/kg every 4–6 hours, up to 15 mg

    4. Oral

      a. Albuterol

        (1) Liquid: 0.1 mg/kg every 4–6 hours for ages 2–6; maximum dose 2 mg (one tsp) three times a day

        (2) Tablets: 2 or 4 mg every 4–6 hours or sustained-release preparation, 4 mg every 12 hours

      b. Metaproterenol

        (1) Liquid: 0.3–0.5 mg/kg every 4–6 hours

        (2) Tablets: 10 or 20 mg every 4–6 hours

  B. Cromolyn sodium (Intal)

    1. Metered-dose inhaler: Two inhalations, two or three times a day

    2. Powder inhaler: One capsule, two or three times a day

    3. Nebulizer solution: One ampule, two or three times a day

  C. Theophylline

    1. Dosage based on serum level; should achieve serum concentration of 5–15 μg/ml

    2. Begin with low dose and increase at 3- to 4-day intervals, depending on clinical response and serum concentration.

    3. Children's dosage should not exceed 400–800 mg/day.

    4. Liquid, extended-release capsules, or tablets

      a. 1–9 years: 16–22 mg/kg/day

      b. 9–12 years: 16–20 mg/kg/day

      c. 12–16 years: 16–18 mg/kg/day

  D. Corticosteroids

    1. Metered-dose inhaler (beclomethasone [Beclovent, Vanceril]): Two inhalations four times a day, or four inhalations every 12 hours

    2. Oral (Liquid [Pediapred] or tablets [prednisone]): 1–2 mg/kg/day

      a. 1 year: 10 mg bid for 5–7 days

      b. 1–3 years: 20 mg bid for 5–7 days

      c. 3–13 years: 30 mg bid for 5–7 days

      d. Over 13 years: 40 mg bid for 5–7 days

      e. Chronic: 20–40 mg one to three times a day. When controlled for 1 month, taper by 5–10 mg every 2 weeks to lowest dose that keeps child symptom-free.

  E. Epinephrine hydrochloride 1:1,000

    1. 0.01 mg/kg

      a. 10 kg: 0.1 ml

      b. 15 kg: 0.15 ml

      c. 20 kg: 0.20 ml

      d. 25 kg: 0.25 ml

      e. 30 kg: 0.30 ml maximum dose

VIII. Education

  A. Do not give antihistamines during an acute attack; they dry respiratory secretions and may produce mucous plugs.

  B. Try to keep child calm during acute attack; anxiety can increase bronchospasm.

  C. Postural drainage: Lie on bed with head hanging over the side.

  D. Side effects of medications

    1. Epinephrine: Tremor, tachycardia, anxiety, sweating

    2. Theophylline: Gastric irritation, nausea, vomiting, diarrhea, headache, palpitations, restlessness, insomnia

    3. Albuterol: Palpitations, tachycardia, tremor, nausea, dizziness, headache, insomnia, drying or irritation of oropharynx

    4. Cromolyn sodium: Cough, wheezing, nasal congestion, dizziness, headache, nausea, rash, urticaria

  E. Theophylline

    1. Metabolism varies among individuals and may be decreased by drugs such as cimetidine (Tagamet), ciprofloxacin (Cipro), and corticosteroids, causing an increase in serum concentrations.

    2. Smoking may increase theophylline metabolism and decrease its effectiveness.

  F. Cromolyn sodium

    1. Prevents and reduces inflammation

    2. Prevents allergen- or exercise-induced bronchoconstriction

    3. Action comparable to that of theophylline or inhaled corticosteroids

    4. No bronchodilating activity; is useful only for prophylaxis and does not work for acute attacks

  G. Albuterol

    1. Produces bronchodilation with less cardiac stimulation than older sympathomimetics

    2. Provides the most rapid relief of acute asthma symptoms with fewest adverse side effects

    3. Improvement should be noted within 15 minutes of use.

    4. Do not exceed recommended dosage; action may last up to 6 hours.

  H. Tablets are less expensive than liquids or chewables.

  I. Metered-dose inhalers

    1. Shake inhaler.

2. Breathe out, expelling as much air from lungs as possible.

3. Place mouthpiece in mouth, holding inhaler upright.

4. While breathing deeply, depress top of metal canister, then remove from mouth.

5. Hold breath as long as possible.

6. If two inhalations are prescribed, wait 5 minutes and repeat steps 1–5.

7. Clean plastic case and cap in warm water after each use.

J. Aerosol-holding chambers (Aerochamber)

1. Consider using Inspirease or Aerochamber with metered-dose inhaler.

2. Improves delivery for children who cannot inhale all medication in one breath and provides more efficient delivery to the lungs

3. Eliminates need to synchronize actuation and inhalation

K. Peak flow meter (see tables in Appendix F)

1. Used to detect airflow obstruction before child is symptomatic

2. PEFR will have decreased by 25% or more before wheezing can be detected by auscultation.

3. PEFR should be measured each morning before taking medication.

4. Monitoring before and after medication in the morning and at bedtime yields the best information.

5. Healthy children generally have a PEFR 90% or above predicted value.

6. Measurements below 80% of predicted value suggest obstruction that requires treatment; measurements 50% or lower herald a severe attack.

L. Avoid offending allergens.

M. Environmental control. See protocol, p.

N. Encourage child to participate in all activities that he or she is capable of.

O. There is no cure for asthma, but child should be symptom-free with proper medication.

P. Without adequate treatment to control asthma, life-threatening pulmonary complications may develop.

Q. Parents or health care provider should maintain working relationship with school personnel.

1. Ensure that school nurse has information on child's medications, including side effects. Request that nurse share this information with teachers.

2. Identify allergen and irritant exposures in the classroom (eg, animals, carpeting, chalk dust, plants).

3. Periodic hearing impairment is common in allergic child. Suggest periodic audiometric evaluations and preferential seating if indicated.

R. Give patient or parent written instructions for plan of care. Include medications, use of peak flow meter, graphs, indications for returning to office, use of metered-dose inhaler, and Aerochamber.

1. *One-Minute Asthma* by Thomas F. Plaut, MD is a highly rated, excellent educational tool.

2. Helpful to give individual informational sheets, which you can develop

IX. Follow-up

A. Call immediately if

1. Breathing difficulty worsens.

2. Skin or lips turn blue.
3. Restlessness or sleeplessness occurs.
4. Cough or wheezing persists, or chest pain or fever develops.
5. There are side effects from medication (eg, nausea, vomiting, irritability, palpitations).

B. Measure theophylline level 2–3 days after initiating oral therapy and every 2–3 months while on medication.

C. Return visit indicated for medication adjustment if asthma is not well controlled

D. Routine follow-up every 6 months

E. When asthma is stable or under control, measure PEFR in office.

X. **Complications**

A. Pulmonary infections (especially in children under 5 years)

B. Status asthmaticus

C. Atelectasis

D. Emphysema (after recurrent attacks)

E. Death

XI. **Consultation/Referral**

A. Severe asthma

B. Initial episode

C. Acute attack unresponsive to treatment

D. Wheezing in an infant or toddler

E. Side effects from medication

F. Persistent wheezing

G. Secondary infection (bacterial, viral, or fungal)

H. For respiratory therapy

I. For allergy testing if indicated

NOTES

BULIMIA

An eating disorder that consists of recurrent episodes of binge eating and subsequent purging or laxative abuse. Most patients are within a normal weight range but can have frequent fluctuations of weight of 10 pounds or more due to alternating binges and fasts.

I. **Etiology**
   A. A complex condition involving biologic, psychological, and social issues
   B. Predisposing factors
      1. Overweight female
      2. Overly concerned with weight
      3. A perfectionist
      4. Difficulty communicating sadness, anger, or fear
      5. Low self-esteem
      6. Difficulty resolving conflict

II. **Incidence**
   A. Occurs primarily in late adolescence or early adulthood
   B. Primarily in females (90%–95% of cases)
   C. An estimated 19% of college females and 5% of college males use purging as a method of weight control. However, not all cases of self-reported overeating and occasional purging are true bulimia. A significant number of cases may be overdiagnosed on the basis of the simple criteria of binge eating and subsequent purging. According to Schotte and Stunkard, the prevalence of bulimia in a sampling of 994 university women was no greater than 1.3%.

III. **Indications of bulimic behavior**
   A. Recurrent episodes of rapid consumption of high-calorie foods
   B. Binge eating done secretly, usually terminated by external factors (eg, abdominal pain, sleep, visitor)
   C. Abdominal pain after binge eating
   D. Purging by vomiting after binge eating; alternating binge eating and fasting
   E. Reasonably normal weight, with periodic fluctuations of about 10 lb
   F. Preoccupation with weight
   G. Attempts at weight loss through rigid dieting, vomiting, laxative or diuretic use, episodes of fasting
   H. Fear of losing control and not being able to stop eating
   I. Depression after binge eating
   J. Awareness of abnormal eating pattern
   K. Poor impulse control, also exhibited in other behavioral aberrations such as substance abuse, self-mutilation, sexual promiscuity, lying, stealing
   L. Excessive exercising
   M. Erosion of tooth enamel
   N. Possible amenorrhea
   O. Electrolyte imbalance

IV. **Subjective data**
   A. Sores in mouth

    B. Dental caries

    C. Heartburn

    D. Chest pain

    E. Bloody diarrhea (with laxative abuse)

    F. Bruising

    G. Muscle cramps

    H. Fainting

    I. Menstrual irregularities

V. Objective data

    A. Weight—normal or overweight

    B. Parotid gland hypertrophy

    C. Dental caries and enamel erosion (from contact with stomach acid)

    D. Pyorrhea

    E. Calluses and abrasions on dorsum of hands (from contact with teeth from self-induced vomiting)

    F. Abdominal distention

    G. Muscular weakness

    H. Intermittent edema

    I. History positive for indications of bulimia. See Appendix J, Are You Dying to Be Thin?

    J. Laboratory abnormalities

        1. Elevated serum bicarbonate (metabolic alkalosis secondary to vomiting)

        2. Hypokalemia, hypochloremia, hyponatremia

        3. Metabolic acidosis (with laxative use)

        4. Hypo- or hypercalcemia

VI. Assessment

    A. Diagnosis of bulimia may be made if three of the following are present:

        1. Consumption of high-calorie, easily digested food during a binge

        2. Inconspicuous eating during a binge

        3. Termination of eating episodes by abdominal pain, sleep, social interruption, or self-induced vomiting

        4. Repeated attempts to lose weight through severely restrictive diets, self-induced vomiting, or use of amphetamines, cathartics, or diuretics

        5. Frequent weight fluctuations of greater than 10 lb due to binges and fasts

    B. See also Appendix K, DSM-IV Diagnostic Criteria for Eating Disorders.

VII. Plan

    A. Interdisciplinary approach incorporating medical management, nutritional counseling, and mental health

    B. Medical management

        1. Visits should be scheduled on an individual basis according to severity of symptoms and physical findings. Initially, they should be frequent, at least every 2 weeks, until patient is medically stable.

2. Include
   a. Physical examination, with particular attention to anticipated physical findings in bulimic patients
   b. Weight
   c. Laboratory tests, depending on physical status
   d. Counseling—include psychosocial issues as well as medical and nutritional. It is unreasonable for the primary health care provider to separate these issues and address medical management alone, as bulimia is a multifaceted problem and generally it is the medical management that "pulls it all together" for the patient.

C. Nutrition
   1. Refer to nutritionist.

D. Mental health
   1. Psychiatrist
      a. Individual counseling
      b. Antidepressants if indicated
   2. Psychologist
      a. Family therapy
      b. Individual therapy to resolve underlying psychological issues, restore normal nutrition, increase self-esteem, help develop self-control

E. Behavior modification

F. Drug therapy
   1. Antidepressants: Sertraline (Zoloft), imipramine
   2. Anticonvulsants (phenytoin): Binge eaters often have an EEG abnormality; anticonvulsants can sometimes control binge eating.

G. For the occasional "binger and purger" whose physical examination and laboratory tests (complete blood count, electrolytes, urinalysis) are within normal limits, office management can be attempted for a short time.
   1. Duration of office treatment must be individualized.
   2. Counseling should concentrate on body image, normal weight for height, nutrition, dental care, excessive exercising, self-control, self-esteem.
   3. Have patient keep careful records of intake and any episodes of binge eating and purging.
   4. Recheck weekly: Weight, dietary history, counseling.
   5. Refer if episodes continue or if depression or despair is present.

VIII. **Follow-up**
   A. Contact after referral for support and encouragement.

IX. **Complications**
   A. Esophagitis
   B. Esophageal tears
   C. Gastric dilatation
   D. Hypokalemia
   E. Depression

X. **Consultation/Referral**
   A. Complications

   B. Failure to respond to treatment (eg, continuing binge eating, purging, laxative abuse)

XI. Resources

   A. National Association of Anorexia Nervosa and Associated Disorders, Inc. (ANAD), P.O. Box 7, Highland Park, IL 60035; (708) 831-3438

   B. Massachusetts Eating Disorder Association, 1162 Beacon St., Brookline, MA 02146; (617) 738-6332

   C. Anorexia Nervosa and Related Eating Disorders, Inc., P.O. Box 5102, Eugene, OR 97405; (503) 344-1144

   D. Center for the Study of Anorexia and Bulimia, 1 W. 91st St., New York, NY 10024; (212) 595-3449

   E. American Anorexia/Bulimia Association, Inc., 418 E. 76th St., New York, NY 10021; (212) 734-1114

XII. List local referral sources.

NOTES

CANDIDIASIS (DIAPER RASH)

Diaper dermatitis characterized by inflammation with a well-defined, scaling border

I. **Etiology**
   A. *Candida albicans* usual causative agent

II. **Incidence**
   A. Most common form of cutaneous candidiasis is in the diaper area of infants.
   B. Most prevalent in infants under 6 months of age

III. **Incubation period**
   A. Unknown

IV. **Subjective data**
   A. Bright-red rash in diaper area
   B. Satellite lesions outside border of rash
   C. Baby does not appear uncomfortable.
   D. History of vaginal infection in mother

V. **Objective data**
   A. Diaper area
      1. Beefy, red, shiny
      2. Sharply demarcated borders
      3. Satellite lesions—erythematous papules or pustules
   B. Inspect entire body; candidiasis may be found in intertriginous areas (eg, neck, axilla, umbilicus).
   C. Inspect mouth for oral candidiasis (thrush).

VI. **Assessment**
   A. Diagnosis is made by a detailed history or the clinical picture.
   B. Potassium hydroxide (KOH) fungal preparation reveals yeast cells and pseudohyphae.
   C. Differential diagnosis
      1. Ammoniacal diaper rash
      2. Chronic mucocutaneous candidiasis reflecting an underlying immunodeficiency

VII. **Plan**
   A. Clotrimazole (Lotrimin) cream: Apply small amount twice daily.
   B. Miconazole (Monistat-Derm): Apply small amount twice daily.
   C. Nystatin (Mycostatin) cream: Apply liberally twice daily.
   D. Nystatin powder: Apply three times daily for concurrent candidiasis in moist intertriginous areas.

VIII. **Education**
   A. Change diapers frequently.
   B. Cleanse diaper area with tepid water at each diaper change.
   C. Keep baby clean and dry, with special attention to warm, moist areas.
   D. Careful hand-washing technique; candidiasis is transmitted by direct contact with secretions and excretions.

   E. Check entire body for rash in intertriginous areas.
   F. Medication
      1. Use sparingly.
      2. Be alert for drug sensitivity—itching, irritation, maceration, secondary infection.
      3. Do not use medication for other rashes.
      4. Continue medication for at least 2 full days after rash disappears.
   G. Do without diapers as often as possible; *C albicans* thrives in warm, moist areas.
   H. Do not use plastic pants.
   I. Do not use cornstarch; it may be metabolized by microorganisms.
   J. If mother is suspect for vaginal candidiasis, refer for diagnosis.

IX. **Follow-up**
   A. Check mouth frequently; call immediately if white spots are present.
   B. Call back in 3 days if no improvement.
   C. Call to report progress in 6–7 days.

X. **Complications**
   A. Overuse of topical corticosteroids may result in striae or telangiectasia.

XI. **Consultation/Referral**
   A. Frequent recurrences: may require oral nystatin therapy to eliminate *C albicans* in intestine; may also reflect an underlying immunodeficiency
   B. Failure to respond to treatment after 1 week

NOTES

CERVICAL ADENITIS, ACUTE

Inflammation of one or more cervical nodes. In children it is most commonly reactive hyperplasia in response to an infection of the ear, nose, mouth, or throat. Pharyngitis or tonsillitis is the most common primary infection. Cervical adenitis is characterized by a 3-cm (or more) enlargement with tenderness and erythema of involved node or nodes.

I. **Etiology**

    A. Group A beta-hemolytic streptococci: 75%–80% of cases

    B. Staphylococci: About 10% of cases

    C. Viruses: Rubella, measles, herpes simplex, and adenoviruses account for remainder of cases.

II. **Incidence**

    A. Seen most frequently in preschool children

    B. 70%–80% of cases are seen in children 1 to 4 years of age.

III. **Subjective data**

    A. Painful swelling of neck—acute onset in 75% of cases

    B. Fever: Variable; may be high

    C. Complaint of malaise, anorexia, or vomiting common

    D. Pertinent subjective data to obtain

        1. History of upper respiratory infection, sore throat

        2. History of toothache, impetigo of face, or severe acne

        3. History of exposure to streptococcal pharyngitis

        4. History of exposure to animals or history of cat scratch

        5. History of exposure to tuberculosis

        6. Duration of swelling, temperature, and concurrent or preceding illness

IV. **Objective data**

    A. Fever

    B. Cervical nodes, generally unilateral

        1. Enlarged—measure size of node; usually 2.5–6 cm

        2. Tender

        3. Erythematous if infection has been present for several days without treatment

        4. Firm, but may become fluctuant

    C. Examine:

        1. Ears: Infection of canal or tympanic membrane

        2. Nose: Rhinitis, infection

        3. Throat: Erythema, exudate, petechiae

        4. Face and scalp: Impetigo, infected acne

        5. Mouth: Gingivostomatitis

        6. Teeth: Examine and percuss each tooth for evidence of infection.

        7. For lymphadenopathy in other areas

        8. Abdomen: Hepatosplenomegaly

    D. Laboratory tests

        1. Elevated white count—20,000/mm^3

        2. Throat culture for streptococcal infection

        3. Heterophil antibody or Monospot test indicated with posterior cervical adenitis or generalized adenopathy

V. Assessment

    A. Consider streptococcal infection with history of acute onset, pain, elevated temperature, history of pharyngitis, petechiae of soft palate, and vomiting.

    B. Consider staphylococcal or viral infection with a sustained high fever and no response to penicillin therapy.

    C. Diagnosis is made by the history, clinical findings, and appropriate laboratory tests.

    D. Differential diagnosis

        1. Infectious mononucleosis: Posterior cervical and generalized adenopathy; heterophil or Monospot positive

        2. Chronic adenitis: By history and presence of smaller, less tender node

        3. Cat-scratch fever: By history and evidence of trauma; generally not acute onset

        4. Tuberculosis: By Mantoux testing

        5. Leukemia: Firm, nontender, more generalized involvement of glands characteristically in posterior triangle or supraclavicular areas; hepatosplenomegaly; peripheral blood changes

        6. Mumps: Location of swelling (crosses angle of jaw) and no clear, palpable border; inflammation of Stensen's duct; leukopenia

        7. Thyroglossal duct cyst: Midline location, movement with protrusion of tongue; may become secondarily infected

VI. Plan

    A. Throat culture

    B. Tuberculin test

    C. Antibiotic therapy: Empiric therapy directed against *Staphylococcus aureus* and group A streptococci. One of the following:

        1. Dicloxacillin: 12.5–25 mg/kg/day in four divided doses (for a child weighing more than 40 kg, 125–250 mg qid, depending on severity of infection)

        2. Cloxacillin: 50 mg/kg/day in four divided doses (for a child weighing more than 20 kg, 250 mg qid)

        3. Cephalexin (Keflex): 25–50 mg/kg/day in two divided doses (for a child weighing more than 40 kg, 250 mg qid or 500 mg every 12 hours)

        4. Erythromycin: 30–50 mg/kg/day in two or four divided doses (for a child weighing more than 20 kg, 250 mg qid)

    D. Antipyretics and analgesics

        1. Acetaminophen (Tylenol): 10–15 mg/kg every 4 hours

        2. Ibuprofen: 5–10 mg/kg every 6–8 hours

    E. Local measures: Warm compresses to enlarged node for 10 minutes five or six times a day for symptomatic relief

VII. Education
A. Call back immediately:
   1. If child seems worse, has difficulty swallowing, or has difficulty breathing
   2. If node enlarges, becomes inflamed, drains, or becomes fluctuant ("pointing" or looking like a pimple)
B. Encourage liquids; do not worry about solid food if child is anorexic.
C. Compresses: Use wet face cloth or other soft cloth with water that feels comfortably warm to wrist; reapply as soon as it cools. Will require the full attention of parent for a full 10 minutes.
D. Give medication for 10 full days.
E. Acetaminophen or ibuprofen is of value only for the relief of discomfort or temperature control. Use only for these indications.
F. Node may not completely resolve for several weeks.

VIII. Follow-up
A. Telephone contact within 24 hours
B. Return to office if no improvement within 48 hours
C. Return immediately if node enlarges or if child seems toxic, dysphagic, or dyspneic

IX. Complications
A. Suppuration of node
B. Rarely, poststreptococcal acute glomerulonephritis or rheumatic fever

X. Consultation/Referral
A. Child under 2 years of age
B. No improvement after 48 hours, or worsening of symptoms at any time
C. Fluctuant node—may require incision and drainage
D. Refer to dentist if dental abscess suspected.
E. Child toxic, dehydrated, dysphagic, or dyspneic
F. Significant enlargement beyond 4–8 weeks for excisional biopsy
G. Child with positive Mantoux (greater than 15 mm of induration)

NOTES

COLIC

Characterized by periods of unexplained irritability and intense crying in healthy infants, apparently associated with abdominal pain

I. **Etiology**
   A. Cause unknown; probably multifactorial
   B. Precipitating factors: Overfeeding, underfeeding, formula intolerance, failure to burp, tension, or emotional problems in the family
   C. Food intolerance may be the cause in 10%–12% of infants.

II. **Incidence**
   A. Occurs during the first 1–2 weeks of life, most often in a first-born infant
   B. Generally subsides by 3 months of age, but may continue for 5–6 months
   C. Occurs with equal frequency in males and females in 10%–20% of infants

III. **Subjective data**
   A. Episodic, intense, persistent crying for periods up to 4–6 hours. Most often occurs in late afternoon and evening.
   B. Legs drawn up to abdomen
   C. Hands tightly clenched
   D. Feet may be cold.
   E. Child passes flatus.
   F. Pertinent subjective data to obtain
      1. Detailed dietary history—include amount and type of feeding.
      2. Detailed history of feeding techniques
      3. If mother nursing, detailed history of her dietary intake
      4. Detailed history of elimination pattern and any changes in elimination
      5. Determine how long this has been going on.
      6. Determine duration and pattern of crying spells—how often do they occur? Do they occur at a particular time of day?
      7. What have parents done to alleviate symptoms, and does anything seem to help?
      8. How are parents coping?
      9. What do parents think is wrong with the infant?
      10. Circumstances prevailing at time of conception
      11. History of pregnancy, labor, delivery
      12. Family interaction: Is father supportive? Is mother depressed? Are parents having marital difficulties?
      13. In addition to being of diagnostic benefit, the history helps the parents unburden and feel supported.

IV. **Objective data**
   A. Temperature, weight, height, head circumference, chest circumference
   B. Complete physical examination; include neurologic (may be marked response to Moro reflex). Abdomen may be distended and tense.
   C. Examine for testicular torsion, anal fissure, intestinal obstruction, incarcerated hernia, open safety pin, hair or thread wrapped around finger, penis, or toe.

D. Observe:
1. Maternal–child interaction
2. Infant's reaction to stimuli (may be marked)
3. Infant's reaction to cuddling

V. **Assessment**

A. Diagnosis is usually made by a history of repeated episodes, normal physical examination, and normal growth and development.

B. Differential diagnosis
1. Anal fissure: Bright blood in stool, fissure visualized in anus
2. Incarcerated hernia: Sudden onset, swelling in groin and ipsilateral scrotum
3. Testicular torsion: Testis tense and tender, cord thickened and shortened
4. Poor feeding practices (over- or underfeeding): Confirmed by history
5. Incorrect formula preparation: Confirmed by history
6. Family tension: May be confirmed by interview
7. Poor coping ability: May be confirmed by interview

VI. **Plan**

Management is varied and may not be successful but should include the following:

A. Immediate response to and understanding of parents' concern. Reassure parents that infant is not ill and that they are not responsible for the colic.

B. Formula
1. No conclusive evidence that formula intolerance is a cause of colic, but consider formula change. A slight difference in the fat source (polyunsaturated versus saturated fats) may help alleviate symptoms.
2. Soy formula may be given on trial basis if attacks are prolonged and there is a positive family history of allergies, although there is a high rate of cross-reactivity to soy protein and baby may develop soy protein intolerance.
3. Nutramigen or Lacto-free: Use if there may be lactose and milk protein intolerance and infant does not improve with soy.
4. Review amount and frequency of feedings and feeding techniques.

C. Breast-feeding
1. Eliminate possible sources of distress from mother's diet—excess tea, coffee, cola, strong-flavored or highly spiced foods, chocolate, shellfish, excess milk.
2. Review frequency of feedings and feeding techniques.
3. Recommend supplementary feedings if weight gain is poor.

D. Abdominal warmth
1. Place warm water bottle wrapped in a soft cloth on infant's abdomen.
2. Put infant to sleep in prone position.

E. Rhythmic movement and singing helps eliminate tension in mother as well—rocking chair, carriage.

F. Feed 1–2 oz of warm water during attack.

G. Counsel parents about:
1. Feelings of inadequacy and guilt
2. Tension or stress in family or parent

   3. Feelings of inability to cope

   4. Changes in lifestyle with birth of infant

   5. Lack of rest and relaxation

   H. Environmental factors

   1. Avoid overstimulation.

   2. Prevent chilling.

   3. Provide soft background noise (eg, music).

   4. Avoid sudden stimulation or startling of infant; approach infant slowly.

   I. Pharmacologic management may be given a trial if other measures are unsuccessful and mother is having a difficult time coping.

   1. Simethicone (Mylicon) drops: 0.3 ml four times a day

VII. Education

   A. Explain natural course of colic; generally subsides at 3 months of age, occasionally lasts until 4 months, rarely until 5–6 months.

   B. Colic will not harm baby physically or psychologically.

   C. No specific treatment is guaranteed to produce an immediate cure.

   D. Feeding

   1. Do not change formulas without consultation.

   2. Do not discontinue breast-feeding; symptoms may worsen.

   3. Adding solid foods will not generally improve symptoms; in fact, it may exacerbate them.

   4. Burp infant frequently during feeding.

   5. Try to maintain a modified demand schedule for the benefit of both mother and infant. Stress consistency in routine. Do not let infant sleep beyond usual feedings during the day.

   6. Be very cautious about overfeeding. Attempts to comfort infant by too-frequent feedings will cause overdistention of the bowel, resulting in more discomfort.

   7. Nipple holes should allow a slow, steady stream.

   E. Give medication only as directed. Call back immediately if vomiting occurs.

   F. Simethicone drops relieve symptoms of excess gas in gastrointestinal tract by freeing gas so that it can be eliminated more easily. Therefore, it may appear that the infant is "gassier."

   G. Try a warm bath at the time baby is usually fussy rather than at the scheduled bath time.

   H. Encourage parents to go out on occasion. A reliable caregiver can cope with a crying baby for a few hours.

   I. Encourage father to participate in care of infant and to relieve mother of some responsibilities.

   J. Infant should not be left in crib to "cry it out," as he or she will become even more inconsolable.

   K. However, it is unnecessary to rush in and pick up the infant the moment he or she cries out. Give the baby an opportunity to go back to sleep. It may be helpful to soothe him or her by sitting by the crib and patting or rubbing the back. It will not spoil the infant to be given love and attention when distressed.

L. Reassure parents that various emotions are normal when they cannot comfort an infant during repeated, prolonged crying episodes. Frustration, guilt, inadequacy, irritability, and even anger or hostility are emotions expressed by the most loving of parents.

VIII. Follow-up

A. Frequent follow-up is necessary to provide support and encouragement to parents and to assess results. Formula changes, elimination diet in mother, and medication should be given an adequate trial and reassessed by telephone or return visit.

B. Daily telephone follow-up may be necessary for the first week if parents are tense and anxious; thereafter, weekly telephone follow-up is sufficient.

C. Return visit in 2 weeks; include detailed interval history, physical examination, assessment of growth and development.

D. If parents have adjusted well and infant is thriving, further return visits are at usual intervals. Weekly or biweekly telephone contact continues to be indicated.

IX. Complications

A. Disruption of the relationship between parents and infant

X. Consultation/Referral

A. Inadequate weight gain

B. Maternal depression

C. Abnormal physical examination

D. Prolonged episodes; little response to treatment

NOTES

CONJUNCTIVITIS

Inflammation of the bulbar or palpebral conjunctiva or both. A self-limited disease in older children and adults.

I. **Etiology**
   A. Viral; predominantly adenoviruses
   B. Bacterial
      1. *Haemophilus influenzae* accounts for 40%–50% of cases of conjunctivitis in older infants and children.
      2. *Streptococcus pneumoniae* is the second most common cause, accounting for 10% of cases, and *Moraxella catarrhalis* is the third most common cause.
      3. *Staphylococcus aureus* is unlikely to be a significant cause of uncomplicated acute conjunctivitis, as it is isolated from eyes with conjunctivitis as well as healthy eyes.
      4. *Chlamydia trachomatis* is a diagnostic consideration in the neonate and sexually active adolescent. *Neisseria gonorrhoeae* should also be considered in the neonate (antimicrobial prophylactic failure rate is about 1% in the neonate).
   C. Allergic: Allergens such as pollens, molds, animal dander, dust
   D. Chemicals and other irritants; commonly seen after silver nitrate prophylaxis in newborns

II. **Incidence**
   A. Common in all age groups; infants and young children particularly susceptible
   B. Bacterial conjunctivitis is highly contagious and therefore prone to epidemics.
   C. In older infants and children, conjunctivitis is twice as likely to be bacterial as viral.

III. **Incubation period**
   A. Viral: 5–14 days
   B. Bacterial: 2–3 days

IV. **Subjective data**
   A. Photophobia
   B. Itching of eyes
   C. Burning of eyes
   D. Feeling of roughness under eyelids
   E. Discharge from eyes
   F. Eyelids stick together
   G. Eyelids swollen
   H. Pertinent subjective data to obtain
      1. History of upper respiratory infection
      2. Any associated signs or symptoms (eg, runny nose, sore throat, earache)
      3. History of exposure to conjunctivitis
      4. Is conjunctivitis prevalent in community?
      5. History of swimming in a chlorinated pool or contaminated pond
      6. History of foreign body or trauma to eye

7. History of exposure to herpes simplex or concurrent cold sore

8. History of exposure to volatile chemicals or other irritants

I. No complaints of decreased vision

V. Objective data

A. Viral conjunctivitis

1. Conjunctiva hyperemic

2. Hypertrophy of lymphoid follicles in lower palpebral conjunctiva

3. Tearing or mild mucopurulent discharge

4. Pupils normal and reactive to light

5. Cornea clear

6. Vision normal

7. May have associated pharyngitis, preauricular adenopathy, or edema of lower eyelids

B. Bacterial conjunctivitis

1. Conjunctiva mildly injected to markedly inflamed; discharge purulent or mucopurulent

2. Pupils normal and reactive to light

3. Vision normal

4. Cornea clear; check for ulcerations.

5. Eyelid margins may be ulcerated.

6. Skin: Occasionally impetigo is found on the face with a staphylococcal conjunctivitis.

7. Examine ears, nose, and throat for concomitant infection.

C. Allergic conjunctivitis

1. Conjunctiva edematous and moderately inflamed

2. Watery or stringy mucoid discharge

3. Vision normal

4. Associated symptoms of allergic rhinitis (see Allergic Rhinitis and Conjunctivitis, p. 227).

5. Symptoms seem worse than inflammation would indicate.

D. Chemical conjunctivitis

1. Conjunctiva inflamed and edematous

2. Tearing

3. Diagnosis made by history of exposure

E. Laboratory studies: Culture of conjunctival exudate should be done on all infants under 1 month of age.

VI. Assessment

A. Diagnosis is made by evaluation of subjective and objective data.

1. Viral conjunctivitis

2. Bacterial conjunctivitis

3. Allergic conjunctivitis

4. Chemical conjunctivitis

B. Differential diagnosis

1. Herpes simplex blepharitis: History of clinical findings of primary or secondary infection; generally unilateral

2. Herpetic keratitis: Corneal inflammation and presence of dendritic figure on staining with fluorescein

3. Trachoma (rare in United States): Upper eyelid and upper portion of globe more severely involved than lower; conjunctiva thickened, with papillary hypertrophy and formation of follicles

4. Dacryostenosis: Chronic tearing with or without discharge; generally unilateral; naris on affected side dry

5. Ophthalmia neonatorum: Diagnosis established by culture of exudate.

6. Corneal abrasion or ulcer: Severe pain and tearing, decreased vision; cornea may be hazy.

7. Iritis: Moderate pain, no discharge, diminished vision, cornea may be cloudy, poor pupillary reaction

8. Uveitis: Light sensitivity, pain, decreased vision

VII. Plan

A. Viral conjunctivitis

1. Usually associated with upper respiratory infection and self-limited

2. Medication of value only to prevent secondary infection

   a. Sodium Sulamyd ophthalmic ointment or solution 10%, five times daily

   b. Cool compresses

B. Bacterial conjunctivitis

1. Sodium Sulamyd ophthalmic ointment or solution 10%, five times daily, or

2. Tobramycin (Tobrex) ophthalmic ointment or solution, two to four times a day, or

3. Polytrim ophthalmic solution, every 3 hours, maximum six doses a day

4. Cool compresses

C. Allergic conjunctivitis

1. Treatment of underlying allergy and allergic rhinitis (see Allergic Rhinitis and Conjunctivitis)

2. Cool compresses

3. 0.5% ketorolac tromethamine (Acular) ophthalmic solution: one drop, four times a day for 5 days

D. Chemical conjunctivitis

1. Immediately flush eye with copious amounts of tepid water or preferably normal saline.

2. Consult ophthalmologist for further treatment.

VIII. Education

A. Viral conjunctivitis lasts about 12–14 days. It is generally self-limited, but secondary bacterial infection may occur.

B. Bacterial conjunctivitis should respond to treatment within 2–3 days. Continue treatment for 1 week or for at least 3 days after symptoms have subsided; otherwise it may recur.

C. Cool, wet compresses: Use cooled boiled water to moisten cotton ball; use a fresh cotton ball each time.

D. Wipe eyes gently from inner canthus to outer canthus to avoid spread to unaffected eye. Eyes should be cleaned before instillation of medication.

    E. To instill ointment or drops, pull down inner canthus of lower eyelid toward center of eye; apply thin ribbon of ointment or drops to the "pocket." Do not allow applicator tip to touch eyelid or fingers.

    F. Instillation of ointment will cause blurring of vision.

    G. Continue medication for at least 2 full days after symptoms have disappeared.

    H. Rubbing of eyes can cause spread to other eye.

    I. Hygiene

        1. Keep child's face cloth and towels separate to avoid spread of infection.

        2. Use careful hand-washing technique to help prevent spread of infection.

        3. Keep child out of school until inflammation and discharge subside.

    J. Ketorolac helps stop the cycle of itching and rubbing that can create substantial irritation of the eyes.

IX. Follow-up

    A. Call back if no improvement in 2–3 days.

    B. Call back immediately if symptoms become worse or child complains of pain.

    C. Call back if child initially responds to treatment but then seems worse; this may be an allergic reaction to the medication.

    D. No routine follow-up is necessary if child responds well to medication. Resolution should be complete in 1 week for bacterial infections, 2 weeks for viral.

X. Complications

    A. Blepharitis or corneal ulcers with bacterial conjunctivitis

    B. Secondary bacterial infection with viral conjunctivitis

    C. Sloughing of cornea or ulcer due to chemical irritation

XI. Consultation/Referral

    A. Corneal ulcer

    B. Corneal inflammation

    C. Suspicion of herpes simplex

    D. No response to treatment within 3 days

    E. Pain, severe photophobia, or decreased vision

    F. Infants under 1 month of age

    G. Irregularities of pupil size or reaction to light

    H. Chemical conjunctivitis

NOTES

NOTES

CONSTIPATION

A decrease in the frequency and bulk or liquid content of the stool. The term "constipation" refers to the character and consistency of the stool rather than to the frequency of bowel movements. Constipation is characterized by stools that are small, hard, and dry.

Encopresis is a syndrome of fecal soiling or incontinence secondary to constipation or incomplete defecation. It occurs in a child over 4 years and may be involuntary or intentional.

I. **Etiology**
   A. Mechanical or anatomic (eg, megacolon, anal stricture, obstruction)
   B. Psychological
      1. Disrupted routine
      2. Improper toilet training, such as early, aggressive training
      3. Encopresis
   C. Withholding: A busy child may ignore the urge to defecate.
   D. Anal fissure
   E. Diet: Too little fiber, too much milk

II. **Incidence**
   A. Frequently seen in childhood and adolescence, as both a chronic and an occasional interruption of normal bowel patterns
   B. Often a familial complaint

III. **Subjective data**
   A. Decrease in frequency of stools
   B. Stools hard, dry, and small, or unusually large
   C. Straining with bowel movement
   D. Pain with stooling
   E. Staining: Intermittent or constant
   F. Recurrent abdominal pain in about 60% of cases
   G. Pertinent subjective data to obtain
      1. Usual pattern of elimination
      2. Description of stools
      3. Duration of constipation
      4. Frequency of episodes of constipation
      5. Detailed dietary history
      6. Use of laxatives
      7. Treatment tried and its effectiveness
      8. History of difficult bowel training
      9. Psychosocial factors
      10. Availability of bathroom facilities and other factors, such as privacy
      11. Enuresis occurs in about 30% of children with encopresis.

IV. **Objective data**
   A. Abdominal examination
      1. Inspect for abdominal distention and bowel sounds.

2. Auscultate for bowel sounds.
3. Percussion
4. Palpation; stool palpable in colon

B. Anus: Fissures
C. Rectal examination
   1. Hard stool in colon
   2. Anal stricture

V. **Assessment**

A. Diagnosis of constipation and its underlying cause is usually made by a detailed history.
B. Differential diagnosis
   1. Normal straining of infancy: Stools soft
   2. Hirschsprung's disease: Staining or soiling rare, ampulla empty on rectal examination, history of constipation since birth
   3. Encopresis: staining, feces in rectal ampulla

VI. **Plan**

A. If constipation is significant when the child presents, a pediatric Fleet enema may be indicated for immediate relief.
B. Retrain bowels.
   1. Encourage child to sit on toilet for 5 minutes, 20 minutes after meals.
   2. Explain gastrocolic reflex.
C. Stool softeners
   1. Docusate sodium (Colace), 5 mg/kg/24 hours, or
   2. Maltsupex
      a. Age 1–12 months, 0.5 tsp bid; may increase to 1 tbsp bid
      b. Age 1–5 years, 1 tsp bid; may increase to 2 tbsp bid
      c. Age 5–15 years, 2 tsp bid; may increase to 2 tbsp bid
   3. Once stools are soft, daily dosage can be reduced.
   4. Continue use for 2–3 months until regular bowel habits are established.
D. Diet: Increase fiber, fluids, fruits, vegetables.
E. If child is toddler and not completely toilet-trained, put him or her back in diapers and eliminate all pressure (eg, from parents, grandparents, other caregivers).
F. Constipation with encopresis
   1. Initial "clean out": Fleet enema for 1–5 consecutive days
   2. Mineral oil, 3 tsp tid or qid. Give until stools are loose to the point of incontinence, then decrease dosage gradually until child has two or three loose stools daily; or
   3. Milk of magnesia (flavored): 0.5 tsp in morning for child under 2 years; 1 tsp in morning for child 2–5 years; 2 tsp in morning for child over 5 years; or
   4. Lactulose: 2.5–10 ml/day in divided doses
   5. Titrate dosages up or down depending on response. It may take 3–4 weeks to determine optimum dose.
   6. Toilet at regular intervals, 20 minutes after meals.

7. Docusate sodium, 5–10 mg/kg/24 hours, as maintenance once regular bowel habits have been established

8. Increase dosage of water-soluble vitamins (vitamin B complex and vitamin C) while on mineral oil.

9. High-roughage diet: Bran, cereals, vegetables, fruits

10. Do not put pressure on child; treatment must be approached in a calm, relaxed manner.

G. Anal fissure

1. Stool softeners as above

2. Sitz baths

VII. Education

A. Avoid laxatives and enemas for simple constipation (except as initial clean out).

B. Every person's bowel habits are unique; a daily bowel movement may not be the norm for everyone.

C. Dietary changes

1. Increase water intake.

2. Increase high-residue foods (green vegetables and fruits).

3. Include bran and whole-grain products in diet.

4. Reduce intake of cheese and milk, which may be constipating.

D. Gastrocolic reflex is a mass movement of colon contents occurring about 20 minutes after a meal.

E. A busy child may not take time to go to the bathroom.

F. Make sure that a bathroom is available for child when he or she needs it. If child is in school, discuss with school nurse and make arrangements for private bathroom time after lunch.

G. Make bathroom time relaxed and unhurried.

H. Keep special books, such as normally forbidden comic books, for relaxation in the bathroom.

I. If child is a small preschooler, toilet may be too big; instead, use a small, portable one.

J. Stool softeners are not laxatives and are not habit-forming. They prevent excessive drying of stool and are ineffective if child is withholding.

K. Mineral oil, lactulose, or milk of magnesia may be administered in juice or cola.

L. If away from home, child may not use bathroom facilities because of unfamiliarity with them or their lack of cleanliness or privacy.

M. Review toilet-training techniques (see p. 192).

1. Start when child indicates readiness.

2. How to proceed

N. Explain physiology of constipation to parent.

1. Because of discomfort from hard stool or anal fissure, child withholds stool.

2. Stool collects in the rectum and, over time, rectum dilates and propulsive peristaltic action decreases.

3. As volume of rectum increases, sensation decreases.

4. Constipation becomes self-perpetuating and often more severe with time.

5. In encopresis, because of the enlarged rectal vault, the external anal sphincter relaxes, allowing loose or mushy stool to leak out around firm stool in rectum. Child has no sense of need to defecate and little or no control over leakage.

O. Water-soluble vitamins are B vitamins (thiamine, riboflavin, nicotinic acid, pyridoxine) and vitamin C. Because excess water-soluble vitamins are excreted in urine, danger of toxicity is low.

VIII. **Follow-up**

A. Telephone call in 1 week to report; repeat telephone contact at intervals indicated by scope of problem.

B. Child who is old enough can make phone calls himself or herself.

C. With chronic constipation or encopresis, recheck every month until rectal vault has returned to normal size.

D. Treatment for constipation or constipation with encopresis may take 6 months to as long as 2–3 years.

IX. **Complications**

A. Encopresis

B. Anal fissure

C. Impaction

X. **Consultation/Referral**

A. Constipation with encopresis: Refer for psychological evaluation if child has poor response to treatment or exhibits emotional problems in other areas.

B. Recurrent fecal impaction

NOTES

DIAPER RASH–PRIMARY IRRITANT

Erythema, scaling, or ulceration of skin in diaper area

I. **Etiology**

   A. Result of prolonged contact of urine and feces with skin, leading to maceration and chemical irritation (from urea and intestinal enzymes)

   B. Consider neglect, carelessness, sensitivity from contact reactions to plastic, rubber, disposable diapers, and laundry products.

   C. Can be the result of overly enthusiastic bathing and inadequate rinsing, resulting in dry skin (xerosis)

II. **Subjective data**

   A. Reddened diaper area

   B. Sores in diaper area

   C. Baby itchy, uncomfortable; cries when voiding

   D. Baby irritable

   E. History of change in or use of inappropriate laundry products, change in diapers (disposable), change in family situation, strong odor of ammonia

   F. Detailed history of treatment used

III. **Objective data**

   A. One or a combination of the following are present in the diaper area:

      1. Erythema

      2. Papules

      3. Vesicles

      4. Oozing

      5. Ulcerations

      6. Burned or scalded appearance

   B. Check urethral meatus in circumcised male; ulceration is frequently present.

   C. Inspect entire child.

      1. Intertriginous areas may be irritated if general hygiene is poor.

      2. Legs and heels may be affected from contact with wet diapers.

      3. Eczema or other skin disease may be present.

IV. **Assessment and differential diagnosis**

   A. Candidiasis: Beefy red, shiny; sharply demarcated borders with satellite lesions. See protocol for identification and treatment.

   B. Atopic dermatitis: By detailed history and involvement of other areas (eg, chest, face, neck, extremities)

   C. Allergic contact dermatitis (sensitivity to disposable diapers, laundry products): By detailed history

   D. Psoriasis: Scaling papules and plaques with inflammation; often a positive family history

V. **Plan**

   A. Treatment determined by type of lesions (oozing, infected, or dry). If it is dry, wet it; if it is wet, dry it.

    B. Mild (erythema only): Apply one of the following at each diaper change:
1. Caldesene medicated powder
2. Dyprotex medicated diaper rash pads
3. Desitin cream

    C. Erythema, papules: Hydrocortisone cream 1%, three times a day

    D. Intense erythema, vesicles, ulcerations
1. Neosporin cream tid.
2. Burow's solution—apply compresses for 20 minutes tid.

    E. Ulcerated meatus: Neosporin cream or gentamicin (Garamycin) cream tid

    F. Corticosteroids should not be used indiscriminately. Begin with the mildest corticosteroid. If child is unresponsive, may increase potency to alclometasone (Aclovate) 0.05% or fluocinolone (Synalar) 0.01%. Do not order refills.

VI. **Education**

    A. Primary concern is prevention.

    B. Frequent diaper changes
1. Wash diaper area at each change.
2. Use a mild, nonperfumed soap such as Dove.
3. Do not use packaged wipes.

    C. Apply petroleum jelly to penis of circumcised male at each diaper change.

    D. Omit diapers as often as possible.

    E. Use plastic pants for social occasions only.

    F. Do not use cornstarch; it can be metabolized by microorganisms.

    G. Use Caldesene medicated powder on a routine basis.

    H. Diaper laundering
1. Diaper service generally acceptable
2. Home laundering
    a. Use mild soap (eg, Ivory Snow).
    b. Do not use bleach, fabric softeners in wash, or softener sheets in dryer.
    c. Put through rinse cycle twice.
    d. Use vinegar (1 oz/gal of water) in final rinse.

    I. Disposable diapers
1. Switch to another brand if sensitivity is suspected.
2. Fold plastic away from body.
3. Tear small holes in plastic to decrease humidity in diaper area.

    J. Diet
1. Increase fluids.
2. Include cranberry juice if child is 12 months of age or older; changes pH of urine, making it less irritating.
3. Exclude all other juices.
4. Do not add any new foods.

    K. Watch for sensitivity to Neosporin cream (erythema, edema, scaling, itching).

    L. Wet dressings cool and dry skin.

    M. Use soft, clean cloth for compresses. Moisten and reapply every 10 minutes.

VII. **Follow-up**

    A. Call if no improvement in 2 days or immediately if rash is worse.

    B. If ulcerated meatus, check for full stream when voiding.

    C. Call if any question of sensitivity to Neosporin.

VIII. **Complications**

    A. Secondary bacterial infection

IX. **Consultation/Referral**

    A. Failure to respond to treatment after 10 days

NOTES

DIARRHEA, ACUTE

Increase in the frequency and fluid content of stools. Usually self-limited in older children and adolescents, but potentially life-threatening in infants.

I. **Etiology**
   A. Causes
      1. Diet
      2. Inflammation or irritation of gastrointestinal mucosa
      3. Gastrointestinal infection
         a. Viral: Rotaviruses, adenoviruses
         b. Bacterial: *Shigella, Salmonella, Campylobacter, Yersinia, Escherichia coli*
         c. Parasitic: Giardiasis
      4. Antibiotic-associated
      5. Psychogenic disorders
      6. Nongastrointestinal disease (parenteral diarrhea)
      7. Mechanical or anatomic conditions
   B. Pathophysiologic reactions
      1. Disturbance of normal cell transport across the intestinal mucosa, as in sugar malabsorption
      2. Increase in intestinal motility due to excess prostaglandins and serotonin
      3. Decrease in intestinal motility causing an increase in bacterial colonization
      4. Decrease in surface area available
      5. Nonabsorbable molecules in intestine
      6. Excessive secretion of water and electrolytes because of increased intestinal permeability

II. **Incidence**
   A. Common symptom throughout childhood
   B. Diet most common cause of acute diarrhea in early infancy
   C. In older infants and children, infections of the gastrointestinal tract and other systems are the most common causes.
   D. Most viral diarrheas are spread by fecal–oral transmission with a 1–3-day incubation period and a 3–7-day duration of illness.

III. **Subjective data**
   A. Temperature may be elevated.
   B. Lethargy
   C. Anorexia
   D. Increase (sudden or gradual) in number of stools
   E. Decreased consistency of stools
   F. Increased fluid content of stools (watery stools)
   G. Crampy abdominal pain
   H. Pertinent subjective data to obtain
      1. Usual pattern of elimination; description of stools
      2. Last accurate weight

3. Type of onset (eg, rapid, with explosive, watery stools)
4. Duration of diarrhea
5. Frequency of stools
6. Description of stools (bloody, purulent, foul-smelling, mucoid)
7. Associated vomiting
8. Localized abdominal pain
9. Antibiotic therapy, concurrent or recent course
10. Epidemiologic data: Exposure to others with gastrointestinal infection (eg, home, day care, school)
11. Detailed dietary history to determine overfeeding, malnutrition, or foods that may cause diarrhea
12. Infant on formula: Type of formula
13. Breast-fed infant: Mother's diet and medication intake
14. Introduction of new foods
15. Previous history of allergic response to foods
16. Family history of atopy
17. Ingestion of suspected contaminated foods
18. History of travel
19. Use of laxatives
20. What treatments have been tried, and how effective have they been?
21. Psychosocial factors creating stress in child's environment
22. Urinary output: Symptoms of urinary tract infection; change in output

IV. **Objective data**

A. Weight
B. State of hydration (see Appendix D, Clinical Signs of Dehydration)
C. Temperature: Elevation may be due to infection or related to degree of dehydration.
D. Abdominal examination
   1. Inspection: Abdominal distention
   2. Auscultation: Hyperactive bowel sounds
   3. Percussion: Increased tympany
   4. Palpation: May be slight, generalized tenderness; no local or rebound tenderness, masses, or organomegaly
E. Ears, nose, throat, chest, glands: Signs of associated infection
F. Skin: Rash

V. **Assessment**

A. Diagnosis of acute diarrhea in children and infants generally can be made with a careful history.
B. Usually a diagnosis of exclusion
C. Stool culture or test for ova and parasites is not indicated unless the history or clinical picture is indicative of a more complex problem.
D. A Hemoccult stool test can be readily done and should be negative for red blood cells.
E. Infectious diarrhea: Diagnosis made by history of exposure and positive stool culture

1. Nonbacterial
    a. Abrupt onset, vomiting common, fever rare, often an associated upper respiratory infection
    b. Stools loose, with an unpleasant odor
2. Salmonellosis
    a. Onset 6–72 hours after ingestion of contaminated foods such as milk, eggs, or poultry or from contact with infected animals
    b. Severe abdominal cramps
    c. Loose, slimy, sometimes bloody, green stools with characteristic odor of rotten eggs
3. Shigellosis
    a. Abrupt onset of fever, abdominal pain, and vomiting
    b. Watery, yellow-green, relatively odorless stools, which may contain blood, occur shortly after onset.
    c. Transmitted by ingestion of infected foods or person-to-person contact
4. *E coli*
    a. Gradual onset of slimy, green, "pea soup" stools with foul odor
    b. Fever and vomiting not predominant symptoms
    c. Major cause of traveler's diarrhea ("Montezuma's revenge")
5. Giardiasis
    a. Commonly waterborne; seen endemically and epidemically in day care centers and communities with inadequate water-treatment facilities
    b. Anorexia, nausea, abdominal distention, crampy abdominal pain
    c. Stools pale, greasy, bulky, malodorous
    d. Onset sudden or gradual
    e. Cysts not always found in stool specimen

F. Parenteral diarrhea: Concurrent infection of another system (respiratory or urinary tract)

G. Diarrhea due to food or drug sensitivities: Indicated by history

H. Starvation diarrhea
    a. Frequent scanty, green-brown stools
    b. History of decreased food intake for 3–4 days

VI. Plan

A. Primary treatment of diarrhea is aimed at resting the intestine and keeping the child well hydrated.

B. Nursing infants
    1. Continue nursing.
    2. Give 120 ml oral rehydration solution after each watery stool.
    3. Do not give any foods or juices.
    4. With concurrent vomiting, give 5 ml water or oral rehydration solution every 5 minutes.

C. Bottle-fed infants 3–18 months of age
    1. First 24 hours
        a. Discontinue formula or milk.

b. Oral rehydration solution (Pedialyte, Ricelyte, Lytren): Give 1–2 oz/lb of body weight divided into frequent feedings of 3–4 oz each.

c. With concurrent vomiting, give 5 ml water or oral rehydration solution every 1–5 minutes.

2. Second day

a. Lactose-free formula: Intestinal lactase levels may be depressed for 7–14 days after acute gastroenteritis; therefore, a lactose-free formula is advisable—or

b. Isomil or ProSobee: Use half-strength; give amount of infant's usual feeding. If infant refuses Isomil or ProSobee, try half-strength formula.

c. Give 120 ml oral rehydration solution after each watery stool.

d. Consult office if diarrhea has not improved. Return for weight and evaluation of hydration.

3. Third day

a. Continue lactose-free formula or

b. Full-strength Isomil or ProSobee or full-strength formula

c. Diet: Slowly introduce usual diet, beginning with bland solids.

(1) Rice cereal

(2) Banana

(3) Jell-O

(4) Soup

d. If diarrhea recurs, resume half-strength formula and proceed again through dietary plan as listed above.

D. Children

1. First 24 hours

a. Give clear liquids only: Water, oral rehydration solution, Pedialyte popsicles, weak tea, Jell-O water, Gatorade, popsicles.

b. Give 1–2 oz every 10–15 minutes.

2. Second day

a. If diarrhea has improved, add bland solids.

(1) Rice cereal

(2) Banana or banana flakes, applesauce

(3) Jell-O

(4) Saltines

(5) Toast and jelly

b. If diarrhea has not improved, consult office. Evaluate for state of hydration.

3. Third day

a. With improvement of diarrhea, gradually add more bland solids; avoid high-fat solids.

b. Avoid milk, fried foods, vegetables, fruits, and meat.

E. Salmonellosis

1. Antimicrobial treatment of mild illness does not shorten clinical course.

2. Consult and treat systemically if disease appears to be progressing systemically in infants, or if child is immunocompromised.

    F. Shigellosis

        1. Trimethoprim–sulfamethoxazole: 8 mg/kg trimethoprim and 40 mg/kg sulfamethoxazole (Bactrim or Septra) per day in two divided doses

        2. Bacteriologic cure achieved in 80% of children after 48 hours

    G. *E coli*: Trimethoprim–sulfamethoxazole: 8 mg/kg trimethoprim and 40 mg/kg sulfamethoxazole (Bactrim or Septra) per day in two divided doses

    H. Giardiasis

        1. Metronidazole (Flagyl)

            a. Children: 15–20 mg/kg/day in three divided doses

            b. Adolescents and adults: 250 mg tid, or

VII. Education

    A. Discontinue milk, juices, and foods.

    B. Do not use boiled skim milk; hypernatremia may result from high solute load.

    C. Too-frequent feedings may exacerbate diarrhea by stimulating the gastrocolic reflex.

    D. Use petroleum jelly or Desitin on perianal area to prevent excoriation.

    E. Use careful hand-washing technique to help prevent spread of infectious diarrhea. Keep child home from school to prevent spread.

    F. Do not continue clear liquids longer than 24 hours.

    G. Childhood diarrhea can be treated effectively by resting the gastrointestinal tract and then slowly resuming a normal diet, but the plan must be followed carefully.

    H. Call back immediately if child is not taking liquids, is vomiting, or has any signs of dehydration (see Appendix D, Clinical Signs of Dehydration).

    I. Sweetened juices and soda can increase the severity of diarrhea, as hyperosmotic fluids draw more fluid into the intestinal lumen.

    J. Incubation period for viral diarrhea is 1–3 days (mean 2 days).

    K. Duration of diarrhea is generally 3–7 days.

    L. Transmission is via fecal–oral route.

VIII. Follow-up

    A. Telephone follow-up in 8–12 hours if child is not dehydrated and retains liquids. Have caregiver call back sooner if child refuses liquids or is vomiting.

    B. Continue to maintain daily telephone contact until diarrhea has subsided, giving caregiver dietary instructions at each stage.

    C. With infants, check weight daily. Continue follow-up until pre-illness weight is re-established.

IX. Complications

    A. With simple diarrhea, dehydration is the major complication.

X. Consultation/Referral

    A. Signs of dehydration

    B. Bloody diarrhea

    C. Diarrhea in a child who is taking antibiotics (eg, ampicillin, erythromycin) or iron

    D. Infant under 3 months of age

    E. Diarrhea persisting longer than 3–4 days

NOTES

| **DYSMENORRHEA, PRIMARY**

Painful menstruation without demonstrable pelvic disease. Occurs 1–3 years after menarche, when ovulation is established.

I. **Etiology**

   A. Recent data demonstrate that prostaglandins released during the breakdown of the endometrium are higher in dysmenorrheic females. The prostaglandins act as pain mediators and stimulate uterine contractility.

   B. Dysmenorrhea is not usually associated with the onset of menses, although some adolescents experience discomfort with the first cycles (generally anovulatory).

II. **Incidence**

   A. An estimated 75% of all adolescent girls complain of one or more symptoms of dysmenorrhea, and an estimated 18% of young women have severe enough symptoms to interfere with normal activities.

   B. Most common gynecologic complaint in this age group

   C. Leading cause of short-term school absenteeism in females

III. **Subjective data**

   A. Onset of one or more of the following symptoms during or before menstruation. Pain usually starts within 1–4 hours of onset of menses but can occur 1–2 days before menses. Symptoms persist for 24–48 hours after beginning of menstrual flow, less frequently for 2–4 days.

      1. Premenstrual tension, including irritability or emotional lability, headache
      2. Abdominal cramps
      3. Nausea, vomiting, anorexia
      4. Constipation, diarrhea
      5. Weight gain
      6. Fluid retention, bloating (3–5 lb in the 4–7 days before onset of menses)
      7. Syncope
      8. Vaginal discomfort
      9. Suprapubic pain radiating to back and thighs

   B. Pertinent subjective data to obtain

      1. Detailed menstrual history
         a. Age at menarche
         b. Regularity of menses
         c. Heaviness of flow
         d. Duration of menses
         e. When cramping started in relation to menarche
      2. Location and description of pain
      3. Timing of pain or cramping
      4. Duration of pain
      5. Presence of premenstrual symptoms (eg, bloating, irritability)
      6. Presence of mittelschmerz
      7. Did patient expect this to happen with menses? Did mother or sisters have dysmenorrhea?

     8. Absence from school due to dysmenorrhea; how often and how many days. Does she miss other activities (eg, parties, sports events)?

     9. Treatment used and effectiveness

    10. Adolescent's understanding of the menstrual cycle

    11. Patient's relationship with mother

    12. Sexual activity; some adolescents use a complaint of dysmenorrhea as an entry to the health care system when they either want, or want to discuss, birth control.

    13. *Note:* Detailed menstrual history should be obtained from every adolescent female presenting for routine health care. Discussion should include questions about discomfort relating to menses.

IV. Objective data

   A. Weight, height, blood pressure

   B. Mild cramps on first day: Complete physical examination, including inspection of external genitalia for hymenal abnormalities, is appropriate for 13–16-year-old girl who is not sexually active.

   C. Moderate to severe cramps: Complete physical examination, including pelvic examination; if unable to complete pelvic exam, rectoabdominal examination should be done to rule out pelvic pathology. Include careful palpation of uterosacral ligaments for tenderness or nodules (suggestive of endometriosis).

   D. Include pelvic examination, Pap smear, and cultures for sexually active adolescents.

   E. Pelvic ultrasound to rule out uterine or vaginal anomalies (will not detect endometriosis)

V. Assessment

   A. Diagnosis of primary dysmenorrhea can be made by history typical for primary dysmenorrhea and negative findings on physical examination.

   B. Differential diagnosis

     1. Secondary dysmenorrhea

       a. Atypical history

       b. Positive findings on physical examination

       c. Adnexal tenderness and masses or nodules on uterosacral ligaments

       d. Pain increases over time.

VI. Plan

   A. Goals of treatment are to allay anxiety and provide symptomatic relief of pain.

   B. Reassurance

     1. Simple explanation of the menstrual process and anatomy

     2. The pain is not "in her head," as may have been suggested.

     3. Pain can be managed; she does not have to anticipate pain every month.

   C. Pharmacologic management

     1. Begin with the simplest treatment and progress to stronger medications as needed. Use one of the following:

       a. Aspirin: 300–600 mg every 4 hours as needed

       b. Anaprox: 550 mg stat, followed by 275 mg every 6 hours or 550 mg bid; maximum dose: 1,375 mg/24 hours.

    c. Ketoprofen (Orudis): 25–50 mg every 6–8 hours. May increase dosage to 75 mg every 6–8 hours; maximum dose: 300 mg/24 hours.

    d. Ibuprofen: 400 mg every 4–6 hours. Increase to 600 or 800 mg every 6–8 hours if necessary; maximum dose: 3,200 mg/24 hours.

    e. Mefenamic acid (Ponstel): 500 mg initially, then 250 mg every 6 hours as needed for pain; do not exceed 1 week of therapy.

2. *Note:* For severe dysmenorrhea associated with vomiting, one of the above medications may be started 1–2 days before menses if not sexually active.

3. Birth-control pills

    a. Pelvic examination and Pap smear before starting treatment

    b. Indicated for severe dysmenorrhea associated with vomiting and with unsatisfactory response to analgesics and antiprostaglandins

    c. Tri-Norinyl #28 or Ortho-Novum 7:7:7 #28: Use for 3 months, discontinue for 3–6 months, and resume for another 3 months. Patient will usually continue to have relief for 1–2 months between use of birth-control pills because of anovulation. If cramps recur, try antiprostaglandin before starting birth-control pills again.

    d. Use of birth control pills helps distinguish organic pathology. If cramps become worse on birth-control pills, refer for laparoscopy to rule out endometriosis.

4. Compazine: 5 mg every 4 hours at onset of menses to control vomiting

D. Local measures: Heating pad on abdomen

VII. Education

A. Dysmenorrhea is not abnormal. It does not mean that there is any physical abnormality or disease present, nor is it a psychosomatic illness.

B. Dysmenorrhea is an indication that ovulation is occurring. Stress the positive future aspects of motherhood.

C. Dysmenorrhea may be more severe during times of stress.

D. If fluid retention or bloating is a problem, decrease salt intake for 10 days before menses.

E. Continue with regular routine as much as possible. Some discomfort may persist once on medication, but if pain is under control, do not forego activities.

F. Increased exercise (eg, jogging, bicycling, ice skating) on a regular basis has been of value in decreasing menstrual pain. Competitive athletes have fewer ovulatory cycles and therefore less dysmenorrhea.

G. Showers, baths, and shampooing during menses will not increase discomfort or cause cramps.

H. Medication

1. Aspirin taken with a cup of coffee or tea may be quite effective; the caffeine potentiates the effects of aspirin.

2. Take antiprostaglandins with food to minimize gastrointestinal side effects.

3. Continue antiprostaglandins for 2–3 days only.

4. Do not use medication longer than necessary.

5. Nonsteroidal anti-inflammatories prevent cramps as well as treat pain.

6. Dysmenorrhea treatment is most effective if treatment is initiated at onset of menstrual shedding or before, if possible.

7. After 1–2 years on a birth-control pill regimen of 3 months on and 3 months off, cramps often improve spontaneously.

8. Do not prescribe antiprostaglandins for anyone with a history of allergy to aspirin or any nonsteroidal anti-inflammatory.
9. When on the birth-control pill, flow will be lighter.
10. Give caregiver and patient complete information on birth-control pill, and have them read the booklet that comes with prescription packet.
11. Stress importance of calling the office immediately if there are any questions regarding side effects.
12. Take all medication as directed. Do not take more than prescribed.

VIII. **Follow-up**

A. Have patient call after next menstrual period to report effectiveness of treatment.
B. Return visit in 3–4 months to evaluate effectiveness of medication and to maintain encouragement and support.
C. Follow-up visit every 3 months while on birth-control pills, with a complete physical, including pelvic examination, every 6 months.

IX. **Complications**

A. Vomiting causing inability to retain medication
B. Psychological stress

X. **Consultation/Referral**

A. Questionable or abnormal findings on physical examination or history
B. Severe dysmenorrhea before institution of pharmacologic therapy
C. No response to prescribed treatment
D. Inability to retain medication because of vomiting

NOTES

| ENURESIS

The involuntary or intentional passage of urine, usually occurring at night (nocturnal enuresis) in a child over 5 years of age into bed or clothes. It is subdivided into two classifications, primary and secondary. Primary enuresis is that occurring in a child who has never been dry at night for a period of greater than a week. Secondary enuresis is that occurring in a child who has been dry at night for a prolonged period and subsequently loses bladder control. Diurnal enuresis is enuresis occurring during the day.

The diagnosis is made when at least two events a month occur in a child under 5 and at least one event a month for older children.

I. **Etiology**
  A. Primary nocturnal enuresis
    1. Immature development of bladder with resultant small capacity
    2. Immature arousal mechanism for non-REM sleep
    3. Psychological problems, such as regression after birth of a sibling
    4. Neurologic causes: Myelomeningocele, mental retardation
    5. Urologic lesions or anomalies
    6. Diabetes mellitus or diabetes insipidus
  B. Secondary nocturnal enuresis
    1. Psychological problems
    2. Developmental delays
    3. Urinary tract infection
    4. Diabetes mellitus or diabetes insipidus

II. **Incidence**
  A. About 10%–15% of 6-year-olds, 5% of 10-year-olds, 3% of 12 year-olds, 1% of 15-year-olds
  B. More common in boys than in girls
  C. Familial tendency toward enuresis; more prevalent in large families and in lower socioeconomic groups

III. **Subjective data**
  A. Primary: Bed-wetting one or more times a night at least once a week without having achieved bladder control at night
  B. Secondary: Bed-wetting one or more times a night at least once a week after having achieved bladder control at night.
     Note: As part of the history obtained at the well child visit, children should be asked if they have any urinary symptoms and if they ever wet their pants or the bed.
  C. Pertinent subjective data to obtain
    1. Has child ever been dry? If so, when did onset of wetting occur?
    2. How frequently does child wet the bed?
    3. When does bed-wetting occur—late evening, early morning?
    4. What do parents do about bed-wetting? How do they feel about it? Do they see it as a problem?
    5. Is there a history of bed-wetting in the family (siblings or parents)?
    6. How does the child feel about wetting the bed?

7. Is there a family history of diabetes mellitus?
8. Has child ever awakened with sore muscles or bitten tongue (suggesting nocturnal seizures)?
9. Does child have a full stream when voiding?
10. Daytime voiding pattern (frequency, volume of urination, dribbling, diurnal enuresis). Frequent, small-volume voidings, dribbling, and diurnal enuresis suggest primary enuresis.
11. Complaints of frequency, urgency, pain, or burning on urination
12. Has the child been dry when sleeping away from home?
13. Presence of psychosocial problems (indicative of secondary enuresis)
    a. New baby in the family
    b. Death of a family member
    c. Illness or hospitalization of child or family member
    d. Divorce or separation of parents
    e. School problems
    f. Loss of a pet
14. Accurate history of hours of sleep and bedtime routine: Regular sleep habits, sufficient sleep, large amount of fluid at bedtime, voiding before going to bed

IV. **Objective data**

A. Physical examination is generally within normal limits. Significant neurologic deficits would present with history or findings in addition to nocturnal enuresis and would probably already have been identified.
   1. Complete physical and neurologic examination
      a. Constant dribbling
      b. Genitalia: External anomalies
      c. Rectal sphincter tone
      d. Skin: Cafe-au-lait spots
      e. Spine: Bony defects, masses, hairy tufts
      f. Abdomen: Masses, enlarged kidneys
      g. Gait
   2. Height, weight, blood pressure to rule out chronic occult urinary tract disease
B. Laboratory tests: Urinalysis and culture of clean-voided specimen

V. **Assessment: Differential diagnosis**

A. Urinary tract infection: Positive urine culture
B. Diabetes mellitus: Urine positive for glycosuria and acetonuria
C. Diabetes insipidus: Specific gravity under 1.006
D. Glomerulonephritis, pyelonephritis, cystitis, urethritis
   1. Urine positive for proteinuria
   2. Microscopic examination positive for erythrocytes and leukocytes

VI. **Plan**

A. Before any treatment for enuresis is attempted, the child must want to be dry and the parents must be willing to participate in the treatment.

B. A voiding volume of less than 200–300 ml is not sufficient for child to remain dry at night.

C. Management should not be attempted until psychosocial issues and pressures within the family have been resolved or ruled out.

D. Do not attempt management when any stress is anticipated, such as a family move or birth of a sibling.

E. Primary enuresis: The following are three commonly used, acceptable methods of management:

  1. Bladder-stretching exercises

    a. Have caregiver measure volume of urine several times.

    b. Once daily, have child hold urine as long as he or she can after desire to void is felt.

    c. Encourage increased fluid intake, particularly during the time child is holding urine.

    d. Measure voiding volume after child has achieved maximum ability to control desire to urinate.

    e. Once child has increased bladder capacity, have him or her practice starting and stopping urine stream.

    f. Make a chart to record bladder capacity, giving gold stars for dry nights.

  2. Pharmacologic therapy

    a. Imipramine (Tofranil)

      (1) Drug most frequently used

      (2) Has an atropine-like effect on the bladder, increasing the capacity by increasing sphincter tone and decreasing tone of the muscle that causes bladder contraction

      (3) An antidepressant; may interfere with natural sleep pattern and depth

      (4) Do not use in children under 6 years of age.

      (5) Initially 15–25 mg at bedtime, increased to a maximum of 50 mg in children under 12 years of age and 75 mg in children over 12 years of age

      (6) Continue treatment for 6–8 weeks, and taper dosage over 4–6 weeks to avoid relapse.

      (7) If child wets during the early night hours, give 25 mg of imipramine at 4 p.m. and repeat dose at bedtime.

    b. DDAVP

      (1) An antidiuretic hormone that decreases urine production

      (2) Used intranasally in children age 6 and older

      (3) Initially 20 mcg intranasally at bedtime. Administer one spray (10 mcg) per nostril.

      (4) Subsequent dosage: If no clinical response, increase by 10 mcg (one spray) at bedtime every 2 weeks, to a maximum of 40 mcg.

      (5) When response is achieved, maintain at dosage for 2 weeks, then titrate down by 10 mcg at bedtime to lowest effective dose (minimum dose: 10 mcg).

  3. Behavioral treatment

    a. Pad and bell technique

(1) Studies report an initial success rate of 75%. The alarm system is a pad of two conductive layers with an insulating cloth in between. The child sleeps on the pad. When he or she wets and soaks through the insulating cloth, an electrical circuit is completed, causing the bell to ring.

(2) When the bell rings, awakening the child, he or she should go to the bathroom to finish voiding.

(3) Child or parent then changes the bed and resets the alarm.

(4) Treatment with this method may take 5–12 weeks.

(5) If no improvement after 10 weeks, stop treatment. Another trial may be undertaken in 3 months.

(6) Relapse rate of 20%–40%. If relapse occurs after cessation of treatment, retreatment with the pad and bell is successful in most instances.

   b. Sleep Dry or Wet Stop

(1) Moisture sensor is attached by Velcro patch sewn on underpants. Alarm unit attaches to pajama top with Velcro.

(2) At onset of voiding, alarm goes off to awaken child.

(3) Sleep Dry program includes instructions and motivational materials (charts, stars).

F. Secondary enuresis: Therapy must be specific to the etiology.

   1. Psychosocial problems or stressful situations

      a. Counseling

(1) Explanation of enuresis to parents and child

(2) Discontinuance of pressure and punishment

(3) Development of a plan with child and parents that will work for them

(4) Contact school principal or nurse regarding school problems

      b. Imipramine: See above for dosage.

   2. Developmental lag

      a. Behavioral conditioning

      b. "Gold star" chart

   3. Urinary tract infection: See Urinary Tract Infection.

   4. Diabetes mellitus or diabetes insipidus: Refer to physician.

VII. Education

A. Do not attempt management unless child is willing and is over 8 years old.

B. Primary enuresis is a self-limited problem. Reassure parents that it is a developmental issue; child is not lazy or refractory.

C. Avoid punishment, embarrassment, or shaming the child.

D. Do not be too aggressive in approach.

E. Avoid causing anxiety in other family members or child.

F. Involve child in treatment plan.

G. Bladder-stretching exercises

   1. When increasing fluid intake, child may have more frequent enuresis and may have daytime accidents.

2. May take several months for child to achieve a voiding volume of 240–300 ml

3. Generally, when voiding volume of 300 ml is achieved, child will be able to sleep through the night without voiding. Some children, however, need a greater volume before becoming dry at night.

H. Do not diaper child.

I. If child is willing, restrict fluids after dinner.

J. Have child void before going to bed.

K. If child has no difficulty going back to sleep, it is sometimes helpful for parents to get child up to void before they go to bed.

L. Make a chart or calendar on which to record bladder capacity and wet and dry nights. Encourage child to keep the chart.

M. Imipramine

1. Most common side effects seen in enuretic children on imipramine are irritability, sleep disorders, fatigue, gastrointestinal disturbances, and nervousness. Other reported reactions include constipation, convulsions, anxiety, emotional instability, syncope, and collapse.

2. Keep imipramine out of reach of small children.

N. DDAVP

1. An antidiuretic hormone that decreases urine production by increasing urine concentration

2. Nasal spray bottle accurately delivers 50 doses of 10 mcg each. Discard remaining medication after 50 doses.

3. Most common side effects are nasal congestion, rhinitis, flushing, and mild abdominal cramps. Symptoms abate with decreased dosage.

4. Restrict nighttime fluid intake to decrease potential occurrence of fluid overload.

O. Pad and bell technique

1. Do not use alarm system that has an electric shock; use only the type that has a bell.

2. Check batteries on apparatus frequently; electrolysis of urine may result from weak batteries, producing topical burns and preventing alarm bell from ringing.

P. Wet Stop and Sleep Dry have moisture sensors in underpants that, when activated by even a few drops of urine, trigger alarms. Child is awakened before bed is wet and voiding is completed. Also, the alarm is located near the child's head so that he or she responds to it more readily.

1. Wet Stop: Palco Labs, 1595 Soquel Drive, Santa Cruz, CA 95065

2. Sleep Dry: Follow instructions with program. Available through Star-Child/Labs, P. O. Box 404, Aptos, CA 95001-0404.

Q. Alarms have the highest cure rate, about 70%.

VIII. Follow-up

A. Primary enuresis

1. Serum electrolytes after 1 week of therapy with DDAVP

2. Telephone contact in 2 weeks. Have child call back to report progress.

3. Return visit in 1 month. Have child bring in chart.

4. Continue follow-up at 2–4-week intervals for encouragement.

5. Follow-up may alternate between telephone calls and office visits.

B. Secondary enuresis

1. Counseling contract should be individualized. Initially, follow-up should be at least every 10–14 days. Encourage child to call and report successes.

2. Return visits at least monthly while on imipramine.

3. With behavioral conditioning and gold star chart, follow recommendations above.

4. Urinary tract infection: See Urinary Tract Infection.

IX. **Complications**

A. A management plan that is too vigorous or stressful may result in psychological problems or increase stress for the family.

X. **Consultation/Referral**

A. Diurnal enuresis, dribbling

B. Significant psychological problems, child abuse

C. Urinary tract infection

D. Genitourinary abnormality

E. Failure to improve with adequate trial of bladder retention or behavioral conditioning

NOTES

| ENVIRONMENTAL CONTROL FOR THE ATOPIC CHILD

With mild or questionable atopy, aggressive environmental control may be disruptive to the family and home environment. The health care professional should select portions of environmental control applicable to the child. In many children, environmental control results in significant improvement.

I.   **Indications for environmental control**
   A. Positive skin tests for environmental allergens
   B. Pollen sensitivity
   C. Clinical history of significant symptoms of allergy, including food sensitivity

II.   **Common allergens in the home**
   A. Animals: Cat, dog, guinea pig, hamster, gerbil
   B. Plants, flowers
   C. Jute, horse hair carpet padding
   D. Kapok: Pillows, upholstery, stuffed animals
   E. Feathers, down pillows, upholstery
   F. Wool: Blankets, clothing
   G. House dust: In addition to containing the allergen, dust contains bacteria, mites, kapok, dander, horse hair.
   H. Cosmetics: Talcum powder, perfumes
   I. Molds: Found in bathroom, shower stall, tile grout, basement, garage, attic, books, wallpaper, foam-rubber pillows
   J. Smoke: Cigarettes, wood stove

III.   **General measures for the home**
   A. Damp dust daily.
   B. Use vacuum cleaner with an effective filtration system (HEPA). Do not vacuum when child is in room.
   C. Steam cleaning of carpeting should be done routinely. Dust mites have sticky feet and vacuuming does not remove them from carpeting.
   D. Use air conditioner rather than fan. Air conditioning allows house to be closed to decrease exposure to outdoor allergens and also lowers humidity.
   E. Hot air ducts and returns should be covered with filters or cheesecloth. Vacuum ducts weekly.
   F. Replace air conditioner and furnace filters regularly.
   G. Shades and cotton curtains are preferable to venetian blinds and draperies.
   H. Avoid wool rugs and blankets.
   I. Paint walls or use washable wallpaper.
   J. Kitchen, bathroom, and laundry should be adequately ventilated. Clean tile, grout, under sink, and behind toilet frequently.
   K. Keep windows closed during pollen season.
   L. Keep humidity below 50%; dust mites thrive at 50% or above.
   M. Use hot water (130°F) laundering to kill mites; they cannot be washed away.
   N. Pet

   1. Recommendation to remove a family pet may be difficult to implement, but it is a sound prophylactic measure even in the absence of a positive skin test because sensitivity often develops in an atopic child.

   2. If giving up the family pet is a problem, try to keep animal outside as much as possible and restricted to one area in the house.

   3. If pet dies, advise parents not to replace it. (Snakes are acceptable for an atopic child.)

O. Do not give child chores such as dusting or mowing the lawn.

P. Plants may harbor mold and should be removed.

Q. Discourage smoking and use of a wood stove or fireplace.

R. Keep child out of attic and cellar.

S. Consider a HEPA air cleaner if symptoms remain severe when other environmental control measures are taken. Dust and dust mites settle quickly, so even HEPA filters are not completely effective for them. They are most effective for airborne particulate material.

T. Cleaning products

   1. Chlorine bleach for bathrooms, cellars, other damp areas

   2. Ammonia for general cleaning

   3. Club soda as a spot remover

   4. Vinegar to remove mold

   5. Baking soda for carpets and refrigerator

IV. Environmental control for child's room

A. Remove everything from room and closet except large pieces of furniture. Rugs should be removed also.

B. Vacuum mattress and box spring, and cover with plastic. Zipper of plastic case can be covered with adhesive tape.

C. Wash walls, woodwork, ceiling, floor, and windows.

D. Paint walls or cover with washable wallpaper. Do not use wall hangings; paint murals on walls instead.

E. Install washable, synthetic window shades.

F. Dust and wax furniture; damp dust drawers.

G. Seal off forced hot air ducts and returns. Use an electric heater if necessary.

H. Carefully screen all items returned to room.

I. Use Dacron pillows. Wash weekly. Replace yearly.

J. Use cotton or Dacron blankets, bedspreads, sheets, and curtains. Do not use mattress pads or quilts.

K. Use wood or plastic chairs and tables. Avoid stuffed or wicker furniture.

L. Do not use venetian blinds or louvered doors.

M. Lamps should have plastic shades.

N. Return clothes to closet and drawers. Do not store woolens, flannels, or unnecessary items of clothing.

O. Books, stuffed animals, sports equipment, old shoes, and collections are dust and mold collectors and should not be in the room the child sleeps in.

P. To maintain a dust-free room

   1. Keep door closed to minimize dust entering room.

   2. Daily, damp dust and damp mop.

   3. Weekly, clean room thoroughly, vacuum mattress and box spring, and wash all bedding and curtains.

V. **School**
   A. Child should not sit near blackboard or handle erasers.
   B. Caged pets such as hamsters or gerbils should not be in school room.
   C. Concrete slab floors covered with carpeting may harbor molds.
   D. Molds may grow on plants or dried arrangements.
   E. Outdoor gym class may be a problem during pollen season.

NOTES

ERYTHEMA INFECTIOSUM (FIFTH DISEASE)

A mild viral illness characterized by a three-stage exanthem. The first is a slapped-cheek appearance, the second is a maculopapular rash on the trunk and extremities that becomes a reticular, lacy rash and in the third stage has periodic evanescence and recrudescence. The disease is important primarily because maternal infection during pregnancy can cause spontaneous abortion, stillbirth, or asymptomatic intrauterine infection. This risk, however, is presumed to be only 1%–2% of those infected.

I. **Etiology**
   A. Human parvovirus B19
   B. Referred to as "fifth disease" because it was the fifth childhood exanthem described, the others being measles, rubella, scarlet fever, and roseola

II. **Incidence**
   A. Community outbreaks are common, most frequently in late winter and in spring.
   B. Highest incidence in schoolchildren 5–15 years old
   C. More than 60% of adults are immune because of prior disease.

III. **Incubation period**
   A. 4–14 days

IV. **Communicability**
   A. Transmitted by droplet infection
   B. Most infectious before onset of rash
   C. Secondary spread occurs in about 50% of close contacts.

V. **Subjective data**
   A. History of mild systemic symptoms of a nonspecific viral illness, often identified only in retrospect
      1. Low-grade fever
      2. Headache
      3. Chills
      4. Malaise
      5. Myalgia
      6. Pharyngitis
      7. Conjunctivitis
   B. Symptoms last 2–3 days and are followed by an asymptomatic period of 4–7 days.
   C. Rash, predominant presenting complaint, seen 17–18 days after exposure. This is the third stage of the disease.

VI. **Objective data**
   A. Objective findings vary according to phase of illness.
   B. Prodromal phase: Duration 1–4 days; mildly erythematous pharynx or conjunctiva
   C. Second stage: Duration 4–7 days; asymptomatic
   D. Third stage: Exanthem appears in three stages.

1. First stage
   a. Typical slapped-cheek appearance 4–7 days after resolution of systemic symptoms. Fiery red rash on cheeks, circumoral pallor.
2. Second stage
   a. 1–4 days after onset of facial rash
   b. Erythematous maculopapular discrete rash on trunk and extremities
   c. Fades as central clearing occurs, leaving a lacy, reticulated rash
3. Third stage
   a. Duration 1–3 weeks
   b. Lacy, reticulated rash characterized by periodic evanescence and recrudescence
   c. Fluctuations in intensity associated with environmental changes such as elevated temperatures and sun exposure

VII. Assessment

A. Diagnosis is generally easily made by appearance of characteristic exanthem.
B. Differential diagnosis. Atypical cases may be confused with other viral exanthems such as measles, rubella, and enteroviruses or with drug reactions or other allergic responses.

VIII. Plan

A. No specific treatment
B. Give acetaminophen or ibuprofen for associated myalgias.

IX. Education

A. Most contagious before onset of rash; therefore, isolation unnecessary once rash appears
B. Avoid contact with pregnant women until rash begins to fade.
C. Erythema infectiosum contracted during pregnancy can result in spontaneous abortion, stillbirth, or asymptomatic intrauterine infection.
D. Fetal abnormalities have not been associated with B19 viral infections during pregnancy.
E. Blood tests to determine diagnosis are generally used only for pregnant women and people who have blood disorders or who are immunocompromised.
F. About 50%–60% of adults have serologic evidence of past infection.
G. Avoid contact with people with hemolytic anemias.
H. In school-related outbreaks, a 25% attack rate is the norm.
I. Exacerbation of rash can be precipitated by exposure to heat or sun.
J. Rash may recur for weeks to months.

X. Complications

A. Generally none

XI. Follow-up

A. None required

XII. Referral

A. Children with hypoplastic anemias

NOTES

EXTERNAL OTITIS

An inflammation of the external auditory canal, commonly known as swimmer's ear, that is characterized by inflammation, pruritus, and pain

I. **Etiology**
   A. Bacterial: *Pseudomonas, Streptococcus, Pneumococcus*
   B. Fungal: *Candida, Aspergillus*
   C. Maceration, trauma, or excessive dryness of the lining of the ear canal causes it to be susceptible to superimposed infection.
   D. Excess cerumen
   E. Secondary to tympanic membrane perforation with purulent drainage

II. **Incidence**
   A. Most often seen in summer, particularly in areas where swimming in fresh water is popular
   B. Seen most often in adolescents who shampoo daily and where year-round swimming pools are available
   C. It is not unusual to find external otitis in an infant who has a bottle in bed because of milk dribbling into the ear canal, keeping it moist and providing a medium for bacterial growth.

III. **Subjective data**
   A. Pain in ear
   B. Pain on movement of earlobe or when ear is touched
   C. Pain when chewing
   D. Sensation of itching or moisture in ear canal
   E. Discharge from ear
   F. Pertinent subjective data to obtain
      1. Has child put anything in ear?
      2. Use of cotton swabs to clean ear canal
      3. History of swimming, particularly in fresh water
      4. Frequent showers or shampoos
      5. Use of hair spray
      6. History of otitis media with perforation
      7. Use of earplugs
      8. Previous history of otitis externa

IV. **Objective data**
   A. Pain on movement of pinna or application of pressure on tragus
   B. Exquisite tenderness of canal on insertion of speculum
   C. Canal edematous, erythematous, exudative; exudate may have foul odor.
   D. Tympanic membrane
      1. May not be clearly visualized because of edema and exudate in canal
      2. May be inflamed with a widespread external otitis
      3. May be perforated if otitis externa is secondary to otitis media
   E. Pinna may be inflamed and edematous.
   F. Adenopathy: Ipsilateral preauricular, postauricular, cervical

   G. Laboratory tests: Bacterial cultures using a calcium alginate nasopharynge͏
   swab to identify causative organism

V. Assessment

   A. Diagnosis confirmed by characteristic inflammation and edema of ear canal
   B. Differential diagnosis
   1. Otitis media with secondary otitis externa: History of acute otitis media with perforation
   2. Foreign body: By history and visualization of foreign body
   3. Abscess in ear canal: Mass visualized in canal
   4. Furunculosis: Discrete furuncle or pustule with surrounding erythema visualized in canal

VI. Plan

   A. External otitis involving only the ear canal
   1. Coly-Mycin S Otic or Cortisporin Otic: Four drops in affected ear tid or qid for 10 days
   2. Aspirin, acetaminophen, or codeine for pain
   3. *Note:* Do not order generic ear drops. They have been associated with increased complaints of pain on instillation, resulting in decreased compliance.
   B. External otitis with fever, tympanic membrane involvement, cellulitis of pinna, or tender postauricular adenopathy should be treated with systemic antibiotics as well.
   1. Ear drops as above. Order suspension if tympanic membrane is perforated or not visualized.
   2. Amoxicillin with clavulanic acid (Augmentin): 45 mg/kg/day divided every 12 hours
   3. If allergic to penicillin, clarithromycin (Biaxin): 15 mg/kg/day in two divided doses
   4. Aspirin, acetaminophen, or codeine for pain
   C. Recurrent external otitis
   1. Follow initial treatment plan above. After final recheck, use as prophylaxis during the swimming season Otic Domeboro Solution or Vosol Otic Solution: Five drops in each ear after swimming.
   2. In external otitis, the pH of the canal changes from acid to alkaline, creating a favorable environment for bacterial and mycotic overgrowth. Domeboro and Vosol are antibacterial and antifungal with an acid pH and are effective in preventing recurrences.

VII. Education

   A. Explain etiology to patient and parent.
   B. Medication
   1. Acute pain should subside within 24–48 hours of treatment.
   2. Call office if no apparent response to medication.
   3. Ear drops contain an antibiotic as well as cortisone to decrease inflammation.
   4. Side effects of ear drops may be a local stinging or burning sensation or a rash where drops have come in contact with the skin.
   5. For instillation of drops, patient should lie on his or her side with the

_ted ear up. Pull tip of auricle up and back, and then instill drops without allowing dropper to touch ear. Remain in this position for at least 5 minutes.

    6. With more extensive involvement and treatment with systemic antibiotics, medication should be taken for 10 full days even if patient seems better.

  C. Ear canal must be kept dry.

    1. No swimming

    2. No shampooing without protection; lamb's wool is water-repellent and can be used to occlude canal for shampoos.

    3. No showers

    4. Do not use cotton in ears; it will retain moisture.

    5. Do not use earplugs.

    6. Silly Putty may be used after the acute phase to keep canal dry while bathing or shampooing; it forms a malleable external plug.

    7. Do not use cotton swabs.

  D. Recurrences are not uncommon, especially in adolescents who swim, shower, or shampoo daily. Many of them also use cotton swabs to dry and clean their ears. Suggest instilling two or three drops of alcohol to dry ears after showering or swimming.

VIII. Follow-up

  A. Recheck in 48–72 hours if there is marked cellulitis and tympanic membrane is not visualized.

  B. Recheck immediately if suspected sensitivity to ear drops or child complains of increased pain.

  C. Recheck in 10 days. If not completely resolved, continue medication and precautions. Recheck again in 10 days.

IX. Complications

  A. Local reaction to ear drops (cutaneous reaction to neomycin)

  B. Recurrent external otitis

X. Consultation/Referral

  A. Symptoms worse after 24 hours of treatment

  B. No response to treatment in 48–72 hours

  C. External otitis not markedly improved at 10-day recheck requires culture and sensitivity.

  D. Foreign body in ear canal not readily removed

NOTES

NOTES

FEVER CONTROL

A common presenting symptom in pediatrics and a cardinal sign of illness. Most fevers in children are seen in conjunction with an acute infectious process. Fever control is secondary to identification and treatment of its underlying cause.

There is controversy over whether all fevers should be actively treated. Fever is actually a protective measure and in itself not harmful. Some experts contend that hyperpyrexia may be helpful in halting replication of a virus, and some studies have demonstrated that fever of a moderate degree can enhance immunologic response. High body temperatures, however, can diminish or reverse this effect, and a rapid increase in body temperature has been implicated as a triggering mechanism in febrile convulsions in susceptible children between 6 months and 5 years of age. Also, a child is generally more comfortable when fever is reduced. For these last three reasons, fevers of over 102°F (38.8°C) rectally should probably be treated once the etiology is established. Elevation of temperature does not correlate with the severity of its cause—for instance, a neonate with sepsis may be hypothermic.

I. **Subjective data**
   A. History of exposure
   B. Diseases prevalent in community
   C. Fever pattern
      1. Continuous
      2. Remittent
      3. Intermittent
      4. Recurrent
   D. How high has the temperature been?
   E. Duration of fever
   F. Determine accuracy of caregiver's method of assessing temperature.
   G. Does child seem sick?
   H. Change in level of sensorium
   I. Other associated symptoms
      1. Respiratory
      2. Gastrointestinal
      3. Genitourinary
      4. Musculoskeletal
      5. Central nervous system
   J. History of drug ingestion
   K. History of decreased liquid intake
   L. Treatment used and its effectiveness

II. **Objective data**
   A. Complete physical examination to determine infectious etiology; include weight.
   B. Activity level
   C. Level of sensorium

   D. State of hydration (see Appendix D, Clinical Signs of Dehydration)

   E. Toxicity

   F. Laboratory tests as indicated by history and physical findings

     1. Urinalysis and culture

     2. Throat culture

     3. Complete blood count

     4. Blood culture

     5. Spinal fluid examination

     6. Stool culture

III. Plan

   A. Assess caregiver's ability to take and interpret temperature correctly.

   B. Oral temperature for most children 5 years and older

     1. Place thermometer under tongue and leave it there for 4 minutes with lips closed.

     2. If child has had anything to eat or drink or has been chewing gum, wait 10 minutes before taking temperature.

   C. Rectal temperature: Lubricate rectal thermometer with K-Y Jelly or petroleum jelly and gently insert 2.5 cm into rectum. Leave in place 3–4 minutes.

   D. Axillary temperature: Place thermometer high in axilla and hold arm close to body; remove shirt so that skin surfaces are touching. Leave in place 4–5 minutes.

   E. Normal temperatures: Oral, 98.6°F; rectal, 99.4°F; axillary, 97.6°F (all ± 0.4–0.5°F)

   F. Fever peaks at about 6 p.m. and is at its lowest point at about 4 a.m.

   G. For each degree of fever:

     1. Pulse increases 10 beats/minute; may be higher in bacterial infections. Increased intracranial pressure, meningitis, and salmonellosis are associated with a decreased pulse rate.

     2. Respirations increase two cycles/minute. Increased intracranial pressure, pulmonary disease, and acid–base disturbance produce greater elevations.

   H. Hydration

     1. Encourage liquids to prevent dehydration; clear liquids are easiest to retain.

     2. Give small amounts frequently.

     3. Try tea, cola, ginger ale, popsicles, ice chips, Jell-O, ices, half- or full-strength juices.

   I. Sponging or bathing

     1. Every 2 hours if necessary for 30 minutes maximum.

     2. Use tepid water (water that feels comfortable to caregiver's wrist). Do not use alcohol or ice water. Chilling effect can cause shivering, which can increase body temperature. Rubbing with alcohol can cause toxicity through inhalation of fumes.

     3. Rub skin briskly with washcloth or towel to dry. Brisk rubbing increases skin capillary circulation and heat loss.

     4. Cold sponging is generally recommended only for heat illness (hyperthermia).

   J. Clothing

1. Clothe lightly to enhance heat loss through skin by radiation.
2. Avoid overdressing or covering with blankets, which will decrease radiation and cause further elevation of temperature.

K. Activity. Encourage rest; activity can increase body temperature.

L. Antipyretics for rectal temperatures over 102°F
   1. Use with caution: Can mask fever, will not cure disease.
   2. Do not use if child is dehydrated.
   3. Acetaminophen: 10–15 mg/kg every 4 hours; do not exceed 60 mg/kg/day. Give adequate dose for weight. Acetaminophen half-life is significantly prolonged in infants and newborns. Use at a reduced dosage and with caution.
   4. PediaProfen or Children's Advil Suspension (100 mg/5 ml)
      a. 5 mg/kg every 6–8 hours for fevers 102.5°F or less
      b. 10 mg/kg every 6–8 hours for fevers over 102.5°F
      c. Maximum daily dose: 40 mg/kg
      d. Do not use for infants under 6 months.

M. Thermometers
   1. Digital: Take about 30 seconds; as accurate as glass
   2. Glass: Record more slowly; more difficult to read
   3. Ear: Rapid (about 2 seconds); accurate

IV. **Follow-up**

A. Depends on degree of fever and etiology. With no established diagnosis, telephone contact should be maintained every 12–24 hours. Even if child does not seem sick, parents may be anxious without definitive diagnosis.

B. Child should be re-evaluated if fever continues beyond 24 hours, if signs of toxicity occur, or if signs or symptoms of infection occur.

V. **Consultation/Referral**

A. Fever persisting more than 5 days (fever of undetermined origin)

B. Acute high fever or prolonged high- or low-grade fever

C. Infant under 6 months of age

D. Stiff neck, petechiae, swollen or inflamed joints, or dehydration

E. Tachypnea out of proportion to temperature elevation

F. Fever associated with seizure

NOTES

NOTES

FROSTBITE

Cellular injury due to cold characterized by pallor and numbness of the affected area

I. **Etiology**
  A. Exposure to cold temperatures, usually for a prolonged period of time
  B. Severity of frostbite influenced by:
   1. Duration of exposure
   2. Intensity of cold exposure (determined both by temperature and wind chill factor)
   3. Rate and method of rewarming

II. **Incidence**
  A. Seen in winter, especially in young children who do not have proper supervision while playing in the snow, in skiers, and in winter sports enthusiasts (eg, mountain climbers, winter campers)
  B. Parts most subject to cold trauma are the hands, feet, and face, particularly the cheeks, nose, and ears.

III. **Subjective data**
  A. Often asymptomatic
  B. Numbness
  C. Prickling sensation
  D. Pruritus
  E. Stiffness
  F. Skin white and cold
  G. Complaints of pain in mild or moderate frostbite
  H. Pertinent subjective data to obtain to aid in assessing degree of frostbite
   1. Previous history of frostbite in same area
   2. Duration of exposure
   3. Cold intensity (temperature and wind velocity)
   4. If treated, method of rewarming

IV. **Objective data**
  A. Degree of frostbite cannot be accurately assessed before thawing.
  B. Mild
   1. Skin pale and cold
   2. Edema
   3. Area feels frozen on the surface, but gentle pressure reveals soft tissue underneath.
  C. Moderate to severe
   1. Skin pale and cold
   2. Edema
   3. Area feels solidly frozen on deep palpation.
   4. Blister and bulla formation 24–48 hours after thawing
   5. Necrosis of subcutaneous tissues 24–48 hours later

V. Assessment

    A. Diagnosis made by history of exposure and appearance of white, cold skin in affected area

        1. Mild: Erythema and edema of part after thawing; sometimes becomes purple. No significant tissue damage.

        2. Moderate to severe: After thawing, area becomes hyperemic, then blue, purple, or black and edematous. Blister and bulla formation occurs in 24–48 hours. With severe frostbite, lack of formation of blebs indicates inadequate circulation and necrosis of underlying tissue.

    B. Investigate possible parental neglect in young children with moderate to severe frostbite.

VI. Plan

    A. Do not attempt rewarming if there is danger of refreezing.

    B. Check body temperature to rule out hypothermia.

    C. Loosen constricting garments.

    D. Remove wet clothing in contact with skin.

    E. Do not rub or massage affected area.

    F. Rewarming. Warm gradually; rapid rewarming increases cell metabolism and without adequate blood supply (due to vasoconstriction) can damage cells.

        1. Immerse part in whirlpool or agitated water at 100°–105°F; monitor water temperature with thermometer.

        2. For face or ears, use warm, moist soaks, changing frequently to maintain temperature at 100°–105°F; monitor water temperature.

        3. Continue rewarming for about 20 minutes, until area is unfrozen.

        4. Use analgesics as necessary (aspirin, acetaminophen, or codeine); rewarming is painful.

        5. Elevate affected part.

    G. General measures

        1. Provide dry clothing.

        2. Adjust environmental temperature.

        3. Encourage warm liquids.

    H. Assess degree of involvement.

        1. Mild or first-degree of small area may be followed at home with a careful follow-up plan.

        2. Mild with extensive involvement or moderate to severe: Consult physician for treatment and admission to hospital.

    I. Sterile, loose dressing to necrotic areas

    J. Assess status of tetanus booster. Administer if necessary with tissue injury.

VII. Education

    A. Never rewarm with dry heat (eg, oven, fireplace).

    B. Do not rub frostbitten area; it will cause further tissue damage.

    C. Protect area from trauma; use padding when indicated.

    D. Avoid smoking, which causes peripheral vasoconstriction, decreasing blood flow to skin.

    E. Keep part elevated.

    F. Watch carefully for blistering or tissue damage.

G. Do not puncture blisters.

H. Do not expose part to extremes in temperature.

I. Paresthesia of injured area is common. Expect some burning, prickling, or tingling sensations.

J. Expect future hypersensitivity to cold and increased susceptibility to repeated frostbite of injured area.

K. Use face mask, earmuffs, mittens, or heavy boots as applicable for protection.

L. Prevention

   1. Avoid alcohol and cigarettes during cold exposure.

     a. Nicotine causes vasoconstriction, inhibiting flow of blood to periphery.

     b. Alcohol causes peripheral vasodilation, which increases rate of heat loss from skin.

   2. If suspicious of potential frostbite, warm by natural body heat (eg, place hands in groin or axilla). Do not use snow, ice, or dry heat.

   3. If frostbite has occurred, do not thaw until possibility of refreezing is eliminated.

   4. Wear several layers of loose, warm clothing. This protects better than one heavy, well-fitting garment.

   5. Do not scrub face, shave, or use aftershave lotion before anticipated exposure.

   6. Mittens generally offer more protection than gloves.

   7. Wet skin increases the cooling and freezing rate. Wet clothing causes conductive heat loss from the part covered.

   8. Use buddy system when out in severe cold; check each other's noses, faces, and ears for evidence of frostbite.

   9. If exposure planned, take extra socks and mittens.

VIII. Follow-up

A. Recheck by phone in 24 hours.

B. Return to office if blisters appear.

C. Return to office if signs of infection.

IX. Complications

A. Necrosis of affected area with subsequent infection

B. Area has increased susceptibility to frostbite.

X. Consultation/Referral

A. Moderate to severe frostbite: Appearance of blisters or bulla

B. Any question of parental neglect

NOTES

NOTES

HAND, FOOT, AND MOUTH DISEASE

A contagious viral disease characterized by fever and vesicular lesions of the mouth, palms of the hands, and soles of the feet

I. **Etiology**
   A. Coxsackie virus A, an enterovirus

II. **Incidence**
   A. Highly infectious disease generally occurring among children in epidemic form
   B. Seen mainly in summer
   C. Enteroviral infections with other manifestations may be prevalent in the community concurrently (herpangina, gastroenteritis).

III. **Incubation period**
   A. 3–6 days

IV. **Communicability**
   A. Highly communicable
   B. Spread by fecal–oral route and possibly by respiratory route
   C. Virus can maintain activity for days at room temperature.

V. **Subjective data**
   A. Abrupt onset of fever, around 101°F
   B. Sore throat, dysphagia
   C. Anorexia
   D. Occasionally headache and abdominal pain
   E. Rash on palms of hands and soles of feet may or may not be noted.
   F. Convulsions may occur with onset of fever.

VI. **Objective data**
   A. Elevated temperature
   B. Hyperemia of anterior tonsillar pillars
   C. Vesicles on an erythematous base on anterior tonsillar pillars; also on soft palate, tonsils, and uvula. Vesicles rapidly ulcerate, leaving shallow ulcers with red areolae.
   D. Maculopapular rash and vesicles on palms of hands and soles of feet, as well as interdigital surfaces

VII. **Assessment**
   A. Diagnosis: Classic case easily diagnosed by clinical picture
   B. Differential diagnosis
      1. Herpangina: Clinical picture similar, but no lesions on hands and feet
      2. Gingivostomatitis (herpes simplex): Gingival and buccal mucosa involved; no lesions on hands and feet

VIII. **Plan**
   A. Treatment is symptomatic.
   B. Warm saline mouth rinses
   C. Acetaminophen: 10–15 mg/kg every 4 hours, or PediaProfen for elevated temperature and discomfort
   D. Tepid baths for elevated temperature

   E. Force fluids.
   1. Cold, bland liquids
   2. Try popsicles, Jell-O, sherbet.

IX. Education
   A. Call back if child will not take fluids or is vomiting.
   B. Fever will last 1–4 days.
   C. Do not overdress; keep child cool.
   D. Be alert for dehydration (see Appendix D, Clinical Signs of Dehydration).
   E. Transmitted by direct contact with nose and throat secretions, stools, and blood of infected child, so keep child isolated until temperature is normal for 24 hours. Highly contagious, at least during acute phase.
   F. There is no prophylaxis.
   G. Carbonated drinks, citrus juices, hot, spicy foods, and the like should be avoided, as they may increase discomfort.
   H. Do not be concerned about dietary intake during acute stage, but do force fluids.
   I. Prognosis is excellent; disease is self-limited.
   J. Immunity to infecting strain is generally conferred after one attack.
   K. Lesions may persist for a week or more.

X. Follow-up
   A. Maintain daily telephone contact if temperature is markedly elevated.
   B. Generally no follow-up visit is necessary.

XI. Consultation/Referral
   A. Signs of dehydration
   B. Hand, foot, and mouth disease in an infant
   C. Prolonged course; no improvement in 5–6 days
   D. Febrile convulsions

NOTES

HERPANGINA

A communicable viral disease characterized by the abrupt onset of fever and vesicular eruptions of the anterior tonsillar pillars

I. **Etiology**
   A. Coxsackie virus A, an enterovirus
II. **Incidence**
   A. Highly infectious disease generally occurring among infants and children in epidemic form
   B. Seen mainly in summer
   C. Other types of Coxsackie viruses may be present in the community at the same time.
III. **Incubation period**
   A. 3–5 days
IV. **Subjective data**
   A. Abrupt onset of fever up to 105°F
   B. Dysphagia occurring within 24–36 hours
   C. Sore throat after temperature elevation
   D. Anorexia
   E. Occasionally headache, vomiting, abdominal pain
   F. Convulsions may occur with abrupt onset of fever.
V. **Objective data**
   A. Elevated temperature
   B. Hyperemia of anterior tonsillar pillars
   C. Grayish-white vesicles on an erythematous base on anterior tonsillar pillars; less frequently on soft palate, tonsils, uvula
   D. Vesicles ulcerate rapidly, leaving shallow ulcers.
   E. No involvement of gingival or buccal mucosa
   F. Mild cervical adenitis
VI. **Assessment**
   A. Diagnosis: Classic case easily diagnosed by the clinical picture
   B. Differential diagnosis
      1. Hand, foot, and mouth disease: Clinical picture similar, but small, grayish papulovesicular lesions on palms of hands and soles of feet
      2. Acute gingivostomatitis (herpes simplex): Gingival and buccal mucosa involved
VII. **Plan**
   A. Treatment is symptomatic.
   B. Warm saline mouth rinses
   C. For elevated temperature or discomfort: Acetaminophen 10–15 mg/kg every 4 hours or ibuprofen 5–10 mg/kg every 6–8 hours
   D. Chloraseptic gargle for children over 6 years of age only; may be used every 2 hours
   E. Tepid baths for elevated temperature

    F. Force fluids (cold, bland liquids); also try Popsicles, Jell-O, sherbet. Avoid carbonated beverages or acidic juices.

    G. Soft, bland diet—try yogurt, puddings.

VIII. Education

    A. Call back if child will not take fluids or is vomiting.

    B. Fever will last 1–4 days; systemic symptoms improve in 4–5 days and recovery is generally complete within a week.

    C. Tepid water for baths; air-dry or rub briskly with towel.

    D. Do not overdress; keep child cool.

    E. Be alert for dehydration (see Appendix D, Clinical Signs of Dehydration).

    F. Transmitted by direct contact with nose and throat secretions, stools, and blood of infected child; keep child isolated until temperature is normal for 24 hours.

    G. Highly contagious, at least during acute phase.

    H. There is no prophylaxis.

    I. Carbonated drinks, citrus juices, spicy foods, and the like should be avoided because they may increase discomfort.

    J. Do not be concerned about dietary intake during acute stage, but do force fluids.

    K. Prognosis is excellent—herpangina is self-limited.

    L. Immunity to infecting strain is generally conferred after one attack.

IX. Follow-up

    A. Maintain daily telephone contact during acute phase.

    B. Generally no follow-up visit is necessary.

X. Complications

    A. Febrile convulsions

    B. Dehydration

XI. Consultation/Referral

    A. Signs of dehydration

    B. Prolonged course (child not improved in 5 days)

    C. Febrile convulsions

NOTES

NOTES

HERPES SIMPLEX TYPE 1

A recurrent viral infection characterized by multiple small, grouped vesicles on an erythematous base on the skin or mucous membranes

I. **Etiology**

　　A. Herpes simplex virus type 1 (HSV-1) in its recurrent form

　　B. The primary herpes simplex infection is often seen in children as acute herpetic gingivostomatitis (see Herpetic Gingivostomatitis).

　　C. The virus remains latent in the sensory ganglia and can be activated by a number of triggering factors or excitants throughout life. Emotional stress, exposure to sun, drugs, menses, trauma, febrile illness, and systemic infections have been identified as factors responsible for activating the virus.

　　D. HSV-1 also causes 5%–15% of initial episodes of genital herpes.

II. **Incidence**

　　A. Seen in all age groups; affects about 7% of the population

　　B. Incidence of herpes simplex lesions is related to susceptibility and exposure to triggering factors.

III. **Incubation period**

　　A. 2–12 days

IV. **Communicability**

　　A. At least as long as lesion is present

　　B. Recurrent herpes lesions shed virus for about 5 days after appearance of lesion. Asymptomatic shedding can occur, also.

V. **Subjective data**

　　A. Burning or tingling sensation several hours before appearance of lesion

　　B. "Cold sore" on lip or anywhere on body

　　C. Generally no systemic symptoms unless fever or infection is the triggering factor

　　D. Often a past history of herpetic gingivostomatitis

　　E. Often a history of a similar lesion after exposure to same triggering factor

　　F. Pertinent subjective data: Symptoms of ocular involvement, such as photophobia, pain (herpetic keratitis), or inflammation of the eyelid (herpes simplex blepharitis)

VI. **Objective data**

　　A. Lesion progresses through the following stages and may be seen at any stage.

　　　　1. Collection of small transparent vesicles on an erythematous base

　　　　2. Vesicles become cloudy and purulent.

　　　　3. Vesicles dry and become crusted; may crack and bleed. Base is edematous and erythematous.

　　B. Lesion is generally found at the mucocutaneous junction of the lips or nose but may be found anywhere on the body; occurs consistently at the same site with recurrent infections.

　　C. Herpetic whitlow (infection of the finger) may be found on finger or thumb of child, particularly one who sucks a finger or thumb.

　　D. Regional, tender lymphadenopathy often present

    E. Inspect entire body.

VII. Assessment

    A. Diagnosis is usually made by characteristic appearance of lesion (grouped vesicles) and history of similar lesion or herpetic gingivostomatitis.

    B. Differential diagnosis

        1. Impetigo: Lesions often similar; presence of yellow or honey-colored crust on lesion indicates bacterial superinfection.

        2. Traumatic lesion

VIII. Plan

One of the following may be tried. There is no documentation that these treatments are of value in decreasing healing time, but they may give symptomatic relief.

    A. Idoxuridine ointment (Herplex): Apply to lesion hourly for 1 day, then four times a day until lesion is healed.

    B. Blistex or petroleum jelly: Apply to lesion as often as desired to soothe and protect from cracking.

    C. Bacitracin or Neosporin ointment: Apply to lesion four times a day to prevent or treat bacterial superinfection.

    D. Acyclovir (Zovirax) ointment is not generally indicated for the treatment of simple, uncomplicated HSV infection in nonimmunocompromised host. It may help select out resistant strains. It can, however, be prescribed to treat large or unsightly lesions or to speed the healing process in certain circumstances (eg, a bride, a health care worker).

        1. Use as soon as lesion appears.

        2. Apply, using finger cot or rubber glove, three to six times a day for 7 days.

    E. Domeboro soaks (Burow's solution)

        1. One packet per pint of cool water

        2. Apply as wet compress for 20 minutes, three times a day.

IX. Education

    A. Latent virus in sensory ganglia can be activated by stress, sun exposure, drugs, menses, trauma, fever, or infection.

    B. Incubation period 2–12 days

    C. Recurrences are common and usually occur at the same site.

        1. Recurrent lesions are less painful than the original herpetic gingivostomatitis.

        2. Recurrent lesions are preceded by a burning or tingling sensation, which may last several hours.

    D. Lesions may be spread by autoinoculation. In a young child, concurrent lesions may be found on fingers or thumb (particularly if child sucks a finger or thumb). Lesions may also be spread to labia via autoinoculation.

    E. Lesion does not leave a scar but may cause temporary depigmentation.

    F. Lesion is self-limited, lasting 8–14 days.

    G. Transmitted through direct contact with saliva

    H. Communicable at least as long as lesion is present

    I. Do not allow child near newborns, children with eczema or burns, or persons on immunosuppressive therapy.

J. Prevention: There is no cure for recurrent herpes simplex, but many methods have been attempted to prevent or abort lesions. The most effective method is to avoid known triggering factors if possible.

1. For lesions activated by sun exposure, liberal use of sunscreen has been effective for some persons.
2. Applying ice may help abort the lesion if used as soon as tingling or burning sensation is felt.
3. Fluorinated corticosteroid creams used at the onset of tingling have been considered useful in diminishing the severity of the lesion by decreasing the inflammatory response. Such creams are contraindicated for use on the face, as they may cause telangiectasia.
4. Acyclovir ointment is not indicated for the prevention of recurrent HSV.

X. Complications

A. Secondary bacterial infection

B. Eczema herpeticum in a child with atopic dermatitis: Characterized by irritability, high temperature (104°F), and generalized lesions (crops of vesicles at site of eczematous skin lesions)

C. Erythema multiforme may occur 3–4 days after a recurrence.

D. Herpetic paronychia: From autoinoculation or in caretaker

XI. Consultation/Referral

A. Neonate or infant

B. Suspicion of herpetic keratitis or herpes simplex blepharitis (photophobia, pain)

C. Child with atopic dermatitis

D. Newborn or child with atopic dermatitis, burns, or immunocompromise who is exposed to HSV

NOTES

HERPES SIMPLEX TYPE 2

One of the most common sexually transmitted diseases; characterized by painful vesicular lesions of the genitals; represents an acute infection or reactivation of latent herpes

I. **Etiology**
   A. Herpesvirus hominis type 2 (HSV-2); occasionally type 1 (HSV-1), especially in primary infections
   B. 75% of HSV-1 infections involve the face and skin above the waist; 75% of HSV-2 infections involve the genitalia and skin below the waist. However, either can be found at either site.
   C. HSV-2 persists in a latent form after infection. Reactivation occurs in about 80% of cases with variable frequency. Recurrence rate generally decreases after the first year.

II. **Incidence**
   A. Primarily seen beyond the age of puberty
   B. One of the most common sexually transmitted diseases

III. **Incubation**
   A. 3–12 days after exposure. Maximum may be several weeks; minimum is 32 hours.
   B. Recurrent herpes: 24 hours after precipitating cause

IV. **Communicability**
   A. Primary infection: 15–42 days
   B. Recurrent infection: 6 days
   C. Virus is present in lesions during the prodromal period and is highly contagious during prodrome. Asymptomatic shedding is a major epidemiologic problem.

V. **Subjective data**
   A. Primary infection
      1. Tenderness of genital area before appearance of lesions
      2. Lesions on vulva or penis
      3. Severe pain in genital area
      4. Swollen glands
      5. Fever may be present, with associated symptoms of headache, malaise, myalgia.
      6. Discharge from lesions of vulva or penis
      7. Inability to void, or burning and stinging on urination
      8. May have lesions or sores at other sites
   B. Recurrent infection
      1. Burning or tingling sensation for several hours before appearance of lesions
      2. Lesions are less painful than in primary infection; may be pruritic.
      3. Urethral or vaginal discharge
      4. Lesions are fewer in number than in primary infection and are generally external.

VI. **Objective data**

  A. Primary herpes

    1. Edema, erythema, and exquisite tenderness of vulva or penis. Uncircumcised males may present with more severe involvement.

    2. Multiple discrete or grouped vesicular lesions with subsequent erosion in 1–3 days, producing gray-white ulcerations

    3. Lesions are found on the labia, vagina, or cervix in females and the external genitalia in males.

    4. Lesions may occur at other sites from autoinoculation (buttocks, thighs, fingers, pharynx, conjunctiva).

    5. Discharge from vagina or penis

    6. Tender inguinal adenopathy

    7. Bladder may be distended.

  B. Recurrent herpes

    1. Discrete or clustered vesicles on an erythematous base; lesions are generally external.

    2. Mucoid discharge if cervical, vaginal, or urethral involvement

    3. Inguinal adenopathy not a significant finding

VII. **Assessment**

  A. Diagnosis is generally made from the history and typical appearance of the lesions. There may be a history of exposure. If diagnosis is in doubt, a culture of the vesicle fluid may be done.

  B. Differential diagnosis

    1. Traumatic lesions

    2. Scabies

    3. Chancroid

VIII. **Plan**

  A. There is no prophylaxis or cure for HSV-2; treatment is aimed at pain control.

  B. Topical: 5% acyclovir ointment (Zovirax) six times a day for 1 week. Begin therapy within 6 days of onset.

  C. Sitz baths

  D. Dry heat (hair dryer)

  E. With urinary retention, females may void with less pain in the tub. Catheterization may be necessary.

  F. Topical anesthetics: Benzocaine aerosol (use as needed) or lidocaine jelly (2%, four times daily)

  G. Betadine 1%, three or four times a day; apply with cotton balls.

  H. Acyclovir (Zovirax) capsules: To treat severe primary herpes or to shorten duration of recurrent episodes

    1. Primary herpes: 200-mg capsule five times a day (every 4 hours) for 10 days

    2. Recurrent herpes: 200-mg capsule five times a day (every 4 hours) for 5 days. Initiate therapy at first sign of recurrence.

    3. Chronic suppressive therapy for recurrent herpes: 400-mg capsule twice a day for up to 12 months

    4. Dosages are for children over 40 kg.

    I. Treatment should include evaluation for other sexually transmitted diseases.

IX. **Education**

    A. Avoid indiscriminate sexual practices.

    B. Avoid sexual contact with person with active lesions. Genital ulcers are of particular concern because they provide a portal of entry for HIV.

    C. Virus is shed during prodrome and can also be shed when entirely asymptomatic.

    D. There is no prevention (other than safe sex) or cure for HSV-2.

    E. Acyclovir ointment speeds healing and in some cases helps decrease the duration of viral shedding and duration of pain. It does not prevent transmission of the virus or prevent recurrences.

    F. Oral acyclovir shortens the viral shedding time. In some patients, it decreases the duration of pain and new lesion formation. With frequent recurrences (six or more episodes a year), administration of acyclovir may prevent or reduce the severity or frequency of recurrences.

    G. Side effects from acyclovir are generally mild and include nausea, diarrhea, headache, and rash.

    H. Although benzocaine aerosol may be used frequently for comfort, caution patient that it may be a skin sensitizer.

    I. Stress hygiene, particularly careful hand washing, to avoid spread of virus.

    J. Use finger cot or rubber glove to apply ointment to avoid autoinoculation of other areas or transmission to other people.

    K. Primary attack lasts 2–6 weeks.

    L. HSV-2 persists in a latent form after infection. Reactivation occurs in about 80% of cases with variable frequency.

    M. Recurrent attack lasts a few hours to 10 days.

    N. Recurrent attacks are less frequent as patient becomes older.

    O. Advise patient that recurrent episodes are heralded by burning or tingling sensation before eruption of lesions. Virus can be transmitted during this time; avoid intercourse.

    P. If HSV-1 caused the initial attack, recurrences are unlikely to occur in genital area.

    Q. Pap smear should be done yearly because of increased incidence of dysplasia and carcinoma of cervix.

X. **Complications**

    A. Secondary infection

    B. Urinary retention

XI. **Follow-up**

    A. Call immediately if unable to void.

    B. Return if possible secondary infection.

    C. Annual Pap smears

XII. **Referral**

    A. Pregnancy

    B. Urinary retention

NOTES

| HERPES ZOSTER

An acute viral infection affecting the dorsal root ganglion cells. It is self-limited and localized and is characterized by a vesicular eruption and neurologic pain.

I. **Etiology**

  A. Varicella zoster virus (VZV): After an attack of chickenpox, the virus remains latent in the dorsal root ganglia. Varicella is the manifestation of the VZV in a nonimmune host, and herpes zoster is the recrudescence of the latent virus in a partially immune host.

  B. Susceptible children who are exposed to cases of zoster often develop chickenpox.

II. **Incidence**

  A. Relatively rare in children under 10 years of age but can occur at any age

  B. Increased incidence in patients with malignancies or on immunosuppressive therapy

III. **Incubation period**

  A. 2–3 weeks

IV. **Subjective data**

  A. Usual history of varicella

  B. History of itching, tenderness, or pain in area about 3–5 days before rash. Prodromal pain can be severe and can mimic cardiac or pleural disease, acute abdomen, or vertebral disease.

  C. Rash: Erythematous maculopapular rash that progresses to vesicles within 24 hours; generally on trunk, face, or back

V. **Objective data**

  A. Rash: Small, grouped vesicles on an erythematous base

  B. Distribution

   1. Appears first at a point near the central nervous system along a dermatome or two adjacent dermatomes

   2. Ends at midline of body

   3. Generally on trunk (over 50%), trigeminal (10%–20%), lumbosacral and cervical (10%–20%)

   4. Generally unilateral; bilateral involvement rare

   5. A few vesicles may be outside the dermatome.

  C. Successive crops of lesions may appear.

  D. Pain with rash is less frequent in children than in adults.

  E. Occasionally a generalized rash occurs.

  F. Regional lymphadenopathy

  G. Sometimes a blistered burn from hot soaks used to relieve pain

VI. **Assessment**

  A. Diagnosis is made by the distribution and characteristic appearance of the rash, as well as by the associated pain. It may be confirmed by cytologic smear of vesicle.

  B. Differential diagnosis

    1. Coxsackie viruses: Distribution of rash differs; lesions do not crust and are not painful.

    2. Multiple insect bites: Generally do not follow path of dermatome or have the characteristic appearance (small group of vesicles), or have herpetic pain

VII. Plan

    A. Treatment is symptomatic.

    B. Calamine lotion

    C. Cool compresses with Burow's solution (one packet dissolved in one quart of cool water, three times a day)

    D. Acetaminophen, 10–15 mg/kg every 4 hours for pain; children do not always have sensory changes, so analgesics may not be indicated.

    E. Infected lesions: Neosporin or bacitracin ointment three times a day

    F. Acyclovir (Zovirax) capsules: 800 mg five times daily for 7–10 days for children over 40 kg

VIII. Education

    A. Successive lesions appear for up to 1 week.

    B. Eruption usually clears in 14–21 days; if vesicles appear over a period of 1 week, clearing may take up to 5 weeks.

    C. Lesions become pustular and dry and crust over.

    D. Transmitted by both direct and indirect contact. About 15% of susceptible (nonimmune) persons will contract varicella.

    E. Avoid exposure of children with malignancies or persons on immunosuppressive therapy.

    F. Postherpetic neuralgia may persist once lesions have healed.

    G. There is no prevention for herpes zoster.

    H. Compresses: Use cool soft cloths four times a day.

    I. Acyclovir reduces viral shedding time and the duration of new lesion formation. It also shortens the time to complete lesion scabbing, healing, and cessation of pain.

IX. Follow-up

    A. Generally not indicated for typical case

    B. Return immediately if any symptoms of ocular involvement.

    C. Recheck in 5 days if there is secondary bacterial infection.

X. Complications

    A. Secondary bacterial infection

    B. Rarely, ocular complications

XI. Consultation/Referral

    A. Lesions on tip of nose (possibility of keratoconjunctivitis)

    B. Hemorrhagic or bullous lesions

    C. Disseminated herpes zoster

    D. Patients on immunosuppressive therapy

NOTES

NOTES

HERPETIC GINGIVOSTOMATITIS

An acute primary herpes simplex infection characterized by painful vesicular lesions and ulcers of the oral mucosa

I. **Etiology**
    A. Herpes simplex virus (type 1) in its primary form
II. **Incidence**
    A. Gingivostomatitis is the most frequent manifestation of the primary form of herpes simplex.
    B. It is the most common cause of stomatitis in children under 5 years of age, with the highest incidence occurring between ages 2 to 4 years.
III. **Incubation period**
    A. 2–12 days (mean 6–7 days)
IV. **Communicability**
    A. Highly infectious throughout course of illness, which takes 4–5 days to evolve and at least an additional 7 days to resolve
    B. Transmitted by saliva and by contact with infected skin or mucous membranes
    C. May also be contracted through contact with an asymptomatic carrier
V. **Subjective data**
    A. History of exposure to a child or adult with cold sores or stomatitis
    B. Fever (104°–105°F)
    C. Irritability
    D. Malaise
    E. Sore throat and mouth
    F. Gums red and swollen
    G. Painful sores in mouth
    H. Drooling
    I. Foul odor to breath
    J. Not eating; taking liquids poorly
VI. **Objective data**
    A. Fever
    B. Vesicular lesions
        1. On or around lips, along gingiva, on anterior tongue, and on hard palate. May be seen over entire buccal mucosa.
        2. On chin and face
        3. Vesicles rupture, leaving a grayish ulceration on an erythematous base, and may coalesce to form large lesions or ulcers.
    C. Gingival edema, erythema, bleeding
    D. Enlarged, tender cervical and submandibular glands
    E. Increased salivation
    F. Foul odor to breath
    G. Occasional vesicular lesion on a sucked thumb or finger
    H. Rarely occurs as a generalized vesicular eruption

   I. May rarely have herpetic vulvovaginitis from handling genital area with contaminated hands

VII. Assessment

   A. Diagnosis is usually made by clinical findings.

   B. Differential diagnosis

   1. Herpangina: No lesions on buccal mucosa; posterior pharyngeal lesions only

   2. Hand, foot, and mouth disease: Oral lesions not on buccal and gingival mucosa; rash present on hands and feet

   3. Varicella: If the rare type of gingivostomatitis with generalized vesicular reaction

VIII. Plan

   A. For fever or pain, acetaminophen, 10–15 mg/kg every 4 hours, or ibuprofen, 5–10 mg/kg every 6 hours

   B. For discomfort, Gly-Oxide Liquid to clean lesions four times a day (after meals and at bedtime); or Viscous Xylocaine, 1 tbsp (15 ml or 300 mg) swished around mouth every 4 hours; or Chloraseptic Mouthwash (for children over 6 years of age) every 2 hours as needed

   C. Force fluids (cold, bland liquids).

   D. Tepid baths every 2 hours as needed

IX. Education

   A. Alert parent to signs of dehydration: Decreased urine output, elevated temperature, decreased tears, dry mucous membranes, increased thirst, lethargy (see Appendix D, Clinical Signs of Dehydration).

   B. Give cold liquids or semisolids.

   1. Try Popsicles, sherbet, ice cream, Jell-O.

   2. Maintain hydration with frequent sips.

   3. Use straw to minimize contact with lips and gums.

   C. Do not give carbonated beverages or citrus juices.

   D. Do not be concerned about solid food intake during acute phase.

   E. Do not allow child to swallow Chloraseptic Mouthwash or Viscous Xylocaine.

   F. Gly-Oxide: Place 10 drops on tongue and swish around mouth; do not swallow or rinse.

   G. Use tepid water for baths; air-dry or rub briskly to increase skin capillary circulation and heat loss.

   H. Dress child lightly.

   I. Duration of illness: 1–3 weeks

   1. Duration of acute phase: 4–9 days

   2. Ulcers heal spontaneously in 7–14 days.

   J. After primary infection, HSV remains latent in sensory neural ganglia innervating sites originally involved. Therefore, recurrences occur in identical regions but are less severe than primary infections.

   K. Recurrent infection appears as a cold sore or fever blister on the mucocutaneous junction.

   L. In adolescents, exudative pharyngitis with typical herpetic lesions on the tonsils may be caused by the HSV-2 virus due to oral–genital sex.

M. *Note:* Highly communicable throughout illness. Do not expose to newborns, children with eczema, children on immunosuppressive therapy, or children with burns.

X. Follow-up

A. Recheck in 2 days by telephone.

B. Call immediately if liquid intake decreases or signs of dehydration or secondary bacterial infection appear.

C. Call immediately if complaints of eye problems.

XI. Complications

A. Dehydration

B. Keratitis

C. Conjunctivitis

XII. Consultation/Referral

A. Newborns and infants

B. Dehydration in child of any age

C. Generalized skin eruption

D. Signs or symptoms of ocular involvement (photophobia, pain, inflammation, or ulceration of cornea)

NOTES

HORDEOLUM (STYE)

Localized infection of a sebaceous gland of the eyelash follicle

I. **Etiology**
   A. Causative organism usually *Staphylococcus aureus*
II. **Incidence**
   A. Occurs frequently in children
III. **Subjective data**
   A. Localized swelling, tenderness, and inflammation of margin of eyelid
   B. Child may complain of a bump or pimple on eyelid.
   C. Generally unilateral
   D. Visual acuity not affected
IV. **Objective data**
   A. Localized erythema, edema, and pain near lid edge
   B. Abscess may point at lid margin.
   C. May be purulent drainage along lid margin
   D. Recurrent lesions may be associated with blepharitis of seborrheic dermatitis.
V. **Assessment**
   A. Diagnosis is made by clinical picture of erythema, pain, and swelling.
   B. Differential diagnosis
      1. Chalazion: A chronic granulomatous infection of the meibomian gland that is relatively painless.
      2. Conjunctivitis: Conjunctival erythema, mucopurulent discharge, foreign body sensation; no localized swelling
      3. Blepharitis: Chronic scaling and discharge with matting of the eyelashes; not localized
VI. **Plan**
   A. Hot, moist compresses for 15–20 minutes every 2–3 hours
   B. Thoroughly cleanse eyelashes with Johnson's Baby Shampoo or CIBA Eye Scrub.
   C. 10% Sodium Sulamyd Ophthalmic Ointment (sodium sulfacetamide) four or five times daily during acute stage
   D. Assess visual acuity. With a refraction error, child may rub eyes repeatedly.
VII. **Education**
   A. For moist compresses, use a soft cloth and water as warm as child can tolerate.
   B. Medication
      1. To instill ophthalmic ointment, gently pull down lower lid and apply a thin ribbon of ointment.
      2. Side effects to ointment are rare, but call back immediately if child complains of burning or stinging.
      3. Vision may be blurred temporarily after administration of ointment.
   C. Use thorough hand-washing technique after soaks and instillation of medication to prevent spread.
   D. Keep fingers away from eyes.

   E. Never squeeze a stye.
   F. Inflammation generally subsides after 5–6 days.
   G. Continue treatment for several days after resolution of lesions.
VIII. Follow-up
   A. Return immediately if symptoms worsen.
   B. Return in 48 hours if no response to treatment.
   C. Return if lesion becomes larger and points.
   D. Return in 6 days if lesion has not resolved.
   E. Return for evaluation if problem is recurrent.
IX. Complications
   A. Conjunctivitis
   B. Cellulitis
X. Consultation/Referral
   A. Well-localized lesion: To assess need for incision and drainage
   B. No response to treatment after 48 hours
   C. Lesion not resolved after 6 days
   D. Recurrent styes may indicate immunologic deficit or systemic disease (eg, diabetes).
   E. Cellulitis may require systemic antibiotics.

NOTES

IMPETIGO

Purulent infection of the skin characterized by honey-colored, crusted lesions or bullae surrounded by narrow margin of erythema.

I. **Etiology**
   A. Most common causative organism: *Staphylococcus aureus*
   B. Earlier research suggested that most crusted impetigo was streptococcal in origin, but it now appears that most crusted as well as bullous impetigo is caused by *S aureus*.
   C. Streptococcal impetigo is always crusted; bullous impetigo is virtually never streptococcal.
   D. Secondary impetigo (superimposed on a preexisting condition such as atopic dermatitis) is nearly always staphylococcal.

II. **Incidence**
   A. Primary bacterial skin infection in children seen in all age groups
   B. Predisposing factors include poor hygiene and antecedent lesions such as chickenpox, scabies, insect bites, or trauma.

III. **Incubation period**
   A. 1–3 days

IV. **Communicability**
   A. Less than 48 hours once therapy is initiated; weeks to months if untreated

V. **Subjective data**
   A. Sores
      1. Occur mainly on the head (particularly around nares and mouth) and extremities, but may occur anywhere on body
      2. Begin as macules, which develop into vesicles and then become pustular
   B. Pruritus, which may spread the infection.
   C. Often a history of minor trauma (eg, insect bites, scratches, scabies, or herpes simplex) providing entry to the organism
   D. History of exposure to impetigo

VI. **Objective data**
   A. Nonbullous
      1. Lesion appears as clear vesicle on an erythematous base and rapidly becomes pustular. Pustule ruptures, enlarges, and spreads. The characteristic honey-colored adherent crust is formed. Satellite lesions are common.
      2. Inspect entire body, as lesions may be multiple.
      3. Check for regional adenopathy.
   B. Bullous
      1. Lesions are rapidly formed and consist of fragile bullae filled with clear fluid, which progresses to cloudy fluid before rupture. These bullae heal centrally, leaving a crusted arcuate or annular formation. Recently ruptured bullae have an erythematous, shiny base; older lesions are dry and not erythematous.
      2. Inspect entire body.
      3. Check for regional adenopathy.

VII. Assessment

    A. Diagnosis

        1. Usually made by clinical picture of oozing vesicles and honey-colored adherent crusts

        2. Routine culturing of lesions not indicated but recommended if lesions are extensive or severe

    B. Differential diagnosis (all of the following may become secondarily impetiginized)

        1. Herpes simplex

        2. Contact dermatitis

        3. Eczema

        4. Seborrhea

        5. Fungal infection

VIII. Plan

    A. Local treatment may be adequate when only one or two lesions are present.

        1. Remove crusts by gentle washing with warm water and an antiseptic soap or cleaner such as Betadine.

        2. Mupirocin (Bactroban) ointment (prescription required): Apply three times a day.

        3. Follow up with a telephone check in 24 hours. If other lesions have appeared or clearing has not begun, institute systemic treatment.

    B. Systemic treatment is needed for multiple lesions, widely separated lesions (eg, one on the face and one on the buttocks), or lesions that are not showing rapid response to local therapy.

        1. Dicloxacillin, 12.5–25 mg/kg/day in four divided doses, or

        2. Erythromycin, 30–50 mg/kg/day in four divided doses

IX. Education

    A. Continue medication for 10 full days; do not stop because lesions have cleared.

    B. Spread occurs cutaneously as well as systemically.

    C. Bullous impetigo is more likely to spread.

    D. Incubation period is 1–3 days.

    E. Not communicable after 48 hours on antibiotic therapy

    F. Use separate towel, washcloth, etc. to prevent spread.

    G. Wash linen and clothing in hot water.

    H. Keep fingernails short to minimize spread caused by scratching.

    I. Check contacts and other family members.

    J. Child should not return to school until lesions are clear or child has been on antibiotics for 48 hours.

    K. Transmitted by direct and sometimes indirect contact

X. Follow-up

    A. Call office if no improvement is noted within 24 hours after treatment has been started.

    B. Call immediately if dark-colored urine, decreased urinary output, or edema is noted.

    C. Return in 3 days if not markedly improved.

XI. Complications

    A. Acute glomerulonephritis, the most important complication, occurs with nephritogenic strains of streptococci. There is no conclusive evidence that early, vigorous treatment will prevent glomerulonephritis.

XII. Consultation/Referral

    A. Signs or symptoms of acute glomerulonephritis

    B. No response to treatment after 4–5 days

    C. Bullous impetigo in newborn or infant

NOTES

INFECTIOUS MONONUCLEOSIS

An acute, self-limited viral infection characterized by fever, malaise, sore throat, generalized lymphadenopathy, splenomegaly, and increased numbers of atypical lymphocytes and monocytes in the peripheral blood

I. **Etiology**

    A. Epstein-Barr virus (EBV), a herpesvirus. Infectious mononucleosis is an initial or primary EBV infection. EBV produces other clinical disorders as well.

II. **Incubation period**

    A. 2–7 weeks

III. **Communicability**

    A. Low to moderate contagion

    B. Transmitted by close contact, especially by oropharyngeal secretions

    C. Because it is spread by the oropharyngeal route, kissing may well be the chief mode of spread in adolescents and young adults.

    D. Viral shedding via saliva occurs in 90% of patients in the first week of illness and continues for many months.

    E. Period of communicability is unknown because 10%–20% of healthy, seropositive persons shed virus intermittently.

IV. **Incidence**

    A. Can occur at any age but is most commonly diagnosed in adolescents and young adults (15–22 years of age)

    B. Equal incidence in males and females

    C. Peak incidence in females 16 years, in males 18 years

V. **Immunity**

    A. One attack is considered to confer immunity, although after the initial EBV infection, the virus regularly produces infection of the B lymphocytes for life.

VI. **Subjective data**

    A. Gradual onset of

        1. Malaise

        2. Fever

        3. Headache

        4. Sore throat

        5. Swollen glands

        6. Abdominal pain

        7. Anorexia, nausea, vomiting

        8. Excessive fatigue

        9. Jaundice (rare)

VII. **Objective data**

    A. Early in disease (first few days)

        1. Tonsils enlarged and erythematous; small areas of patchy gray exudate

        2. Pharynx inflamed

        3. Petechiae at junction of hard and soft palate (seen at the middle to end of first week of illness)

   4. Bilateral posterior cervical adenopathy, nontender
   5. Fever (101°–103°F)
   6. Periorbital edema
B. After 3–5 days of presenting complaints, the following may be found in addition to the above.
   1. Tonsillar exudate becomes more extensive, with large patches.
   2. Pharyngeal edema
   3. Tender anterior and posterior cervical adenopathy
   4. Axillary and inguinal adenopathy
   5. Erythematous maculopapular rash
   6. Jaundice
   7. Splenomegaly (in about 75% of patients)
   8. Hepatomegaly (in about 50% of patients)
C. Laboratory tests
   1. White blood cell count generally 10,000–20,000/mm³
   2. Lymphocytes over 50%, with numerous atypical lymphocytes and monocytes
   3. Monospot test: Positive after 7–10 days of illness
   4. Heterophil antibody test: Titer of 1:112 significant, 1:160 diagnostic (may be negative for first 7–10 days of illness and in young children). Heterophil titers are highest during first 4 weeks; anti-EBV reach peak titers within 2–4 weeks and persist probably through life.
   5. Throat culture to rule out streptococcal pharyngitis, seen concurrently in about 20% of children with infectious mononucleosis

VIII. **Assessment**
A. Diagnosis is made by the history, clinical findings, and positive laboratory results.
B. Differential diagnosis
   1. Streptococcal pharyngitis: Positive throat culture; may occur concurrently
   2. Blood dyscrasias, especially leukemia: Pancytopenia and blast cells present
   3. Measles: Preceded by a 3–4-day prodrome of cough, coryza, and conjunctivitis; pathognomonic Koplik's spots present; negative immunization history
   4. Viral exanthems: Clinical course differs; extensive lymphadenopathy rare
   5. Viral hepatitis: Clinical picture similar, but fewer atypical lymphocytes and lacks positive heterophil; liver function tests abnormal

IX. **Plan**
A. Symptomatic
   1. Rest, according to degree of illness, until afebrile
   2. Liquids
   3. Acetaminophen or ibuprofen for elevated temperature or discomfort
   4. Warm saline gargles
   5. No contact sports
B. Treat concurrent streptococcal pharyngitis with penicillin or erythromycin (see protocol, p. 404). Do not use amoxicillin: it causes an allergic-type rash in about 80% of patients treated.

C. Corticosteroids do not generally affect the course of the disease but are indicated if upper respiratory obstruction by enlarged, infected tonsils is impending or if pharyngitis is so severe that child is not taking liquids.

   1. Prednisone dosage

      a. Adolescent: 20 mg three times daily for 5 days

      b. Child: 1–2 mg/kg three times daily for 5 days

D. *Note:* Acyclovir has not been proven to modify the clinical course of uncomplicated infectious mononucleosis although it has good in vitro activity against EBV.

X. Education

A. Infection is self-limited.

B. Treatment is symptomatic.

C. Isolation is unnecessary.

D. Throat may be very sore.

E. Gargle: 1 tsp salt in a glass of warm water, as often as necessary

F. Encourage fluids.

   1. Avoid orange juice or carbonated beverages if sore throat is a problem.

   2. Use cool, bland liquids.

G. Rest

   1. Encourage bed rest when febrile.

   2. Encourage frequent rest periods.

H. Patient may feel an overwhelming fatigue, which may persist for 6 weeks.

I. Strenuous activity and contact sports should be avoided while splenomegaly persists.

J. Avoid alcoholic beverages because of the possibility of liver involvement.

K. Encourage a well-balanced diet as soon as anorexia subsides.

L. Acute phase lasts 1–2 weeks; fatigue generally resolves in 2–4 weeks.

M. Complete recovery may take 3–6 weeks.

N. Call office if rash or jaundice appears.

O. Patient should not donate blood.

XI. Follow-up

A. Diagnosis may not be confirmed on the first visit, even with a high index of suspicion; therefore, patient may need to be seen in 24–48 hours for confirmation of the diagnosis or reevaluation.

B. Monospot or heterophil antibody test becomes positive 1 week after onset of illness.

C. Recheck weekly until patient is completely recovered and splenomegaly no longer persists.

D. More frequent telephone contacts may be necessary during acute phase, particularly if throat is so sore that drinking is a problem.

XII. Complications

A. Splenic rupture

B. Neurologic

   1. Guillain-Barré syndrome

   2. Aseptic meningitis

XIII. **Consultation/Referral**
  A. Marked toxicity, splenomegaly, or respiratory compromise (may require prednisone)
  B. Markedly enlarged tonsils and difficulty swallowing (may require prednisone)
  C. Jaundice

NOTES

INTERTRIGO

An inflammatory dermatosis occurring where two moist skin surfaces are in opposition

I. **Etiology**
   A. Skin rubbing on skin in the presence of heat and moisture leads to maceration and inflammation.
   B. *Candida albicans* can be causative agent or may be secondarily involved.

II. **Incidence**
   A. Seen most often in summer, but can be present at any time of year in obese children and overdressed infants

III. **Subjective data**
   A. Complaints of red rash (mild to severe) in body folds
   B. Complaints of soreness or itching
   C. May be no presenting complaint; nurse practitioner may find on routine physical examination.

IV. **Objective data**
   A. Inspect entire body; areas most often involved in infants and children are neck creases, axillae, umbilicus, inguinal area, and crease of buttocks.
   B. Mild
      1. Moist
      2. Mild erythema
   C. Moderate
      1. Oozing
      2. Moderate erythema
   D. Severe
      1. Oozing and crusting
      2. May be purulent
      3. Intense erythema

V. **Assessment: Differential diagnosis**
   A. Eczema: By detailed history and appearance of rash
   B. Candidiasis: By detailed history and typical appearance of moist, red, sharply demarcated borders with satellite lesions
   C. Bacterial: Culture of pustules, if present

VI. **Plan**
   A. Wash area with mild soap and water three or four times a day; gently pat dry.
   B. Mild to moderate
      1. Caldesene Medicated Powder: Apply liberally; gently brush away excess, or
      2. Calamine lotion (soothing and drying)
   C. Moderate to severe
      1. Domeboro (Burow's) solution compresses to exudative areas three or four times a day for 2–3 days
      2. 1% hydrocortisone cream three times a day

    D. Candidiasis

        1. Nystatin cream three times a day, or if areas are very moist, nystatin powder three times a day

        2. Domeboro solution compresses three or four times a day for 2–3 days

    E. Secondary infection

        1. Mupirocin (Bactroban) ointment, three times daily

VII. Education

    A. Dry carefully after bathing.

    B. With a drooling baby, keep neck dry; avoid plastic bibs.

    C. Clothing

        1. Use loose cotton clothing.

        2. Avoid wool, nylon, synthetics.

        3. Do not overdress, but use cotton undershirt to help keep body folds separated.

    D. Do not let plastic on disposable diapers come in contact with skin.

    E. Try to keep environment cool and dry. Use dehumidifier, fan, air conditioner.

    F. Laundry

        1. Use mild soap (eg, Ivory Snow).

        2. Do not use bleach or fabric softeners.

    G. Powder

        1. Use powder with caution to avoid inhalation by infant or child. Do not shake on from can; shake into hand and apply.

        2. Do not let powder accumulate in creases.

        3. Do not use cornstarch; it may be metabolized by microorganisms.

    H. Medication

        1. Avoid prolonged use of corticosteroid creams.

        2. Apply hydrocortisone cream sparingly.

        3. Dissolve 1 packet of Domeboro powder in one pint of warm water; keep in covered container.

        4. Use soft cloth for compresses.

    I. Separate skin folds with soft cotton cloth.

    J. Dietary counseling if obesity is a problem

VIII. Follow-up

    A. Telephone follow-up in 5–7 days

    B. Return in 1 week if no improvement noted. May require a fluorinated corticosteroid cream (eg, Kenalog) if severely inflamed.

IX. Consultation/Referral

    A. No response to treatment after 2 weeks

    B. Recurrent or persistent intertrigo for evaluation of diabetes

NOTES

NOTES

IRON-DEFICIENCY ANEMIA

A hypochromic, microcytic anemia that is characterized by a lowered hemo-globin content of red blood cells and decreased numbers of red blood cells. It is the most common hematologic disease of infancy and childhood.

I. **Etiology**

    A. Insufficient available iron for hemoglobin synthesis because of

        1. Inadequate iron stores at birth due to prematurity, maternal or fetal bleeding, or maternal iron deficiency

        2. Insufficient dietary iron to meet requirements of expanding blood volume during periods of rapid growth

        3. Iron loss

            a. Occult gastrointestinal blood loss (eg, in cow's milk intolerance)

            b. Hemorrhage

II. **Incidence**

    A. Rarely seen in the full-term infant under 6 months of age because the iron stores available at birth are adequate to meet the infant's needs for the first 3–6 months

    B. Iron-deficiency anemia is the leading cause of anemia in children 6 months to 2 years old. It is also common during the adolescent years because of rapid growth and often inadequate dietary iron.

III. **Subjective data**

    A. Mild

        1. Pale appearance

        2. Diminished energy level

        3. May be asymptomatic and discovered in routine screening

    B. Moderate to severe

        1. Pallor

        2. Listlessness, fatigue, irritability

        3. Anorexia

        4. Weight gain usually satisfactory in early deficiency ("milk baby"); poor growth rate in chronic, untreated cases

        5. Delayed development

        6. Slow growth of nails

        7. Pica (especially of ice)

        8. Increased incidence of infections

    C. Pertinent subjective data

        1. History of prematurity

        2. Detailed dietary history may reveal the following:

            a. Excessive milk intake (more than 1 quart/day)

            b. Lack of iron-fortified formula or iron supplement in first year of life

            c. Diet low in solid foods with high iron content

            d. Poor appetite; picky eater

            e. Increased intake of junk foods

      3. History of iron-deficiency anemia or other types of anemia in siblings or parents

      4. History of blood loss

      5. History of chronic infection (eg, diarrhea)

IV. **Objective data**

  A. Mild

      1. Palpebral conjunctiva may be pale.

      2. Physical findings normal

  B. Moderate to severe

      1. Pallor

      2. Listlessness

      3. Splenomegaly in 10%–15% of children

      4. May be obese or underweight

  C. Marked

      1. Poor muscle tone

      2. Heart murmur

      3. Spoon-shaped nails

  D. Laboratory tests

      1. Complete blood count with red cell indices

      2. Reticulocyte count

      3. Blood smear

      4. Lead level

      5. Findings in iron-deficiency anemia (see Appendix E for normal red blood cell values)

         a. Hematocrit below normal value for age

         b. Low hemoglobin: Less than one third the hematocrit

         c. Low serum iron: Below 30 μg/100 ml (normal 90–150 μg/100 ml)

         d. Elevated total iron-binding capacity: 350–500 μ/100 ml (normal 250–350 μg/100 ml)

         e. Red cells on smear microcytic and hypochromic

         f. Reticulocyte count low, normal, or slightly elevated

         g. Decreased mean corpuscular hemoglobin: 12–25 μg

         h. Decreased mean corpuscular volume: 50–80 μ3

         i. Low mean corpuscular hemoglobin concentration: 25%–30%

V. **Assessment**

  A. Diagnosis is made by blood values consistent with findings identified as diagnostic for iron-deficiency anemia and by the response to therapeutic doses of iron.

  B. Differential diagnosis

      1. Thalassemia trait: Normal or increased serum iron; no response to iron therapy

      2. Lead poisoning: Elevated lead level and FEP

      3. Chronic infection: Evidence of infection on history or physical examination.

VI. Plan

A. Establish etiology: deficient diet, blood loss, intestinal malabsorption.

B. Aim of therapy is to achieve normal hemoglobin values and to replenish iron stores in the marrow.

C. Pharmacologic therapy

    1. Elemental iron: 4–6 mg/kg/day

        a. Ferrous sulfate is the most effective and least expensive oral therapy: Fer-In-Sol (15 mg elemental iron/0.6 ml) or Feosol Elixir (44 mg elemental iron/5 ml).

        b. Continue treatment for at least 3 months after normal hemoglobin level is reached to replenish body stores.

    2. Vitamin C: 35 mg/day for infants, 40 mg/day for children. Supplement if child is not on multivitamins and if dietary history is deficient in vitamin C (no citrus fruits, potatoes, or vegetables such as cabbage, cauliflower, broccoli, spinach, tomatoes).

D. Dietary recommendations

    1. Iron-fortified formula (supplemented with 12 mg/l) for infants

    2. Foods high in iron

        a. Best sources: Liver; dried pinto and kidney beans; cream of wheat; dry baby cereal

        b. Good sources: Beef, veal; dried prunes, apricots, raisins; spinach and other leafy, dark-green vegetables; egg yolks; nuts; fortified cereals

    3. If milk intake is excessive, decrease to 24 oz/day.

VII. Education

A. Give iron in three divided doses between meals; absorption of iron is decreased if given with meals or with milk. Iron may be given with juice.

B. Iron can stain teeth; give through a straw if possible. Follow medication with water, rinsing mouth, or tooth brushing.

C. Iron may cause gastrointestinal upset (cramps, nausea, diarrhea, or constipation). It is best to give on an empty stomach, but if it is causing distress, consider giving with meals.

D. Stools may be black or green.

E. Keep iron out of reach of children. It is highly toxic in large doses.

F. Strive for a diet high in vitamin C to ensure optimal absorption of iron from foods.

G. Iron intake is a function of caloric intake. There is about 6 mg of iron per 1,000 calories.

H. Avoid whole cow's milk in infants under 1 year. Blood loss induced by protein in cow's milk is not related to lactose intolerance or milk allergy.

I. Iron losses increase in rapid pubertal growth and with heavy menses.

J. Athletes are particularly vulnerable: 20% of runners have positive tests for fecal blood. Also, excessive perspiration produces increased loss of iron in perspiration.

K. Iron therapy generally produces rapid recovery.

L. Continue iron therapy for 3 months after hemoglobin and hematocrit return to normal to replace marrow iron stores. A medication reminder chart may be helpful.

VIII. Follow-up

- **A.** Marked or symptomatic anemia (hemoglobin 2 g or more below lower limits of normal)
    - **1.** Repeat reticulocyte count and hemoglobin in 1–2 weeks. Reticulocyte count should rise in 3–5 days and peak 7–10 days after therapy is initiated. Hemoglobin begins to increase during the first 7–10 days of therapy.
    - **2.** Repeat hemoglobin and hematocrit after 1 month.
        - **a.** If normal, continue treatment for 3 months, and recheck at completion of therapy.
        - **b.** If below normal, continue treatment (stress dosage and compliance), and recheck in 1 month. Consult physician if below normal at this time. If normal, continue treatment for 3 months, and recheck at completion of therapy.
- **B.** Mild anemia (hemoglobin 1–2 g below lower limits of normal): Repeat reticulocyte count and hemoglobin in 1 month.
    - **1.** If normal, continue treatment for 3 months, and recheck at completion of therapy.
    - **2.** If below normal, continue treatment (stress dosage and compliance), and recheck in 1 month. Consult physician if below normal at this time. If normal, continue treatment for 3 months, and recheck at completion of therapy.

IX. Complications

- **A.** Progressive anemia
- **B.** Intercurrent infection

X. Consultation/Referral

- **A.** Marked, symptomatic anemia
- **B.** Infants under 6 months of age
- **C.** Noncompliance with oral pharmacologic therapy
- **D.** Normal hemoglobin levels not achieved after 2 months of therapy

NOTES

LYME DISEASE

A tick-borne illness associated with widespread immune-complex disease. It has three stages, each with multiple clinical features, not all of which are apparent in each patient. It can affect the dermatologic, cardiac, neurologic, and musculoskeletal systems. The hallmark of the disease is erythema chronicum migrans (ECM), an annular expanding skin lesion. This protocol deals primarily with the identification and treatment of stage 1, as recognition of the clinical picture and treatment at this stage prevents subsequent manifestations.

I. **Etiology**

A. A spirochete, *Borrelia burgdorferi*, which is transmitted by *Ixodes dammini*, a tiny deer tick. The cycle of transmission depends on the interaction of immature deer ticks and the white-footed mouse, their primary host.

II. **Incidence**

A. Primarily occurs in northeastern, midwestern, and western parts of the United States

B. Onset of illness generally between May and November, with most cases seen in June and July

C. All ages and both sexes are affected.

D. Disease is endemic in areas where the adult female deer tick can feed on deer, virtually the sole blood source for the adult tick. The larval ticks subsequently feed on infected mice. After feeding for a 2-day period, which is when infection by *Borrelia* is suspected to occur, they lie dormant over the winter. They molt to the nymph stage in the spring; this is the stage when the ticks tend to bite humans.

E. The risk of developing Lyme disease after a tick bite in an endemic area is low (about 5%).

III. **Incubation period**

A. 3–32 days

IV. **Subjective data**

A. History of tick bite may not be reported because of the tiny size of the tick (no larger than a pinhead). Child or parent may not realize child has been bitten.

B. First stage (7–10 days after inoculation)

1. Rash

a. Round, red rash that enlarges

b. Clear in center

c. May have one or several lesions

d. Nonpruritic, nonpainful

2. Associated symptoms

a. Chills, fever

b. Headache, backache

c. Malaise

d. Fatigue, often severe and incapacitating

e. Conjunctivitis

       f. Arthralgia

  C. Second stage (2 weeks to months after bite)

     1. Heart palpitations, chest pain

     2. Dizziness

     3. Shortness of breath, dyspnea

     4. Generalized swollen glands

     5. Neurologic complications (meningitis, cranial neuritis, peripheral neuropathy, encephalitis)

  D. Third stage (weeks to years after onset if untreated; generally 2–6 months after vector bite)

     1. Joint pains, particularly knees

     2. Less commonly, memory loss, mood swings, inability to concentrate

V. Objective data

  A. Characteristic rash (ECM)

     1. Seen at site of tick bite 3–30 days after inoculation

     2. Occurs most commonly on thighs, groin, axillae

     3. Occurs in 80%–90% of cases

     4. An annular, expanding lesion 6–60 cm in size

     5. As lesion expands, it looks like a red ring and generally has central clearing.

     6. Center may be intensely erythematous and indurated in early lesions.

  B. Secondary and migratory annular lesions

     1. Smaller

     2. Centers not indurated

     3. May occur anywhere on body but generally spare palms, soles, and mucous membranes

  C. Regional lymphadenopathy

  D. Neck pain and stiffness

  E. Hepatosplenomegaly

  F. Malar flush

  G. Urticaria

  H. Bell's palsy

  I. Except for ECM or Bell's Palsy, physical examination of limited value

VI. Assessment

  A. Diagnosis

     1. Clinical diagnosis is most readily made by evaluation of ECM (the hallmark of Lyme disease), history of associated flulike symptoms, epidemiologic data, and serologic testing.

     2. Lyme titer not accurate until 3 weeks after exposure. Indirect fluorescent antibody and an ELISA test are available but tests are not standardized. ELISA has slightly greater specificity and sensitivity. Both false-positive and false-negative results occur. Diagnostic help is most needed during stage 2 or 3 when patient has attained a peak antibody rise. Because antibodies remain elevated for years, missing the diagnostic rise in stage 1 can be problematic in making an association between positive titer and symptoms in stages 2 and 3.

VII. Plan

A. Prophylactic antimicrobial therapy is not routinely indicated after a tick bite in endemic areas. In most cases, experts advise judiciously waiting for symptoms of Lyme disease or the appearance of ECM unless patient is immunocompromised.

B. Antimicrobial treatment at stage 1 shortens the stage and aborts stages 2 and 3. Regardless of treatment, signs and symptoms disappear in 3–4 weeks. However, dermatologic manifestations often recur. Duration of treatment depends on clinical response. All patients with Bell's palsy or early arthritis should be treated for the maximum duration.

C. Children through age 9
   1. Phenoxymethyl penicillin (Pen-V), 250 mg every 6 hours for 21–30 days (50 mg/kg/day in divided doses), or
   2. Amoxicillin, 250 mg every 8 hours for 21–30 days (30–50 mg/kg/day in divided doses, maximum 1–2 g/day)
   3. If allergic to penicillin, give erythromycin, 250 mg every 6 hours for 21–30 days (30 mg/kg/day in divided doses).

D. Ages 9 and up
   1. Tetracycline (preferred therapy), 250 mg orally every 6 hours for 21–30 days, or
   2. Doxycycline, 100 mg orally every 12 hours for 21–30 days, or
   3. Amoxicillin, 500 mg orally every 8 hours for 21–30 days

E. Stages 2 and 3 should be treated with antibiotics as indicated above. Persistent arthritis, carditis, meningitis, or encephalitis require intravenous or intramuscular antibiotics and hospitalization.

VIII. Education

A. Prompt removal of ticks is the best method of prevention. A minimum of 24 hours of attachment and feeding is necessary for transmission to occur.

B. Examine children's bodies after playing outside, hiking, and so forth.

C. Shower or bathe after expected exposure.

D. Scalp, axillae, and groin are preferred sites for tick attachment.

E. Avoid tick-infested areas.

F. Areas of risk must be suitable for both mice and ticks to live in (generally wooded areas and overhanging brush), although they have been found in grass.

G. Dress for protection.
   1. Light-colored clothing so that ticks can be easily spotted
   2. Long-sleeved shirts
   3. Tuck cuffs of pants into socks or boots.
   4. Check clothes for ticks.

H. Wash and dry clothing in high temperatures.

I. Use tick repellent containing DEET or permethrin.

J. Use DEET sparingly in young children, as seizures have been reported coincident with its use.

K. Identify tick.
   1. *Ixodes dammini*: Size of a pinhead
   2. Oval body with no apparent segmentation and no antennae

  3. Body covered with leathery, granulated cuticle

  4. Deer ticks have a scutum, or hard shield, on their backs.

  5. Stages

   a. Larvae: Less than 2–3 mm long with six legs

   b. Nymphs: 4–8 mm long with eight legs (stage at which they generally infect humans)

  6. Unfed ticks are flat; ticks that have recently fed are engorged.

 L. Tick removal

  1. Do not handle tick with bare hands; infectious agents may enter through breaks in the skin.

  2. Use blunt tweezers.

  3. Grasp tick close to skin and pull with steady, even pressure.

  4. Do not squeeze, crush, or puncture tick; body fluids may contain infected particles.

  5. Disinfect bite site.

  6. Flush tick down toilet or submerse in alcohol.

 M. Rash

  1. ECM and secondary lesions generally disappear within days once treatment is started.

  2. If untreated, lesion may persist for months and recur for up to 1 year after onset.

 N. Pets may bring ticks into the house, but pets themselves do not transmit disease to humans.

IX. Follow-up

 A. Recheck in 24–48 hours by telephone.

 B. Call immediately if symptoms worsen.

 C. Recheck Lyme titer if unresponsive to medication.

 D. Convalescent titers may be done to monitor progress of disease.

X. Complications

 A. Cardiac complications: Seen 4–83 days (median 21 days) after onset of ECM in about 8% of untreated cases

 B. Lyme arthritis

 C. Neurologic: Bell's palsy, Guillain-Barré syndrome, polyradiculitis

XI. Consultation/Referral

 A. Stages 2 and 3

NOTES

NOTES

MARGINAL BLEPHARITIS

Chronic inflammation of the eyelid margins with accumulation of yellowish scales; often associated with seborrheic dermatitis

I. **Etiology**
   A. Seborrhea (see Seborrhea of the Scalp)
   B. May be associated with *Staphylococcus aureus*

II. **Incidence**
   A. Seen in all age groups, but most common in infants and adolescents
   B. Often occurs in conjunction with seborrhea of the scalp

III. **Subjective data**
   A. Scaling and inflammation of eyelid margins
   B. Crusting, itching, or burning may be present.
   C. May be asymptomatic and identified on routine physical examination

IV. **Objective data**
   A. Yellowish, oily scales on eyelashes
   B. Lashes often matted
   C. Eyelashes may not grow.
   D. Inflammation, scaling, and exudate on eyelid margins
   E. Mild conjunctivitis may be present.
   F. Ulcerations of lid margins if severe
   G. Check entire body for seborrhea elsewhere, particularly on scalp and eyebrows.

V. **Assessment**
   A. Diagnosis easily made by typical appearance.

VI. **Plan**
   A. Warm, moist compresses four times a day to remove crusts and scales
   B. Use CIBA Eye Scrub or Johnson's Baby Shampoo to cleanse lashes daily.
   C. Sodium Sulamyd Ointment (sodium sulfacetamide) at bedtime; use four times a day if inflammation is present, or
   D. Ilotycin Ophthalmic (erythromycin) at bedtime; use four times a day if inflammation is present.
   E. Treat concurrent seborrhea of scalp according to protocol.

VII. **Education**
   A. Use warm, moist compresses for 10 minutes.
   B. Use soft face cloth for compresses.
   C. Pull down lower eyelid and apply a thin ribbon of ointment along inner margin of lower lid.
   D. Continue treatment for 1 week after symptoms have cleared.
   E. Use of ointment may cause temporary blurring of vision.
   F. Sodium Sulamyd may cause stinging or burning if child is sensitive to it. Discontinue use and call office.
   G. Problem is chronic.
   H. Treatment controls the condition but generally does not effect a complete cure.

    I. Once cleared, teach parent or child to be alert for symptoms of recurrence so treatment can be instituted early. Warm compresses should be used immediately if symptoms recur.

    J. Does not affect visual acuity

VIII. Follow-up

    A. Return in 3–4 days if no improvement is noted or symptoms seem worse.

    B. Call back immediately if any reaction to medication occurs.

IX. Consultation/Referral

    A. No response to treatment after 1 week

    B. Refer to ophthalmologist for monitoring of intraocular tension with intermittent or chronic use of steroid therapy.

NOTES

| **METATARSUS ADDUCTUS**

A positional deformity characterized by a concavity of the medial border of the foot

I. **Etiology**
   A. Caused by uterine position

II. **Incidence**
   A. Frequently seen in newborns, most commonly as a flexible deformity
   B. If uncorrected, metatarsus adduction corrects spontaneously in 85% of children; 10% will have a mild adduction and 5% a severe adduction.

III. **Subjective data**
   A. Generally detected on physical examination of the neonate
   B. If missed in the newborn, subjective findings include a complaint by the parents of toes turning in and often a concurrent complaint of bowlegs.

IV. **Objective data**
   A. Forefoot adducted on the hind foot with the heel in a normal position
   B. Lateral border of the foot angulated at the base of the fifth metatarsal, a convex lateral border
   C. Flexible deformity: Foot assumes a normal position when lateral border of the foot is scratched.
   D. Rigid deformity: Deformity cannot be corrected past the midline.
   E. Carefully check hips and legs for other postural deformities (eg, tibial torsion).

V. **Assessment: Differential diagnosis**
   A. Talipes equinovarus: Includes plantar flexion of the foot at the ankle joint, inversion deformity of the heel, and forefoot adduction

VI. **Plan**
   A. Rigid deformity: Refer to orthopedist for probable serial casting.
   B. Flexible deformity
      1. Exercising by parent six times a day
         a. Place thumb along lateral border of foot, and with other hand on distal medial border, apply pressure to straighten lateral border.
         b. Hold in position for a slow count of 10.
      2. Use equinovarus prewalkers or reverse-last shoes if deformity persists despite exercise or if parent does not do exercising routinely. Order for involved foot only, and leave on 24 hours a day initially. Gradually decrease time as deformity improves.
      3. Straight-last shoes: Persistence of deformity on weight bearing is an indication for straight-last shoes once child is walking.
      4. Spontaneous correction occurs in 85% of infants without treatment.

VII. **Education**
   A. Problem was caused by intrauterine position.
   B. Correctable, but treatment plan must be followed.
   C. Demonstrate exercise, and have parent do return demonstration.
   D. Equinovarus prewalkers or reverse-last shoes
      1. Leave on for prescribed length of time.

2. Remove for bath.

3. Remove several times a day to check foot for pressure and to exercise.

4. Buy pajamas slightly large so that shoe will fit underneath.

5. Use white cotton sock under shoe. Buy correct size so there will be no wrinkles under shoe.

6. Shoe must be firmly laced and securely strapped if it is to be effective.

E. A busy parent may feel pressured by the additional time it takes to do the exercises; provide support and encouragement.

VIII. Follow-up

A. First recheck should be at office visit at 2–3 weeks of age. If easily corrected, continue exercises until next visit. If no improvement is noted, stress exercising.

B. Second recheck should be at 6–7 weeks of age. If no improvement is noted at this time, reverse-last shoes should be used.

C. Routine follow-up should be included at each well child visit. Check carefully for persistence of deformity, both at rest and on weight bearing. Reverse-last shoe may be used for several months. If there is marked improvement after 1 month of use, shoe may be left off for longer periods of time.

IX. Consultation/Referral

A. Refer to orthopedist if rigid deformity (one that cannot correct past the midline).

B. Refer to orthopedist at 4–6 months of age if no improvement of flexible deformity with conscientious exercising by parent.

NOTES

MILIARIA RUBRA

Also known as heat rash or prickly heat; characterized by an erythematous papular rash, distributed in areas where sweat glands are concentrated

I. **Etiology**

   A. Heat and high humidity from external environment cause sweating, which leads to swelling and plugging of the sweat gland orifice. The duct becomes distended and ruptures, leaking sweat into the skin, thereby causing the irritation.

II. **Incidence**

   A. Infants and children are most prone.

   B. Seen most often in the summer and in obese and overdressed infants

III. **Subjective data**

   A. Pruritus

   B. Fine, red, raised rash

   C. Pustules may be present in neck and axillae.

   D. History of overdressing

   E. History of predisposing environmental factors (eg, hot spell in summer or house kept too warm)

IV. **Objective data**

   A. Rash is erythematous and vesiculopapular. Lesions are pinhead size and may coalesce on an erythematous patch or remain isolated.

   B. Distribution: Found in areas of sweat gland concentration and areas of friction (eg, neck, axillae, face, shoulders, chest, antecubital and popliteal fossae, diaper area)

   C. Check entire body; intertrigo may be present as well.

V. **Assessment**

   A. Diagnosis is made by appearance and history (hot, humid environment).

   B. Differential diagnosis

   1. Contact dermatitis: Distribution different according to contact; edematous; erythematous; vesicular; history of contact

   2. Viral exanthems: Accurate history would reveal elevated temperature and other prodromal signs or symptoms.

   3. Candidiasis: Shiny, intensely inflamed, sharply defined border with satellite lesions

VI. **Plan**

   A. Treatment is symptomatic.

   1. Keep environment cool and dry; use air conditioner, fan, or dehumidifier if possible.

   2. Tepid to cool baths three times daily; may use baking soda in bath

   3. Caldesene powder: Apply frequently.

   4. Clothing

   a. Light, absorbent cotton clothing

   b. Do not overdress baby.

   c. Use a cotton shirt to keep body folds separated.

      d. Omit plastic pants, disposable diapers, and plastic bibs.

    5. Use cotton mattress pad over plastic-covered mattress.

    6. Calamine lotion can be used on toddlers or older children.

  B. Severely inflamed miliaria: 1% hydrocortisone cream three times a day

VII. Education

  A. Prevention is of prime importance.

  B. Powder

    1. Do not allow child or baby to play with powder.

    2. Use powder with caution near face to avoid inhalation.

    3. Shake into hand to apply. Do not shake from can directly onto infant or child.

    4. Do not let powder accumulate in creases.

    5. Do not use cornstarch; it encourages bacterial and fungal overgrowth.

  C. Use hydrocortisone cream sparingly.

  D. Use mild or hypoallergenic soap (Neutrogena or Lowila).

  E. Laundry: Avoid harsh detergents, bleach, and fabric softeners.

  F. Keep baby's fingernails short.

  G. If rash is on back of neck, advise mother not to wear irritating fabrics (wool, nylon, synthetics) when feeding baby.

  H. Do not put baby to sleep in the sun.

VIII. Follow-up

  A. Telephone follow-up in 4–6 days

  B. If no improvement is noted by parents, try calamine lotion four times a day for soothing and drying effect.

  C. Return for reevaluation if above measures are unsuccessful.

IX. Consultation/Referral

  A. No improvement with treatment, or exacerbation of rash

NOTES

MOLLUSCUM CONTAGIOSUM

A benign viral disease of the skin with no systemic manifestations. It is characterized by waxy, umbilicated papules.

I. **Etiology**
   A. Poxvirus

II. **Incubation period**
   A. Generally 2–7 weeks
   B. May be as long as 6 months

III. **Communicability**
   A. Period of communicability unknown
   B. Infectivity is low, although occasional outbreaks have occurred.
   C. Contracted by direct contact, fomites, and autoinoculation
   D. Humans are the only known source of the virus.

IV. **Subjective data**
   A. Complaints of "warts" or bumps
   B. May be one or two to hundreds of lesions
   C. Occasional complaints of infected lesions
   D. Often asymptomatic and found on physical examination

V. **Objective data**
   A. Papules 1–5 mm in diameter
      1. Pearly white or skin-colored
      2. Waxy
      3. Umbilicated
      4. Isolated or in clusters
   B. Distribution
      1. Face
      2. Trunk
      3. Lower abdomen
      4. Pubis, penis
      5. Thighs
      6. Mucosa
   C. Check for secondary infection.
   D. No associated systemic manifestations

VI. **Assessment**
   A. Diagnosis is usually made by the characteristic appearance of the lesions.
   B. Diagnosis can be confirmed by scraping lesions and viewing molluscum bodies under magnification.
   C. Warts are the most common differential diagnosis.

VII. **Plan**
   A. Curettage: Remove each lesion with a sharp curette.
   B. Trichloroacetic acid 30%: Apply to base of each lesion, avoiding surrounding skin.

    C. Salicylic acid (Occlusal-HP)

       1. Apply to lesion.

       2. Cover with tape.

       3. Remove tape after 12 hours.

    D. Tretinoin (Retin-A) gel 0.01%: Apply to lesions once daily.

    E. Infected lesions

       1. Hot soaks five or six times a day for 10 minutes

       2. Neosporin ointment

    F. Genital lesions: Rule out sexual abuse.

    G. Cryosurgery if only a few lesions and at least 1 cm apart

    H. *Note:* Some physicians recommend no treatment, but the lifespan of the lesions can be months to years and they are distressing to parents and children. Therefore, a treatment trial should be attempted using the least traumatic method for the numbers of lesions present.

    I. Sometimes children effect a cure themselves by picking at the lesions, causing them to disappear.

VIII. Education

    A. Lesions are generally self-limited. They may last 6–9 months but can last for years.

    B. Trauma to or infection of a lesion may cause it to disappear.

    C. Treatment prevents spread by autoinoculation.

    D. Restrict direct body contact with infected child to prevent spread.

    E. Can be spread by contact with contaminated surfaces

    F. Children with atopic dermatitis are prone to develop widespread lesions.

    G. Although many lesions can be and are picked off by children, they may become secondarily infected.

IX. Follow-up

    A. Recheck in office in 1 week.

    B. Call if inflammatory reaction to local medication.

X. Complications

    A. Secondary infection

    B. Reaction to local treatment

XI. Consultation/Referral

    A. Question of sexual abuse

    B. Multiple, widespread lesions unresponsive to treatment: Refer to dermatologist.

NOTES

NOTES

MYCOPLASMAL PNEUMONIA

An acute infection of the lungs characterized by cough and fever. Symptoms are generally milder than those of bacterial pneumonia. Mycoplasmal pneumonia is the so-called walking pneumonia.

I. **Etiology**

   A. *Mycoplasma pneumoniae*, the smallest known pathogen that can live outside of cells

II. **Incidence**

   A. The most common cause of pneumonia in school-age children and adolescents, occurring in about five per 1,000 school-aged children annually
   B. The most common cause of nonbacterial pneumonias in all age groups
   C. Peak incidence is in the fall and early winter, but it does occur sporadically year round.

III. **Incubation period**

   A. 14–21 days

IV. **Subjective data**

   A. Insidious onset
   B. Headache
   C. Chills
   D. Low-grade fever
   E. Malaise
   F. Cough: Initially nonproductive, dry, hacking
   G. Sore throat
   H. Occasionally, ear pain
   I. Anorexia
   J. History of exposure to mycoplasmal pneumonia or other respiratory illness (pharyngitis, cough, earache)

V. **Objective data**

   A. Fever: Variable, generally low-grade
   B. Lethargy
   C. Does not appear particularly ill
   D. Chest findings are variable.
      1. Decreased percussion note (rare)
      2. Decreased tactile and vocal fremitus (rare)
      3. Diminished breath sounds
      4. Few scattered rales or crackles to severe bilateral involvement
      5. Expiratory wheezing may be heard.
      6. Lower lobes are involved more commonly than are upper lobes.
   E. X-ray findings are variable but are more extensive than would be expected from clinical signs.
      1. Increase in bronchovascular markings
      2. Unilateral peribronchial infiltrate or lobar consolidation, although multi-lobe involvement does occur.

F. Laboratory tests

   1. Cold agglutinins are helpful in diagnosis but are nonspecific.

      a. Cold agglutinins are seen in influenza, infectious mononucleosis, and other nonbacterial infections.

      b. Cold agglutinin titer develops in about 50% of children with mycoplasmal pneumonia.

      c. Titer rises 8–10 days after onset and peaks in 12–25 days.

      d. Titer of 1:256 is suggestive of mycoplasmal pneumonia.

   2. Culture and serologic testing take too long to be useful in determining treatment.

VI. Assessment

A. Diagnosis is based on typical features; generally an "informed clinical judgment"

   1. Patient age

   2. Patient nontoxic

   3. History of slowly evolving symptoms: Indolent course, fatigue, cough

   4. Fine rales heard on auscultation

   5. Low-grade fever

B. Differential diagnosis: Mycoplasmal pneumonia cannot be distinguished from other atypical pneumonias by clinical signs. (See also Differential Diagnosis of Viral Croup, Bronchiolitis, Pneumonia, and Bronchitis.)

VII. Plan

A. Antibiotics: Because *M pneumoniae* is the predominant cause of antibiotic-responsive pneumonia in school-aged children, therapy should be instituted if the diagnosis is suspected.

   1. Erythromycin, 40–50 mg/kg/day in four divided doses (more than 20 kg, 250 mg four times daily), or

   2. Tetracycline (in children over 12 years of age), 250 mg four times daily, or

   3. Clarithromycin (Biaxin), 15 mg/kg/day in divided doses every 12 hours (more than 33 kg, 250 mg twice daily). Drug of choice if uncertain whether mycoplasmal or pneumococcal pneumonia.

B. Acetaminophen for temperature over 101°F; use sparingly, because temperature in part indicates response to pharmacologic therapy.

C. Rest

D. Increased fluids

E. Cool mist vaporizer

F. Cough suppressant as indicated (Benylin Cough Syrup)

VIII. Education

A. Give antibiotic for 10 full days.

B. Antibiotics shorten the course of the illness but generally do not produce a dramatic response as in bacterial pneumonias.

C. Clarithromycin or erythromycin can be given with or without food.

D. Do not give antihistamines.

E. Encourage fluids to help keep secretions from thickening.

F. Transmitted directly by oral and nasal secretions and indirectly by contaminated articles

    G. Use careful hand-washing technique.

    H. An attack probably confers immunity for a year or longer, but no permanent immunity is conferred.

    I. If child has trouble coughing up secretions, place child prone with head lower than feet and percuss chest with cupped hands.

    J. Call immediately if child has difficulty breathing or if he or she becomes restless or anxious; these symptoms indicate anoxia.

    K. Duration of illness is about 2 weeks. A night cough persists longer.

IX. Follow-up

    A. Call back daily until improvement is noted.

    B. Recheck if no improvement in 48 hours.

    C. Recheck in 10 days.

    D. Call if any question of sensitivity to medication.

    E. Repeat chest X-ray in 2 weeks if

        1. Signs of respiratory difficulty persist.

        2. Previous history of pneumonia

        3. Child has cardiopulmonary disease.

X. Complications

    A. Rare

XI. Consultation/Referral

    A. Infant

    B. Toxic child

    C. Respiratory distress or cyanosis

    D. No clinical improvement after 48 hours of therapy

NOTES

OTITIS MEDIA, ACUTE

An acute infection in the middle ear characterized by middle ear effusion leading to partial or complete obstruction of the eustachian tube. It is associated with acute signs of illness.

I. **Etiology**

    A. Major causative organisms: *Streptococcus pneumoniae* (about 31%), *Haemophilus influenzae* (22%), and *Moraxella catarrhalis* (7%). A few cases are due to beta-hemolytic streptococci.

    B. Middle ear aspirates have identified a virus in 16% of cases of acute otitis. It is unclear whether the viruses are a primary cause of acute otitis or whether they promote bacterial superinfection.

II. **Incidence**

    A. Otitis media is the second most common organic disease seen in pediatric practice (upper respiratory tract infection is the most common).

    B. Incidence corresponds to the incidence of acute upper respiratory infection.

    C. Peak prevalence is in children 6–36 months old.

    D. Increased incidence in children with cleft palate and with Down's syndrome

    E. About 93% of all children have at least one episode by age 7.

    F. Diagnosis, treatment, and follow-up of otitis media comprises up to 33% of pediatric office visits.

    G. Incidence declines at about 6 years of age.

III. **Subjective data**

    A. Rhinorrhea

    B. Malaise

    C. Irritability

    D. Restlessness

    E. Pulling or rubbing ear

    F. Pain in ear

    G. Purulent discharge from ear

    H. Temperature may be elevated (101°–102°F).

    I. Diarrhea or vomiting

    J. Pertinent subjective data to obtain

        1. History of upper respiratory infection

        2. Previous history of ear infections

        3. Family history of allergies

        4. Does hearing seem normal?

        5. Does the child take a bottle to bed, or is he or she fed supine with a propped bottle or flat on adult's lap?

IV. **Objective data**

    A. Fever

    B. Rhinorrhea

    C. Tympanic membrane

        1. Discharge suggests perforation of eardrum.

2. Contour: Fullness, bulging, or loss of concavity, which results in diminished or absent landmarks

3. Color

    a. Intense erythema

    b. Abnormal whiteness can result from scarring or the presence of pus in the middle ear.

4. Luster: Generally dull with loss of light reflex, but dullness in itself is not indicative of otitis media.

5. Bulla may be seen on eardrum.

6. Perforation or scarring may be present.

7. Mobility decreased or absent

B. Evaluate for:

1. Mastoid tenderness

2. Adenopathy

3. Pharyngitis

4. Lower respiratory tract involvement

V. **Assessment**

A. Diagnosis is confirmed by the characteristic findings of the tympanic membrane.

B. Differential diagnosis

1. Hyperemia of tympanic membrane from crying or high temperature: Tympanic membrane is bright, landmarks are evident, and mobility is normal.

2. Eustachian tube obstruction: Causes transient pain, but tympanic membrane is normal.

3. Serous otitis: Tympanic membrane is not inflamed and will not move inward with positive pressure, although it may move outward on negative pressure. Air bubbles may be visualized behind tympanic membrane.

4. External otitis: Diffuse inflammation of the ear canal with or without exudate; pain on movement of pinna. Tympanic membrane may be inflamed with widespread involvement.

VI. **Plan**

A. Antimicrobials: Usual duration of treatment is 10 days.

1. Amoxicillin, 40 mg/kg/day in three divided doses every 8 hours (more than 20 kg, 250 mg three times a day) for 10 days

2. If allergic to amoxicillin or two prior treatment failures in one respiratory season, trimethoprim (TMP)–sulfamethoxazole (SMX) (Bactrim or Septra), 8 mg TMP and 40 mg SMX/kg/day in divided doses every 12 hours (10 kg, 5 ml every 12 hours; more than 40 kg, one DS tablet every 12 hours) for 10 days

3. If nonresponsive to above after 48 hours of therapy or previous otitis during same season has not responded to above, amoxicillin with clavulanic acid (Augmentin), 45 mg/kg/day in two divided doses every 12 hours (more than 20 kg, 400 mg every 12 hours) for 10 days (dosage based on amoxicillin component). Do not use regular 250- or 500-mg tablets for a child less than 40 kg; instead, use chewables or suspension.

4. Cefuroxime (Ceftin), 30 mg/kg/day in divided doses every 12 hours (more than 20 kg, 250 mg every 12 hours), or

5. Loracarbef (Lorabid), 30 mg/kg/day in divided doses every 12 hours (more than 26 kg, 400 mg every 12 hours),or

6. Cefprozil (Cefzil), 30 mg/kg/day in divided doses every 12 hours (more than 20 kg, 250 mg every 12 hours)

7. *Note:* In an acute episode of otitis media, amoxicillin is the drug of choice for initial therapy. However, about 17% of *H influenzae* and *M catarrhalis* organisms are ampicillin resistant (usually beta-lactamase-producing organisms). The rationale for the subsequent antimicrobial therapy, if otitis media does not respond to amoxicillin, is that these antimicrobials are beta-lactamase inhibitors. Because they are generally more expensive and have more side effects than amoxicillin, these antimicrobials are not generally used as a first line of defense.

8. Cephalosporins are best reserved for children with amoxicillin and sulfa allergies. They are very effective but are also more expensive and have more potential for significant hypersensitivity reactions.

B. Antihistamines and decongestants

1. These drugs have been widely used in attempts to open the eustachian tube, but efficacy has not been proved. They are not recommended for treatment of otitis; therefore, order them only for symptomatic relief, not routinely.

2. Use an antihistamine and decongestant such as Actifed or Dimetapp for children with known allergic rhinitis.

3. Use a decongestant such as Sudafed for children with acute nasal congestion.

C. Acetaminophen: For elevated temperature or pain, 10–15 mg/kg every 4 hours

D. Auralgan Otic Solution four times a day for relief of pain and reduction of inflammation if tympanic membrane is not perforated

E. Do a record review with each incidence of otitis. Question caregiver about interval visits to emergency room or other health care provider. Follow-up plan may need to include prophylaxis.

VII. Education

A. Encourage fluids. Baby may not suck because of pain. Offer small amounts frequently by teaspoon or shot glass.

B. Medication

1. Give medication for 10 full days.

2. If child cannot retain medication, call back immediately.

3. Side effects of antimicrobials are diarrhea, rash, and fever.

4. Side effects of antihistamine and decongestant preparations are lethargy and hyperactivity.

5. If using Auralgan, fill canal with medication; do not touch ear with dropper; use cotton pledget in meatus after instilling. Use only for pain; discontinue use once pain has subsided. Do not use if eardrum is ruptured. Do not use for future ear infections until ear has been evaluated.

C. Improvement should be noted within 24 hours of treatment.

D. Child may return to school once temperature has been normal for 24 hours.

E. There is no evidence that otitis media is transmitted from person to person; rather, the viral infections predisposing a child to otitis are transmitted person to person.

   F. Child may have temporary difficulty hearing. Notify school if applicable.

   G. Complete resolution of middle ear effusion may require 8–12 weeks.

   H. Explain disease process to caregiver. Reassure him or her that earache did not occur because child went out without a hat or because the ears got wet during shampooing.

   I. Explain postural factors implicated in otitis media. Discontinue bottle in bed or horizontal feedings.

   J. Stress importance of follow-up. Recognize that treatment of an episode of otitis media can be expensive. If there are recurrences or if two children in the same family have otitis media, parents may be concerned about the cost and may not return unless they understand why it is necessary.

   K. Explain that there will be an increased incidence of otitis with new exposures when child enters day care or kindergarten.

   L. Concurrent viral infections significantly interfere with the resolution of otitis media.

VIII. Follow-up

   A. Call back if child vomits medication or if side effects to medication occur.

   B. Return if child is not improved in 24 hours or if there is persistent fever, pain, or discharge.

   C. Return in 10 days for recheck. Include otoscopic examination, pneumatic otoscopy, and audiogram, as well as tympanometry or acoustic otoscopy if available.

   D. If symptoms have not improved within 48 hours or otitis has not resolved in 10 days, re-treat for resistant organisms. Include subsequent follow-up in another 10 days in plan.

   E. General guidelines for chemoprophylaxis

   1. Three episodes in 6 months or four in 1 year

   2. Chemoprophylaxis should be continued during period of peak incidence of viral respiratory infections.

   3. Recheck every 3–4 weeks (according to office protocol) if child is on chemoprophylaxis.

   4. Chemoprophylaxis: Half the therapeutic dose once daily, preferably at bedtime

   a. Sulfisoxazole, 50 mg/kg/day, or

   b. Amoxicillin, 20 mg/kg/day in a single daily dose

   F. If otitis media recurs while on chemoprophylaxis, discontinue chemoprophylaxis and treat with another antibiotic.

IX. Complications

   A. Recurrent otitis media

   B. Perforation of tympanic membrane

   C. Mastoiditis

   D. Meningitis

   E. Reaction to medication

X. Consultation/Referral

   A. Infants under 3 months of age

   B. No improvement within 24 hours

C. Failure of tympanic membrane to regain normal appearance after 20 days of treatment

D. For frequent recurrences (eg, three in one season), consult or refer for chemoprophylaxis. Give half the therapeutic dose of amoxicillin, sulfisoxazole, or TMP–SMX to suppress colonization.

E. Persistent diminished hearing

F. Myringotomy with tube insertion must be considered in a child with

1. Persistent middle ear effusion between recurrent episodes of acute otitis media

2. Consistent hearing loss of more than 15 dB for longer than 3 months

3. Effusion present for greater than 3 months

NOTES

PEDICULOSIS CAPITIS, CORPORIS, AND PUBIS

Pediculosis capitis are human lice that live in the hair. Pediculosis corporis live on the body and in seams of clothing. Pediculosis pubis live in the pubic hair and may also infest the eyebrows, eyelashes, beard, moustache, and hair of the trunk.

I. **Etiology**
    A. Capitis: *Pediculus humanus capitis* (head louse)
    B. Corporis: *Pediculus humanus corporis* (body louse)
    C. Pubis: *Phthirus pubis* (pubic or "crab" louse)
    D. These lice, which are in the order Anoplura, are ectoparasites. They are sucking lice and are completely dependent on their host's blood for nourishment.
    E. They are transmitted by close personal contact as well as by clothing and bedding.
    F. Because they are obligate parasites, they cannot survive away from their hosts for more than 10 days. However, most pubic or head lice that are on fomites are dead or dying, so the danger of spread from toilet seats, for example, is minimal.

II. **Incidence**
    A. Occurs without regard to socioeconomic status, age, or sex
    B. Infestation is seen most frequently in areas of overcrowding where sanitation facilities and hygiene are poor.
    C. In general, lice are more common among children than adults and females than males.
    D. Pubic lice are commonly found on adolescents who are engaged in multiple sexual relationships.
    E. Head lice are common among elementary school children.
    F. Blacks are rarely infested.

III. **Incubation period for ova**
    A. Varies depending on temperature; average 8–9 days
    B. Ova may lie dormant for up to 35 days.
    C. Ova develop to adulthood in 10–15 days and generally live for 30 days.
    D. Newly hatched nymphs must feed within 24 hours to survive.

IV. **Subjective data**
    A. Pediculosis capitis
        1. Pruritus of scalp
        2. "Bugs" in head
        3. "Dandruff" that sticks to hair
        4. History of exposure
    B. Pediculosis corporis
        1. Pruritus of body
        2. Multiple bite and scratch marks, particularly on upper back, around the waist, and on upper arms
        3. History of exposure

    C. Pediculosis pubis

        1. Pruritus of pubic area; most intense at night

        2. Multiple bite and scratch marks in pubic area

        3. "Bugs" in pubic hair, in eyebrows, or in axillae

V. Objective data

    A. Pediculosis capitis

        1. Lice on scalp; most commonly found behind the ears and on the back of the head

        2. Ova visualized as whitish ellipsoids on hair shafts, firmly attached and difficult to remove. These are the usual signs of infestation.

        3. Bites on scalp

        4. Scratch marks on scalp; may be secondarily infected

        5. Occipital and cervical adenopathy

    B. Pediculosis corporis

        1. Body lice are rarely found.

        2. Lice in seams of clothing

        3. Bite marks where lice have fed, generally on upper back, waist, and axillae

        4. Excoriations from scratching

        5. Secondary infections in areas of excoriations

        6. Regional adenopathy

        7. Occasionally, nits on body hair

    C. Pediculosis pubis

        1. Lice attached to pubic hair

        2. Lice may also be found in eyebrows, axillae, thighs, and beard

        3. Ova visualized as whitish ellipsoids firmly attached to hair shaft

        4. Bite marks on abdomen, lower thighs, and genital area (bluish-gray, faint purpuric-like lesions)

        5. Excoriations from scratching

        6. Secondary infections in areas of excoriation

        7. Inguinal adenopathy

        8. Rule out sexual abuse if found in child.

VI. Assessment

    A. Diagnosis is made by the characteristic signs and symptoms and by history of exposure.

    B. With head and pubic lice, diagnosis is generally made by observation alone.

VII. Plan

    A. Follow selected treatment plan. Do not overtreat. Chemical irritation from medication or hypersensitivity to the bite of the louse may result in persistent itching and may be misinterpreted as treatment failure. Order only enough medication for the treatment schedule.

    B. For all infestations, all family members and other close contacts should be examined and treated if any evidence of lice or nits is found. All sexual contacts should be treated simultaneously.

    C. Pediculosis capitis

        1. Nix Creme Rinse (permethrin 1%)

    a. Shampoo and rinse hair; towel dry.

    b. Apply Nix Creme Rinse, thoroughly saturating hair and scalp.

    c. Allow Nix to remain on hair for 10 minutes, then rinse.

    d. Nits may be combed out for cosmetic reasons (Nix is ovicidal).

    e. Advantages

        (1) Ovicidal

        (2) Active for 14 days after treatment

        (3) Action of rinse is not affected by shampooing.

        (4) 99.2% effective

        (5) Generally a single treatment suffices, but a second application may be made in 10–14 days.

        (6) Minimal systemic absorption

        (7) No potential for sensitization

  2. Kwell shampoo (gamma-benzene hexachloride). Do not prescribe for pregnant women or children under 2 years of age.

    a. Thoroughly wet hair and scalp with Kwell shampoo.

    b. Add small amount of water and work in shampoo until good lather forms.

    c. Continue shampooing for 4 minutes.

    d. Rinse thoroughly.

    e. Towel dry.

    f. Comb nits from hair after treatment using a fine-toothed comb.

    g. Repeat application in 7 days (Kwell is not ovicidal).

D. Pediculosis corporis: Because body lice are rarely found on the body except when they are feeding, clothing and bedding are the main foci of treatment.

  1. Kwell cream or lotion (gamma-benzene hexachloride)

    a. Bathe or shower thoroughly.

    b. Apply cream or lotion to affected hairy areas and surrounding skin and to suspect areas.

    c. Leave medication on for 12–24 hours.

    d. Shower or bathe thoroughly with soap and warm water.

    e. Bed linen and clothing must be changed and laundered or dry cleaned.

    f. Application may be repeated in 4 days if necessary.

  2. RID

    a. Bathe or shower thoroughly.

    b. Apply RID to all infested areas and suspect areas until wet; do not apply to eyelashes or eyebrows.

    c. Leave on for 10 minutes.

    d. Bathe or shower thoroughly with soap and warm water.

    e. Bed linen and clothing must be changed and laundered or dry cleaned.

    f. If necessary, treatment may be repeated once only in 24 hours.

  3. Clothing (see Education below)

E. Pediculosis pubis

  1. Kwell lotion (gamma-benzene hexachloride)

      a. Shower and towel dry.

      b. Apply sufficient quantity to cover thinly skin and hair of pubic area and, if involved, the thighs, trunk, and axillae.

      c. Rub into skin.

      d. Leave lotion on for 12–24 hours.

      e. Shower thoroughly.

      f. Repeat treatment in 7 days.

    2. Kwell shampoo

      a. Apply sufficient shampoo to wet thoroughly hair and skin of affected and adjacent hairy areas.

      b. Add small amount of water, working shampoo into hair and skin until lather forms.

      c. Continue shampooing for 4 minutes.

      d. Rinse thoroughly.

      e. Towel dry.

      f. Repeat application after 7 days if living lice were found on examination.

F. Oral antihistamine

    1. Rarely indicated if treatment has been effective

    2. Diphenhydramine (Benadryl), 12.5–25 mg three times daily

G. Infected lesions: Follow protocol for Impetigo (see p. 328).

VIII. Education

A. Infestation with lice can be a traumatic emotional experience for child and family. Education and support are important in helping them cope with the problem.

B. Lice are highly contagious and can affect all social classes.

C. Most head and pubic lice that are on inanimate objects are dead or dying.

D. Human lice are not transmitted by animals; they live and breed only on humans.

E. Lice cannot jump or fly from one person to another.

F. Head lice

    1. Transmitted by direct contact with an infested person's hair or by contact with hats, brushes, combs, or bedding. Head lice can crawl from one place to another.

    2. Head lice do not normally live on the hair shafts of blacks.

    3. Head lice leave the body if the host temperature rises due to fever or drops due to death. (Ova cannot hatch at temperatures below 22°C.)

    4. Eggs are laid close to the scalp. Because hair grows about 1/4″ each month, any eggs found a greater distance from the scalp are probably empty shells.

    5. Do not borrow combs, barrettes, ribbons, hats, helmets, scarves, or pillows.

    6. Do not stack or hang coat or hat so that it touches other persons' clothing.

    7. Nits must be removed manually or with a fine-toothed comb.

G. Body lice

    1. Transmitted by direct contact or by contact with infected clothing or bedding

    2. Lice usually cling to clothing, particularly in the seams, and are least prevalent in areas where hygiene is good.

  H. Pubic lice

    1. Transmitted through close personal contact and through clothing, bedding, and, less commonly, toilet seats

    2. Particularly common among persons aged 15–25, probably because of close physical contact, especially sexual intercourse

  I. Do not use lice spray on a person or a pet.

  J. Laundry

    1. Use hot water and detergent.

    2. Use hot dryer.

    3. Use hot iron.

    4. Change all clothing and bed linen daily.

  K. Woolens

    1. Dry clean.

    2. Press with hot iron, paying particular attention to seams of clothing if infestation with body lice.

    3. If expense of dry cleaning is prohibitive, place articles in sealed plastic bag for 35 days (ova generally hatch in 8–9 days but may remain dormant for up to 35 days, and newly hatched nymphs must feed within 24 hours to survive).

  L. Furniture

    1. Vacuum.

    2. Use R&C Spray (lice control insecticide) or hot iron on upholstered furniture.

    3. Damp-dust or wash other furniture.

  M. Kwell

    1. Avoid unnecessary skin contact. If treating more than one child, use rubber gloves for applying.

    2. Do not use on open cuts or extensive excoriations.

    3. Has no residual effects; therefore, should not be used for prevention

    4. Requires a prescription

  N. Notify school nurse; most schools have a "no nit" policy.

  O. Examine all contacts.

IX. Follow-up

  A. Recheck in 3–5 days if child presents with secondary infection.

X. Complications

  A. Secondary bacterial infection

  B. Concomitant sexually transmitted diseases seen with pediculosis pubis

XI. Consultation/Referral

  A. Concomitant sexually transmitted disease (eg, gonorrhea, syphilis, trichomoniasis, chlamydia)

NOTES

NOTES

PERTUSSIS

An acute communicable respiratory illness; commonly known as whooping cough. The "whoop" is a classic manifestation caused by a sudden massive inspiration following episodes of severe repetitive coughing.

I. **Etiology**
   A. *Bordetella pertussis*
II. **Incidence**
   A. Becoming increasingly important in the differential diagnosis of cough
   B. Incidence is increasing most rapidly among young adults because of lack of exposure to the disease and waning immunity. This group of young adults serves as a reservoir for the organism and transmits the disease to infants and young children, most of whom contract it because of underimmunization.
   C. Protection after the last dose of DTP wanes and is generally absent 12 years after the last dose.
   D. Occurs worldwide, with about 1 million deaths in children every year. Half the reported cases in the United States are in children under 1 year of age, and 12% occur in children older than 15 years.
   E. Most commonly seen vaccine-preventable disease (except for varicella). If allowances are made for underreporting and misdiagnosis, the rate would be even higher.
III. **Incubation period**
   A. 7–10 days after exposure
IV. **Communicability**
   A. Transmission occurs from person to person by respiratory droplet infection.
   B. Highly communicable in the beginning of the catarrhal stage. Communicability decreases over time and lasts until 3 weeks after onset of paroxysmal cough.
V. **Subjective data**
   A. History of upper respiratory infection that becomes progressively worse
   B. Cough that becomes increasingly persistent over a period of 1–2 weeks
   C. Generally afebrile
   D. Classically presents in three stages
      1. Phase I (catarrhal stage): 2-week duration
         a. Cough
         b. Coryza
      2. Phase II (paroxysmal stage): 2–4-week duration
         a. Episodic, sudden coughing
         b. Whooping with cough (pathognomonic)
         c. Vomiting with cough
      3. Phase III (convalescent stage): Lasts for months
   E. Paroxysms may be precipitated by eating, drinking, or activity.
   F. Paroxysms may occur 20 or more times a day.
   G. Whoop and paroxysms may be mild or absent in children and young adults who have been immunized.
   H. History of exposure to person with a chronic paroxysmal cough

VI. **Objective data**

    A. Generally no significant physical findings to confirm diagnosis

    B. Cough

        1. Episodic, paroxysmal

        2. Whoop may be heard.

    C. Subconjunctival hemorrhages

    D. Petechiae

    E. Check for signs of secondary infection in ears and lungs.

    F. Hernia (inguinal or umbilical)

    G. Laboratory tests

        1. Children under 11 years of age

            a. Nasopharyngeal culture for *B pertussis*. (Use alginate swab, leave in place for 20 seconds, inoculate special media.)

            b. Most sensitive during catarrhal stage and during the first 14 days after onset of cough.

        2. Children over 11 years of age

            a. Nasopharyngeal culture during catarrhal phase, 14 days or less of illness

            b. Serology for IGG antibody to *B pertussis* during paroxysmal stage, after 14 days of illness

                (1) Very specific

                (2) Sensitivity increases with duration of cough.

                (3) *Note:* Serology is not interpretable in children under 11 years of age because of antibody levels persisting after immunization.

VII. **Diagnosis**

    A. If a whoop is present, the diagnosis is easily considered and confirmed by nasopharyngeal culture or serology.

    B. Because most cases are atypical or modified by immunization, pertussis should be a diagnostic consideration in children or adolescents with a persistent cough.

VIII. **Plan**

    A. Preferred treatment: Erythromycin, 40–50 mg/kg/day in four divided doses (child more than 20 kg, 250 mg four times daily) for 14 days. Adult dosage, 500 mg four times a day for 14 days.

    B. Alternative treatment: Trimethoprim (TMP)–sulfamethoxazole (SMX), 8 mg TMP and 40 mg SMX/kg/day in two divided doses (10 kg, 5 ml every 12 hours; more than 40 kg, one DS tablet every 12 hours) for 14 days. Adult dosage, 160 mg TMP and 800 mg SMX/day in two divided doses (one DS tablet every 12 hours) for 14 days.

    C. Treat all household and close contacts (eg, day care, classmates, school personnel, sports contacts) regardless of age, history of disease, or immunization status.

    D. Report to local Board of Health.

    E. Contacts under 7 years of age who are unimmunized or have received fewer than 5 doses of DTP should be immunized.

    F. Children who received their third dose of DTP more than 6 months before exposure should be given the fourth dose.

G. Children who received four doses of DTP should have a booster unless given within the last 3 years.

IX. **Education**

A. Do not return to school or work until receiving 5 days of treatment.

B. Partially immunized or unimmunized infants are at high risk.

C. Cough may persist for 6 months or more and is aggravated by subsequent upper respiratory infections.

D. Avoid situations that trigger attacks.

E. Maintain hydration and nutrition.

X. **Follow-up**

A. Maintain telephone follow-up in uncomplicated cases.

B. Return to office with any suspicion of complications.

XI. **Complications**

A. Respiratory
   1. Bronchopneumonia: Significant fever, tachypnea
   2. Atelectasis
   3. Bronchiectasis
   4. Pneumothorax
   5. Interstitial or subcutaneous emphysema

B. Otitis media

C. Central nervous system complications
   1. Seizures
   2. Coma
   3. Hemiplegia, paraplegia
   4. Ataxia
   5. Blindness
   6. Deafness

D. Secondary pressure effects during paroxysmal stage
   1. Epistaxis
   2. Melena
   3. Petechiae
   4. Subdural hematoma
   5. Hernia (umbilical, inguinal)
   6. Rectal prolapse

XII. **Consultation/Referral**

A. Consult for all children with pertussis.

B. Refer all infants for hospitalization.

NOTES

NOTES

| PINWORMS

Infestation by intestinal parasite; generally benign; characterized by anal pruritus, especially at night

I. **Etiology**

   A. *Enterobius vermicularis,* a 4-mm worm; inhabits rectum or colon and emerges to lay eggs in the skin folds of the anus. Ingested eggs hatch in the duodenum, mature in the small intestine, and reproduce in the cecum. The worms then migrate to the rectum and eventually to the perianal skin, where eggs are laid. The eggs become infectious within 2–4 hours.

   B. Entire cycle, from ingestion of eggs to egg-laying phase, takes 4–6 weeks.

II. **Incidence**

   A. Most common parasitic infestation in children in the United States

   B. All ages are susceptible.

   C. Autoinfection is common.

   D. Humans are the only host.

III. **Incubation period**

   A. 3–6 weeks after ingestion of eggs

IV. **Communicability**

   A. Transmissible through fecal–oral route as long as viable worms are present

V. **Subjective data**

   A. Perianal pruritus, especially at night

   B. Restlessness during sleep

   C. Females may complain of pain or itching of genitals.

   D. If anus is inspected during the night, ova or white, threadlike worms, about 0.5–1.0 cm long, may be seen.

VI. **Objective data**

   A. Rectal excoriation may be seen

   B. Inflammation of vulva may be seen

   C. Pinworms or ova almost never observed in the office

VII. **Assessment**

   A. Diagnosis is made by microscopic identification of ova on transparent Scotch tape that has been applied to the perianal area and placed on a glass slide. Before microscopic examination, place a drop of toluene between tape and slide.

VIII. **Plan**

   A. Mebendazole (Vermox) chewable tablets, 100 mg orally, one time, for all ages over 2 years

   B. Treat all family members simultaneously, except pregnant women and children under 2 years of age.

   C. Sitz baths for rectal or vulvar irritation

   D. Desitin to perianal area if irritated from scratching

   E. Retreatment: Mebendazole removes young larvae as well as adult worms, but it does not destroy eggs. Retreatment can be done in 2–3 weeks, before the worms originating from eggs at the time of initial treatment progress to the egg-laying phase.

IX. **Education**

A. Teach caregiver how to prepare slide.

1. Use clear Scotch tape wrapped around finger, sticky side out.

2. Spread buttocks and tap firmly around perianal area during the night or in the early morning, preferably before the child gets up but at least before toileting.

3. Apply tape, sticky side down, to clear glass slide.

4. *Note:* Slides for diagnosis may be purchased, but the above method is less expensive and works just as well.

B. Communicability is high.

C. Transmitted directly by autoinfection: Child scratches anus, gets eggs under fingernails, and then puts fingers in mouth.

D. Pinworms are contracted through human contact only; they are not worms from dogs or cats.

E. Eggs remain viable in a humid environment for several days.

F. Stress personal hygiene to avoid autoinfection.

1. Bathe daily.

2. Wash hands after toileting and before eating.

3. Keep fingernails short and clean.

4. Wear tight cotton underpants.

5. Change underpants twice a day, in the early morning and at bedtime.

6. Change bedding nightly.

7. Laundry should be washed in hot water and dried in a hot dryer. Avoid shaking bedding and clothing before laundering.

G. Perianal itching is caused by gravid worm crawling out of anus and laying eggs.

H. Mebendazole

1. Side effects: Abdominal pain, diarrhea

2. Tablet may be chewed, swallowed, or crushed and mixed with food.

3. 95% cure rate

I. Recurrences are common, particularly in large families and dormitories.

J. Reassure caregiver that course is benign and infestation is easily treated. Pinworm infestation can be very upsetting to caregivers, who may go to extremes in environmental control.

X. **Follow-up**

A. Not generally indicated

B. Call or return to office in 3 weeks if symptomatic.

C. Treatment with mebendazole may need to be repeated.

XI. **Complications**

A. Vulvovaginitis from migration of worms to vagina

B. Secondary bacterial infection from excessive scratching

C. Occasionally, symptoms of appendicitis

XII. **Consultation/Referral**

A. Pregnancy

B. Children under 2 years of age

NOTES

PITYRIASIS ROSEA

An acute, self-limited disease characterized by a superficial scaling eruption. Seen classically on the trunk in a "Christmas tree" configuration.

I. **Etiology**
   A. Unknown; presumed to be viral in origin
   B. No definite evidence of contagion, although small epidemics have been reported

II. **Incidence**
   A. Seen frequently in children, adolescents, and young adults; rare in infants
   B. Occurs most often in spring and fall

III. **Subjective data**
   A. May be asymptomatic until rash appears
   B. Initially a single scaling, erythematous maculopapular patch with central clearing; generally found on the trunk
   C. Mild prodromal symptoms occasionally (headache, malaise, sore throat, swollen glands)
   D. Rash appears 3–10 days after initial lesion.
   E. Pruritus of varying degrees

IV. **Objective data**
   A. Herald patch ("mother spot") precedes the generalized rash by 2–10 days.
      1. Initial lesion
      2. Scaly with central clearing; salmon-colored
      3. Round or oval plaque 3–6 cm in diameter
      4. Spreads peripherally
      5. Border erythematous
   B. Rash
      1. Salmon-colored, oval lesions
      2. Lesions smaller than herald patch; vary in size
      3. Lesions scaly, generally macular and papular. Vesicular lesions may be present.
      4. Generally seen on normally clothed areas (i.e., trunk), but occasionally a reverse distribution is seen with prominent involvement of the face and proximal extremities.
      5. In typical case, long axis of lesions are seen along cleavage lines, parallel to the ribs, and a Christmas tree configuration can be seen on the back.
   C. Mild regional lymphadenopathy

V. **Assessment**
   A. Diagnosis. Usually readily diagnosed by appearance and distribution of rash, particularly if herald patch is present
   B. Differential diagnosis
      1. Tinea corporis: Primary lesion is very similar in appearance, but child is not usually seen with primary lesion alone.
      2. Seborrheic dermatitis: Lesions may appear similar but do not have characteristic distribution.

3. Secondary syphilis: Generalized rashes of secondary syphilis and pityriasis are strikingly similar except for pruritus. A serologic test is often indicated to rule out syphilis in patients who are sexually active.

4. Psoriasis: Lesions have silvery scales and are on elbows, knees, scalp as well; more insidious onset.

5. Guttate psoriasis: Acute onset after streptococcal infection. If initial lesions appear on trunk, they are similar to those of pityriasis without the herald patch.

VI. **Plan**

Symptomatic treatment

A. Aveeno oatmeal baths

B. Calamine lotion, applied three times daily

C. Benadryl, 12.5–25 mg t.i.d. to q.i.d.
or
Periactin, 2–6 years: 2 mg po, b.i.d. or t.i.d.; 7–14 years: 4 mg po, b.i.d. or t.i.d.

D. Exposure to sunlight relieves itching and enhances resolution of rash.

E. Severe pruritus: Prednisone, 1–2 mg/kg/day in three divided doses for 5 days

VII. **Education**

A. No need to isolate; low communicability

B. Typically, the rash develops over a 2-week period, persists for 2 weeks, and then fades over another 2 weeks. The duration of the rash can be as long as 3–4 months, but it commonly disappears within 6 weeks.

C. Rash disappears in the reverse order in which it appeared.

D. Recurrences are uncommon.

E. Antihistamine may cause drowsiness.

F. Prognosis is excellent; disease is self-limited.

VIII. **Follow-up**

A. None indicated as a rule. However, with a severe inflammatory reaction, it is advisable to keep in contact by telephone.

B. Recheck in 5 days if on prednisone.

IX. **Complications**

A. Lesions excoriated from scratching may be secondarily infected.

X. **Consultation/Referral**

A. Extensive rash

B. Severe pruritus

NOTES

NOTES

POISON IVY OR POISON OAK DERMATITIS

An acute, intensely pruritic vesicular dermatitis characterized by a linear eruption

I. **Etiology**
   A. *Rhus* toxins produced by poison ivy and poison oak
   B. The eruption is a delayed hypersensitivity reaction to urushiol, which is present in the poison ivy and poison oak plants and is released with trauma to the leaves.
   C. Dried leaves, stems, and roots as well as burning vines may release particles, affecting sensitive persons.

II. **Incidence**
   A. Most common contact dermatoses seen in a physician's office
   B. Most common in the summer but can occur at any time of year

III. **Communicability**
   A. Dermatitis cannot be transmitted to another person. However, if the oil from the plant is on the skin of the affected person, a susceptible person could contract it in that manner.

IV. **Subjective data**
   A. Rash
      1. Vesicular
      2. Intensely itchy
      3. Continues to occur over a period of several days
   B. History
      1. Playing in the woods, skating on bogs or ponds, camping, fishing, other outdoor activities
      2. Weeding, burning brush
      3. Previous episode of poison ivy or oak dermatitis

V. **Objective data**
   A. Classic eruption is a vesicular, linear rash; however, linear and nonlinear erythematous papules are found as well.
   B. Face may be erythematous and edematous.
   C. Inspect entire body, as rash may be found anywhere on body.
   D. Rash commonly found on genitals
      1. From exposure to the plant when voiding in the woods
      2. From failure to wash hands before using bathroom inside
   E. Check for secondary infection or ulceration from scratching.

VI. **Diagnosis**
   A. Diagnosis is generally made by characteristic vesicular rash in a linear distribution that is intensely pruritic.
   B. Differential diagnosis
      1. Scabies
      2. Contact dermatitis from primary irritants: By distribution of rash and history

   3. Psoriasis: Dry patches with silvery scales
   4. Eczema: By distribution of rash and history
VII. Plan
   A. Mild
   1. Domeboro (Burow's solution) soaks
      a. Dissolve on packet in one quart of cool water.
      b. Apply for 20 minutes two or three times a day.
   2. Diphenhydramine (Benadryl), 12.5–25 mg three or four times a day, or chlorpheniramine (Chlor-Trimeton), 2–5 years: 1 mg every 4–6 hours (maximum 4 mg in 24 hours); 6–12 years: 2 mg every 4–6 hours (maximum 12 mg in 24 hours); over 12 years: 4 mg every 4–6 hours
   3. Calamine lotion–use as needed.
   4. 1% hydrocortisone cream four times a day for inflammation
   5. Aveeno oatmeal baths
   B. Extensive
   1. As above, plus prednisone, 1–2 mg/kg/day in three divided doses for 5 days
   C. Secondary infection
   1. For small area: Bacitracin ointment four times a day
   2. For extensive involvement: Treat as for impetigo with mupirocin (Bactroban) or systemic antibiotics.
VIII. Education
   A. Rash may appear within hours if very sensitive or a lot of contact with the plant.
   B. Rash continues to appear over several days on areas where contact was minimal.
   C. Domeboro soaks should be used as long as there are blisters and oozing.
   D. Use of antihistamine helps break the "itch–scratch" cycle.
   E. Vesicular fluid does not spread infection. Child cannot spread it to other parts of body or give it to anyone else.
   F. If contact with poison ivy or poison oak is suspected, immediate scrubbing of areas suspected to have contact may help prevent, or at least modify, the course.
   G. Clothing should be washed in hot, soapy water after exposure to remove allergenic resin.
   H. Rash may last 2 weeks.
   I. Poison ivy cannot be contracted from an animal per se, but if the urushiol adheres to the animal's fur, a person may get it from contact with the fur.
   J. Barrier creams such as Hydropel and Stokogard may decrease incidence if used before anticipated exposure.
IX. Follow-up
   A. Mild: Generally none necessary
   B. Extensive: Telephone follow-up after 4 days before discontinuing prednisone
   C. Secondary infection: Return to office if suspected.
X. Consultation/Referral
   A. Extensive dermatitis in a child under 2 years of age
   B. Severe reactions (for consideration of desensitization)

NOTES

ROSEOLA (EXANTHEM SUBITUM)

An acute disease of infants and young children characterized by a high fever that lasts 3–4 days and the appearance of a faintly erythematous maculopapular rash after defervescence

I. **Etiology**

   A. Confirmation not available, but evidence suggests human herpes virus 6.

II. **Incidence**

   A. Most common in spring and fall, although it does occur throughout the year.

   B. Infants and preschoolers are the most susceptible: 95% of cases are seen between 6 months and 3 years of life.

   C. Peak incidence is seen in the second year of life, with 80% of cases seen before age 18 months.

III. **Incubation period**

   A. Estimated to be 7–17 days; average 10 days

IV. **Communicability**

   A. Probably for duration of illness

V. **Subjective data**

   A. Abrupt onset of high fever (up to 103°–105°F) for 3–4 days

   B. Irritability

   C. May present with a febrile convulsion

   D. Generally, symptoms are minimal.

VI. **Objective data**

   A. Child appears nontoxic.

   B. Slight edema of eyelids

   C. Mild pharyngitis

   D. Suboccipital and cervical lymphadenopathy may be present.

   E. Typical clinical course

      1. Spiking high fever and irritability for 3–4 days

      2. Fever falls by crisis to normal or subnormal.

      3. Exanthem appears just before or shortly after temperature returns to normal. It is a faintly erythematous macular or maculopapular eruption, first appearing at the nape of the neck and behind the earlobes. It spreads mainly to the trunk, rarely on the face, and disappears within 24 hours.

   F. Physical examination findings are generally unremarkable.

   G. Laboratory findings

      1. Progressive leukopenia to 3,000–5,000 white blood cells on the third to fourth day of illness, with a relative lymphocytosis of up to 90%

      2. Urinalysis and culture should be done to rule out urinary tract infection.

VII. **Assessment**

   A. Diagnosis is based mainly on clinical findings, particularly if other cases are present in the community.

   B. Differential diagnosis

      1. Rubella: Prodromal period of mild catarrhal symptoms and low-grade fever; rash concurrent with fever

2. Rubeola: Prodromal period with variable fever, which elevates to 103°–104°F with appearance of rash and remains elevated. Also, cough, coryza, and conjunctivitis are present during prodrome, and Koplik's spots appear on second to fourth day of prodromal period.

3. Meningococcemia: Fever, chills, headache, nuchal rigidity, nausea, vomiting, and petechial rash are present. In children over 2 years of age, Brudzinski's and Kernig's signs are positive. Lumbar puncture is positive.

4. Urinary tract infection (before onset of rash): Do urine culture.

5. Other acute febrile illnesses

VIII. Plan

A. Treatment is symptomatic.

B. Acetaminophen, 10–15 mg/kg every 4 hours, or ibuprofen, 5–10 mg/kg every 6–8 hours

C. Tepid baths

D. Encourage fluids.

IX. Education

A. Do not overdress child.

B. Try to keep environment calm and quiet.

C. Use tepid water for bath; allow to air dry, or rub skin briskly to increase skin capillary circulation, facilitating heat loss.

D. Bathe every 2 hours as necessary.

E. Keep child well hydrated. Encourage liquids; do not worry about decreased appetite for solids.

F. Give small amounts of liquids frequently; try Popsicles, Jell-O, juice, sherbet.

G. Do not expose to other children until well.

H. One attack probably confers permanent immunity.

I. Disease is self-limited.

X. Follow-up

A. Maintain daily contact with parents until diagnosis is confirmed.

XI. Complications

A. Febrile convulsions

XII. Consultation/Referral

A. Prolonged high fever (after rash appears)

B. Febrile convulsions

C. Signs of meningeal irritation

NOTES

NOTES

SCABIES

A skin infestation of a mite; causes an intractable pruritus that is particularly intense at night when the patient is warm and the mite more active. It is characterized by a generalized excoriated eruption.

I. **Etiology**

    A. Female mite, *Sarcoptes scabiei*, burrows into stratum corneum to lay eggs. Larvae hatch within 2–4 days and move to the surface of the skin. After 14–17 days, the process is repeated by the now-mature larvae.

    B. Sensitization to the ova and feces of the mite occurs about 1 month after the initial infestation, producing the symptom of intense pruritus.

II. **Incidence**

    A. Pandemic

    B. Cyclic in nature; believed to occur in 30-year cycles, an epidemic lasting 15 years

    C. Scabies affects all ages and both sexes without regard to socioeconomic status, but it is most common in urban areas where crowded conditions enhance the spread of the mite.

    D. It also occurs as a nosocomial outbreak.

III. **Incubation period**

    A. Usually 1–3 weeks, but can be as long as 2 months

IV. **Communicability**

    A. Highly communicable

    B. Spread by skin-to-skin contact

V. **Subjective data**

    A. Rash

    B. Itching, most intense at night

    C. Restlessness; poor sleep

    D. History of similar rash in other family members or other exposure to similar rash

    E. Symptoms noted 3–4 weeks after infestation

VI. **Objective data**

    A. Characteristic lesions

        1. Linear, threadlike, grayish burrows 1–10 mm long; burrows may end in a vesicle or papule.

        2. Most predominant in finger webs, flexor surface of wrists, and antecubital fossae

    B. Other lesions

        1. Vesicles, papules (pale pink, pinpoint size), excoriations

        2. Pustules present with secondary infection

        3. Bullous lesions are often present on face, palms, and soles of infants and small children.

    C. Distribution

        1. Generally below the neck, but palms, soles, head, and neck may be involved in infants and children.

2. Most common sites of lesions
   a. Finger webs
   b. Wrists
   c. Extensor surfaces of elbows and knees
   d. Lateral aspect of feet
   e. Axillae
   f. Buttocks
   g. Intergluteal folds
   h. Waist
   i. Penis and scrotum in males
   j. Nipples in females
   D. Many lesions are secondarily infected.

VII. Assessment

A. Diagnosis
   1. Scrapings of the burrow or papules using a surgical blade may reveal the mite, eggs, or a black speck of feces when viewed under the microscope. These scrapings are best obtained from interdigital areas or the flexor surface of the wrists.
   2. Scrapings are often negative, so scabies must then be diagnosed by the clinical signs and symptoms as well as by the epidemiologic data.
   3. Scabies should be ruled out in any generalized, excoriated eruption.
B. Differential diagnosis
   1. Impetigo: Secondary bacterial infection often occurs and obscures the lesions of scabies. There is a high index of suspicion, however, with widespread impetiginous lesions involving the most frequent sites of involvement of scabies; a history of intense pruritus, especially on retiring; or a positive history of exposure.

VIII. Plan

A. Follow selected treatment plan; do not overtreat. Chemical irritation from medication or a hypersensitivity reaction to the mite may result in persistent itching, which may be seen as a treatment failure. Order only enough medication for treatment schedule.
B. Children under 2 years
   1. Bathe thoroughly with soap and warm water using a rough washcloth. Towel dry.
   2. Apply crotamiton (Eurax) cream—order 60 g—to entire body from chin down. Apply to facial and scalp lesions, if present.
   3. Repeat application in 24 hours. (Child may shower after 24 hours before reapplication.)
   4. Bathe 48 hours after last application.
   5. Use clean clothing, sheets, and towels after each application and at completion of therapy.
C. Children and adults
   1. Permethrin 5% (Elimite)—order 30 g for average adult.
      a. Safe and effective in children age 2 months and older
      b. Thoroughly massage into skin from head to soles of feet.

    c. Wash off after 8–14 hours.

    d. One application usually is curative, but a second application can be repeated in 1 week.

  2. Kwell lotion (not recommended for infants or pregnant women)

    a. Bathe thoroughly with soap and hot water using rough washcloth or scrub brush. Towel dry.

    b. Apply Kwell lotion from chin down. Apply to facial and scalp lesions, if present.

    c. Leave lotion on for 12 hours, then bathe thoroughly again.

    d. Use clean clothing, sheets, and towels after application and after bathing.

    e. Repeat application in 1 week (scabicides are not ovicidal, so a repeat application is needed to kill newly hatched larvae).

D. Alternative treatment for all ages: Precipitated sulfur (6%–10%) applied every 24 hours for 3 days. It is effective but less commonly used because it is messy and smells like sulfur.

E. Secondary bacterial infections

  1. Neosporin or bacitracin ointment three or four times a day 24 hours after treatment with Kwell or after treatment regimen with crotamiton for one or two infected lesions

  2. If infection is extensive, penicillin G for 10 days

F. Pruritus

  1. 1% hydrocortisone cream

  2. Diphenhydramine (Benadryl), 5 mg/kg/day in four divided doses as needed, if intense

G. It is reasonable to treat all close contacts (family members, babysitters, sexual contacts) prophylactically to prevent reinfection.

  1. Order 2 oz Kwell (maximum) per adult, 1 oz per child, and 60 g crotamiton (maximum) per person; do not give refills.

  2. Crotamiton is the primary alternative therapy. It is an antipruritic as well as a scabicide, although its cure rates are lower than those of Kwell.

IX. Education

A. Recognize that infestation by scabies can be a traumatic emotional experience for many persons. Support, education, and reassurance are vital to assist them in coping with and eradicating the parasite.

B. Scabies are acquired by close personal contact. They may also be transmitted through clothing or linens.

C. Treat close family and personal contacts if indicated.

D. Female mite can survive 2–3 days without human contact.

E. Lack of cleanliness does not cause scabies, but scrupulous hygiene can help eradicate and prevent reinfestation.

F. Low economic classes are not the only victims; scabies affects all socioeconomic groups and all ages.

G. Transmission is unlikely 24 hours after treatment is instituted.

H. Symptoms may persist for several weeks after the mites have been killed. Symptoms may be due to persistent infestation, sensitivity to the scabicide, or hypersensitivity to the mite. Patient should call back for an evaluation.

I. Notify school so nurse can be alert for symptoms of infestation in contacts.

J. Laundry

1. Use hot water and detergent.
2. Use hot dryer.
3. Use hot iron.
4. Change all clothing daily.

K. Woolens

1. Dry clean.
2. Press with hot iron.
3. If expense of dry cleaning is prohibitive, place woolens in plastic bag and seal for 2 weeks.

L. Furniture

1. Use R&C Spray for upholstered furniture.
2. Damp-dust or wash other furniture.

M. Teach parent the signs and symptoms of secondary bacterial infection.

N. Scabicide

1. Reapply to hands after washing.
2. Do not use on face or scalp unless lesions are present there.
3. Do not get in eyes or on mucous membranes.
4. Be sure to cover all areas of body, paying special attention to interdigital areas. If any areas are missed, treatment may not be successful.
5. Poisonous if ingested
6. Side effects: Eczematous eruptions
7. Do not apply to acutely inflamed skin or raw, weeping surfaces.

X. **Follow-up**

A. Check babies and small children in 7–10 days.
B. Recheck in 3–5 days if child presented with secondary infection of lesions.
C. If persistent pruritus after 2 weeks, repeat scraping of lesion to determine presence of mites.

XI. **Complications**

A. Secondary bacterial infection
B. Reaction to scabicide

XII. **Consultation/Referral**

A. Infants under 2 months and pregnant women
B. Failure to respond to therapy
C. Secondary bacterial infection

NOTES

NOTES

SCARLET FEVER

A streptococcal infection characterized by fever, pharyngitis, and a fine, sandpapery, erythematous rash

I. **Etiology**

   A. Erythrogenic strain of group A beta-hemolytic streptococci

II. **Incubation period**

   A. Average 1–3 days

III. **Communicability**

   A. Weeks or months without treatment

   B. Generally noninfectious within 24 hours after therapy is started

IV. **Subjective data**

   A. Acute onset of sore throat

   B. Fever: 102°–104°F (39°–40°C)

   C. Listlessness

   D. Abdominal pain

   E. Vomiting

   F. Rash

   G. Child appears toxic.

   H. History of exposure to streptococcal pharyngitis

V. **Objective data**

   A. Fever

   B. Toxic child

   C. Circumoral pallor

   D. "Strawberry tongue"—protruding red papillae showing on coated surface, which then desquamates

   E. Tonsils and pharynx intensely erythematous and edematous; purulent yellowish exudate on tonsils

   F. Palatal petechiae

   G. Anterior cervical nodes enlarged and tender

   H. Exanthem

      1. Appears 12–48 hours after onset of illness

      2. Bright-red, punctate rash with a sandpapery feel; begins in skin creases and rapidly spreads to involve the trunk, extremities, and face. Rash blanches with pressure.

      3. Lasts 3–6 days, after which desquamation occurs (particularly on fingertips and deep creases)

   I. Pastia's lines: Linear streaks of rash in antecubital fossa that do not blanch with pressure

   J. Objective findings are similar in all respects to those of streptococcal pharyngitis, except for the exanthem and the strawberry tongue.

VI. **Assessment**

   A. Diagnosis is usually made by clinical appearance and a throat culture strongly positive for group A streptococcus.

   1. Throat culture positive for group A beta-hemolytic streptococcus
   2. White blood count usually elevated (12,000–15,000)
   B. Differential diagnosis
      1. Rubeola: Koplik's spots; characteristic rash; prodrome of cough, coryza, conjunctivitis; epidemiology
      2. Rubella: Postauricular adenopathy, mild illness, epidemiology
      3. Fifth disease: "Slapped cheek" rash, no pharyngeal signs or symptoms
      4. Roseola: Fever of 3 days; child is not toxic; rash appears after temperature drops.
      5. Enterovirus: Gastrointestinal symptoms; negative throat culture; epidemic locally.
      6. Kawasaki syndrome: Engorged conjunctival vessels; hands and feet erythematous and edematous; prolonged fever (5 or more days); fever starts high and remains high.

VII. Plan

   A. Penicillin G 200,000–400,000 U four times a day for 10 days
      1. *Note:* Buffered penicillin G is less expensive, but consider treating with penicillin V, 250 mg four times a day. The latter can be given with meals if it would enhance compliance.
   B. If child is allergic to penicillin, erythromycin 40 mg/kg/day in four divided doses (more than 20 kg, 400 mg every 12 hours) for 10 days
   C. Acetaminophen for elevated temperature and discomfort, 10–15 mg/kg every 4 hours
   D. Warm saline gargles
   E. Treat contacts at risk (eg, child who has had rheumatic fever).
   F. Cephalosporins are effective in the treatment of streptococcal pharyngitis. Penicillin, however, is safe, effective, and inexpensive and is the one agent proven in controlled studies to prevent acute rheumatic fever.

VIII. Education

   A. Medication
      1. Antibiotic must be given four times a day for 10 days. Continue drug even if child seems better.
      2. Give penicillin G 1 hour before or 2 hours after meals.
      3. Side effects of medication include nausea, vomiting, diarrhea, and rashes (maculopapular to urticarial).
   B. Isolation is unnecessary after 24 hours of antibiotic therapy.
   C. Do not send child back to school until temperature has been normal for 24 hours. Child may then resume normal activities.
   D. Encourage fluids.
      1. Try Popsicles, sherbet, Jell-O, apple juice.
      2. Avoid orange juice and carbonated beverages; they may be difficult for child to swallow.
   E. Sucking hard candies may help relieve discomfort of sore throat.
   F. Expect child to improve within 48 hours once on medication.
   G. Second attacks are rare.
   H. Generally transmitted by direct contact

IX. **Follow-up**

A. Call immediately if any symptoms of adverse reaction to penicillin.

B. Call immediately if child cannot retain medication; return to office for administration of intramuscular penicillin.

C. Call immediately if family members complain of sore throat. Cultures should be done on those with symptoms.

D. Call if no improvement within 48 hours, sooner if child seems worse.

E. Call if child improves and then 7–14 days later complains of malaise, headache, fever, anorexia, abdominal pain, edema, dark urine, decreased urinary output, or migratory joint pains.

F. Ideally, child should return for throat culture and urinalysis after completion of penicillin therapy. Follow-up at this time should include a careful cardiac examination.

X. **Complications**

A. Complications and sequelae are less likely to occur if treatment is instituted early. However, they may occur despite early, vigorous treatment.

1. Otitis media

2. Pyoderma

3. Cervical adenitis

4. Rheumatic fever

5. Acute glomerulonephritis

XI. **Consultation/Referral**

A. Prolonged course or no improvement once on medication for 48 hours

B. Any signs of complications

NOTES

SEBORRHEA OF THE SCALP (CRADLE CAP)

Inflammatory, scaling eruption of the scalp

I. **Etiology**
   A. Presumed to be accelerated epidermal growth
   B. Although it occurs in an area with large numbers of sebaceous glands, there is no documented proof that it is caused by increased sebum production.

II. **Incidence**
   A. Occurs predominantly in newborns and adolescents

III. **Subjective data**
   A. Pruritus
   B. Scaling of the scalp
   C. Dandruff
   D. Often no presenting complaints; may be found on routine physical examination

IV. **Objective data**
   A. Scalp is primary site.
      1. Slight to severe erythema
      2. Yellowish, greasy scales
      3. Excoriations from scratching
   B. Check entire body, as seborrhea may progress to other areas.
      1. Face: Erythema and scaling may progress to forehead, eyebrows, eyelashes (marginal blepharitis), and cheeks.
      2. Ears: Dryness, scaling, erythema, and cracking in postauricular areas
      3. Back of neck, groin, umbilicus, and gluteal crease may also have erythema and fine, dry scaling.
      4. Secondary infection may occur.

V. **Assessment**
   A. Diagnosis is generally made by the typical clinical picture of a yellowish, greasy, crusted dermatosis of the scalp in an infant; in an older child by erythema and scaling of the scalp.
   B. Differential diagnosis
      1. Tinea capitis: Lesions round; broken hair stumps in lesions
      2. Tinea corporis: Erythematous, circinate or oval scaling patches
      3. Psoriasis: Erythematous macules or papules covered with dry, silvery scales

VI. **Plan**
   A. Infants (cradle cap)
      1. Rub petroleum jelly into scalp to soften crusts 20–30 minutes before shampooing.
      2. Shampoo daily with baby shampoo, using a soft brush.
      3. If lesions are inflammatory or extensive, use 1% hydrocortisone cream twice a day; if nonresponsive, use betamethasone (Valisone) lotion daily for scalp only.
   B. Toddlers or adolescents (seborrhea of scalp)
      1. Antiseborrheic shampoo every other day (Selsun, Exsel, or Nizoral)

    2. If lesions are inflammatory or extensive, use topical corticosteroid lotion (Valisone) daily.

  C. Seborrheic blepharitis: See Marginal Blepharitis.

  D. Lesions on areas other than scalp: 1% hydrocortisone cream three or four times a day

VII. Education

  A. Stress prevention.

  B. Teach mothers of newborns how to shampoo and rinse hair.

  C. Reassure that it is all right to wash over "soft spot."

  D. Daily shampooing is recommended.

  E. Keep shampoo out of eyes.

  F. Do not use prescription shampoos if child is not cooperative or any sensitivity results.

  G. Continue treatment for several days after lesions disappear.

  H. Shampoo at least weekly once resolved.

  I. If lesions have spread to forehead and eyebrows, vigorous successful treatment of scalp generally results in clearing of the face.

  J. Seborrhea generally disappears by 6 months but may recur at puberty.

  K. Seborrhea cannot be cured, but it can be controlled.

  L. Seborrhea does not cause permanent hair loss or baldness unless it becomes grossly infected.

VIII. Follow-up

  A. Telephone call in 5–6 days to report progress; return to office if no improvement.

IX. Consultation/Referral

  A. Secondary impetigo

  B. No response to treatment in 10–14 days

NOTES

SEROUS OTITIS MEDIA

Accumulation of fluid in the middle ear, characterized by decreased or absent mobility of the tympanic membrane and varying degrees of hearing loss

I. **Etiology**
   A. Eustachian tube obstruction or dysfunction resulting in decreased pressure in the middle ear. The causes of eustachian tube obstruction include allergic rhinitis, upper respiratory infection, enlarged adenoids, and cleft palate.
   B. Bacteriology closely mimics that of acute otitis media.
   C. Also seen as sequela of otitis media when fluid becomes sterile but does not resolve
   D. May be caused by increased secretions of mucosa of middle ear

II. **Incidence**
   A. Most frequent cause of air conduction hearing loss in school-aged children; seen most often in 5–7-year-olds
   B. About 10% of children will have middle ear effusion persisting for 3 months or longer after an episode of acute otitis media.

III. **Subjective data**
   A. Complaints of
      1. Ears popping
      2. Ears feeling plugged or full
      3. Own voice sounding strange or hollow to child
   B. Subjective hearing loss
      1. Child may say he or she does not hear well.
      2. Parents may notice diminished hearing.
      3. Child does not respond well.
      4. Child "never listens."
      5. Child sits close to television.
      6. School grades go down.
      7. Hearing loss may be noted on school audiologic examination.
   C. May have history of otitis media, upper respiratory infection, or allergic rhinitis
   D. Condition may be asymptomatic and found on routine well child visit.

IV. **Objective data**
   A. Tympanic membrane
      1. Dull
      2. Opaque
      3. Color varies from white to bluish to orange-blue.
      4. Fluid level may be visualized behind tympanic membrane.
      5. Air bubbles may be visualized (suggesting intermittent eustachian tube function).
      6. Mobility absent or diminished (does not move inward with positive pressure but may move outward with negative pressure)
   B. Rinne test reveals bone conduction greater than air conduction.
   C. Other positive objective findings would be those associated with causes of eustachian tube obstruction.

   1. Mouth breathing
   2. Thin, watery nasal discharge
   3. Nasal turbinates pale and boggy
   D. Audiogram generally shows a 15- to 30-dB air conduction loss with normal bone conduction.
V. Assessment
   A. Diagnosis is made by pneumatic otoscopy, which reveals decreased mobility or immobility of the tympanic membrane in the absence of acute inflammation.
   B. Tympanometry and examination by acoustic otoscope confirm the diagnosis by demonstrating decreased compliance of the tympanic membrane.
VI. Plan
   A. Antimicrobials
   1. Recent studies have indicated that middle ear effusion is not a sterile process, and a course of antibiotic therapy is indicated.
   2. Treat children who have had a course of antibiotics with a second antibiotic.
   3. Antibiotic intervention may be used for 2–4 weeks.
   4. Amoxicillin, 40 mg/kg/day in three divided doses (more than 20 kg, 250 mg three times a day) for 10 days
   5. If child is allergic to penicillin and is over 2 years of age, trimethoprim (TMP)–sulfamethoxazole (SMX), 8 mg TMP and 40 mg SMX/kg/day in two divided doses (every 12 hours) for 10 days. For a child weighing 10 kg, 5 ml every 12 hours; for a child more than 40 kg, one DS tablet every 12 hours.
   6. Follow-up in 10 days as for acute otitis media
   B. Eustachian tube autoinflation: Purpose is to build up positive pressure in nasopharynx.
   1. Have child hold nose, keep lips closed, puff cheeks out, and swallow.
   2. Have child chew sugarless gum.
   C. Oral decongestants are not indicated as treatment for otitis media with effusion.
   D. Corticosteroids have not been proven effective in the treatment of middle ear effusion.
VII. Education
   A. Do not feed infant supine or give bottle in bed.
   B. Explain that it is a temporary hearing loss and common in children; normal hearing will return.
   C. Speech development may be affected.
   D. Speak slowly and distinctly to child when you have his or her full attention, preferably face to face.
   E. Do not punish for assumed inattentiveness, but be aware that manipulation may occur.
   F. Habit of asking "What?" may be formed.
   G. Notify school of problem.
   H. It may take 2–4 months for problem to resolve.
   I. Serous otitis may recur as sequela to otitis media or seasonally in an allergic child.

J. With frequent recurrences in an allergic child, allergic rhinitis should be treated.

K. Recommend that child chew sugarless gum for eustachian tube autoinflation.

VIII. **Follow-up**

A. There has been much controversy over the surgical treatment of serous otitis over the past several years, and treatment has changed from aggressive therapy to a more conservative watch-and-wait approach.

B. Child can be followed for 4 months or longer with a unilateral serous otitis.

C. Referral for a myringotomy may need to be made after 1 month of observation if child has bilateral serous otitis, especially if it is interfering with speech development or school progress.

D. Follow-up must be individualized for each patient. Psychosocial factors and development, as well as tympanic membrane mobility and audiogram, must be assessed at each visit.

E. General guidelines

1. Recheck in 2 weeks. Discontinue antibiotics if tympanic membrane mobility and audiogram are normal. If examination is not within normal limits, continue treatment and recheck in another 2 weeks.

2. Recheck in 2 weeks. The presence of air bubbles behind the tympanic membrane indicates intermittent functioning of the eustachian tubes. If child is not handicapped by hearing loss, continue to recheck at 2–4-week intervals.

3. Rechecks should include audiometric evaluation in addition to otoscopic examination.

4. Refer for evaluation for myringotomy with tube insertion if

a. Persistent effusion between episodes of acute otitis media

b. Consistent hearing loss of more than 15 dB for longer than 3 months

5. *Note:* Tube insertion decreases scarring of tympanic membrane and middle ear space and diminishes cholesteatoma formation and chronic conductive hearing loss in these children.

IX. **Complications**

A. Delayed speech development

B. Poor school progress

C. Problems with social adjustment

X. **Consultation/Referral**

A. Bilateral hearing loss (30–50 dB) interfering with speech development and school progress

B. No improvement after 2 months

C. No resolution after 3 months

D. For evaluation for respiratory allergy, obstructive adenoidal hypertrophy, immunodeficiency, submucous cleft palate

NOTES

NOTES

SINUSITIS, BACTERIAL

An acute inflammatory process involving one or more of the paranasal sinuses

I. **Etiology**

   A. *Streptococcus pneumoniae, Haemophilus influenzae,* and *Moraxella catarrhalis* are the bacteria most commonly responsible for acute bacterial sinusitis (70%). Other organisms implicated are *Staphylococcus aureus, Streptococcus pyogenes,* gram-negative bacilli, and respiratory viruses.

   B. Acute sinusitis usually follows rhinitis, which may be viral, allergic, or vasomotor in origin. It also may result from abrupt pressure changes (eg, airplane travel, diving) or from dental extractions or infections.

II. **Incidence**

   A. The incidence of sinusitis closely parallels the incidence of upper respiratory tract infections because the paranasal sinuses are lined with epithelium that is contiguous with the rest of the respiratory tract; therefore, it is seen most often in winter.

   B. If associated with allergic rhinitis, incidence increases at times of high pollen counts.

III. **Subjective data**

   A. History of upper respiratory infection or allergic rhinitis

   B. History of pressure change (eg, airplane, diving, bungee jumping)

   C. Sensation of pressure over sinuses followed by local pain and tenderness

   D. Pain increases in intensity 1–2 hours after arising and subsides in late afternoon.

   E. Malaise

   F. Low-grade fever

   G. Purulent nasal discharge

   H. Postnasal drip

   I. Cough

   J. History of previous episodes of sinusitis

IV. **Objective data**

   A. Nasal mucosa edematous and hyperemic

   B. Percussion or palpation tenderness over a sinus

      1. Maxillary sinusitis: Over cheek and upper teeth

      2. Frontal sinusitis: In forehead above the eyebrow

      3. Sphenoid sinusitis: Headache in occipital area

      4. Anterior ethmoidal sinusitis: In the temporal area

      5. Posterior ethmoidal sinusitis: Over trigeminal nerve distribution

   C. Purulent nasal discharge in corresponding nasal meatus

   D. Postnasal discharge visualized in posterior pharynx

   E. Periorbital swelling

   F. Examine for other respiratory tract involvement.

   G. History positive for upper respiratory infection of greater than 7–10 days' duration

   H. Laboratory studies

1. Culture of sinus puncture aspirates
   a. Most reliable indicator other than sinus biopsy
   b. Indicated if child is not responsive to therapy, in an immunocompromised child, or with life-threatening complications
2. X-ray is not a reliable indicator: Most children with an uncomplicated upper respiratory infection have abnormal x-rays, as do many children without upper respiratory infections.
3. CT scan is often abnormal in patients without clinical signs of sinusitis.

V. **Assessment: Differential diagnosis**

A. Viral upper respiratory infection: Low-grade fever, pharyngitis, conjunctivitis; typically presents with 2–3 days of purulent nasal discharge that then turns clear again
B. Group A streptococcal infection: Nasopharyngeal or throat culture positive for group A streptococci
C. Nasal foreign body: Unilateral, foul-smelling discharge, often bloody

VI. **Plan**

A. Antimicrobials: Treat for 2–3 weeks, depending on severity, with one of the following:
   1. Amoxicillin, 20–40 mg/kg/day in three divided doses (more than 20 kg, 250 mg three times a day)
   2. Amoxicillin and clavulanic acid (Augmentin), 25–45 mg/kg/day in two divided doses (more than 20 kg, 400 mg every 12 hours). Do not use regular 250- or 500-mg tablets for a child less than 40 kg; use chewables or suspension.
   3. Clarithromycin (Biaxin), 15 mg/kg/day in two divided doses (more than 30 kg, 250 mg every 12 hours)
   4. Cefprozil (Cefzil), 15 mg/kg/day in two divided doses (more than 35 kg, 250 mg twice a day)
   5. Loracarbef (Lorabid), 30 mg/kg/day in two divided doses (more than 26 kg, 400 mg twice a day)
B. Budenoside (Rhinocort) nasal spray, two sprays in each nostril every 12 hours for children over 6 years

VII. **Education**

A. Moist heat over affected sinus may ease discomfort.
B. Prolonged shower (for as long as hot water lasts) helps promote drainage.
C. Avoid deep diving or jumping into deep water with an upper respiratory infection.
D. Sinus inflammation occurs as a normal part of a cold; antibiotics are not always indicated.
E. Budenoside nasal spray
   1. Blow nose gently before use.
   2. Gently inhale with actuation of spray.

VIII. **Follow-up**

A. Call in 48 hours if not improved.
B. Recheck in 2 weeks.

IX. **Consultation/Referral**
   A. Chills and fever
   B. Persistent headache
   C. Edema of forehead, eyelids
   D. Orbital cellulitis

NOTES

STREPTOCOCCAL PHARYNGITIS

An acute pharyngitis seen in about 10% of all children who present with a sore throat

I. **Etiology**
   A. Group A beta-hemolytic streptococcus (*Streptococcus pyogenes*)
II. **Incubation period**
   A. 1–3 days
III. **Communicability**
   A. Weeks or months without treatment
   B. Generally noninfectious within 24 hours once treatment has started
IV. **Subjective data**
   A. Acute onset of sore throat
   B. Fever 102°–104°F (39°–40°C)
   C. Vomiting, abdominal pain
   D. Listlessness
   E. Dysphagia
   F. Voice thick or muffled, not hoarse
   G. Anorexia
   H. Urticaria
   I. History of exposure to streptococcal pharyngitis
   J. May have few presenting symptoms
V. **Objective data**
   A. Typical clinical findings
      1. Elevated temperature
      2. Tonsils and pharynx intensely erythematous
      3. Purulent, yellowish exudate on tonsils
      4. Petechiae or "doughnut lesions" (raised red lesions with pale centers) on soft palate
      5. Edematous, beefy-red uvula
      6. Anterior cervical nodes enlarged and tender
      7. Infant may present with excoriated nares.
   B. May not present with typical picture
      1. A throat culture should be done to confirm or deny diagnosis of group A beta-hemolytic streptococcus in any child with pharyngitis.
      2. This author has seen many instances when the presenting complaint has been an urticarial rash with no history of pharyngitis. However, in examining the child and finding erythema of the anterior pillars, I found a markedly positive rapid strep test for group A streptococcus.
VI. **Assessment**
   A. Diagnosis
      1. Rapid direct antigen test (DAT) or throat culture positive for group A beta-hemolytic streptococcus

2. *Note:* Current data on rapid strep tests suggests that the specificity is 95%–99% and the sensitivity is 85%–95% and higher when more than 10 colonies of streptococcus are present.

3. If the rapid strep test is negative, a conventional throat culture should be done if clinically warranted.

B. Differential diagnosis

1. Viral pharyngitis: Negative rapid strep test or negative throat culture

2. Infectious mononucleosis: Positive heterophil antibody or Monospot test; more generalized adenopathy; tonsillar exudate generally thicker and whiter. 20% of children with infectious mononucleosis have concurrent streptococcal pharyngitis.

VII. Plan

A. Penicillin G, 200,000–400,000 U four times a day for 10 days

1. *Note:* Although buffered penicillin G is less expensive, consider treating with penicillin V 250 mg four times a day, which can be given with meals, if this treatment schedule would enhance compliance.

B. If allergic to penicillin, erythromycin, 40 mg/kg/day in four divided doses for 10 days

C. For fever, headache, and general discomfort, acetaminophen, 10–15 mg/kg every 4 hours, or ibuprofen, 5–10 mg/kg every 6–8 hours

D. Warm saline gargles

E. Treat contacts at risk (eg, child who has had rheumatic fever).

F. Cephalosporins are effective in the treatment of streptococcal pharyngitis. Penicillin, however, is safe and inexpensive and is the one agent proven in controlled studies to prevent acute rheumatic fever.

VIII. Education

A. Medication

1. Antibiotic must be given four times a day for 10 consecutive days.

2. Give penicillin G 1 hour before or 2 hours after meals.

3. Continue antibiotic even if child seems better.

4. Side effects of medication include nausea, vomiting, diarrhea, and rashes (maculopapular to urticarial).

B. Isolation is unnecessary after 24 hours of antibiotic therapy.

C. Clinical improvement is generally noted within 24 hours after initiating treatment.

D. Do not send child back to school until temperature has been normal for 24 hours. Child may then resume normal activities.

E. Force fluids.

1. Try popsicles, sherbet, Jell-O, apple juice.

2. Avoid orange juice and carbonated beverages; they may be difficult for child to swallow.

3. Do not be concerned about solid food intake.

F. Sucking hard candies may help relieve discomfort of sore throat.

G. Expect child to improve within 48 hours once on medication.

H. Immunity is not conferred, but some resistance is built up.

I. Streptococcal pharyngitis is transmitted by direct or close contact.

IX. **Follow-up**

    A. Call immediately if any symptoms of adverse reaction to medication.

    B. Call immediately if child cannot retain medication; return to office for intramuscular medication.

    C. Call back if child is not improved within 48 hours.

    D. Call immediately if other family members complain of sore throat. Those with symptoms should have a throat culture.

    E. Call if after 7–14 days child complains of malaise, headache, fever, anorexia, abdominal pain, edema, dark urine, decreased urinary output, or migratory joint pains.

    F. Ideally, child should return for throat culture and urinalysis after completion of antibiotic therapy. Follow-up should include a careful cardiac examination.

    G. Follow-up throat culture and eradication of carrier state are indicated:

        1. When family has a history of rheumatic fever

        2. When "ping-pong" spread of group A beta-hemolytic streptococcus has occurred within a family

        3. When outbreaks occur in closed or semiclosed communities

        4. When tonsillectomy is considered because of chronic group A beta-hemolytic streptococcus

        5. When family is inordinately anxious about group A beta-hemolytic streptococcus

        6. Treatment for eradicating carrier state

            a. Rifampin, 20 mg/kg every 24 hours for four doses during the last 4 days of penicillin therapy

            b. Clindamycin, 20 mg/kg/day orally in three divided doses for 10 days

X. **Complications**

    A. Complications and sequelae are less likely to occur if treatment is instituted early, but they may occur despite early, vigorous treatment.

        1. Otitis media

        2. Pyoderma

        3. Cervical adenitis

        4. Rheumatic fever (risk about 0.3%)

        5. Acute glomerulonephritis (risk 10%–15% if infecting strain is nephritogenic)

XI. **Consultation/Referral**

    A. Prolonged course

    B. Any signs of peritonsillar abscess (eg, asymmetric swelling of tonsils, uvula shifted to one side, edema of palate)

    C. Any signs or symptoms of acute glomerulonephritis or rheumatic fever

    D. Frequent recurrences of streptococcal pharyngitis

NOTES

NOTES

SUICIDE PREVENTION

Suicide is the act of taking one's own life. Suicide attempts are acts of life-threatening behavior that fall short of completion. Suicidal ideas are thoughts or plans about self-destruction. Death by suicide is by nature secretive.

Because suicide is such a strong social taboo, many health care workers are reluctant even to ask patients about it. Many persons feel that suicide is a sign of craziness, weakness, lack of courage, possession by the devil, or moral inadequacy. Health care workers often miss opportunities to interview or help persons considering suicide.

I. Etiology

    A. The causes of suicide are many, but the most common is the turmoil of adolescence, that critical period during which a person is establishing his or her identity, learning to be independent, growing physically and intellectually, choosing a career, and developing love relationships. For some persons, adolescence is a time of great unhappiness, rebellion, confusion, and disturbance.

II. Incidence

    A. Because of family instability and mobility, children may be deprived of the nurturing and love they need to withstand the pressures of growing up.

    B. It used to be that suicide affected primarily adolescents, but in recent years there has been an increase of 150% in the incidence of suicide among persons aged 10–24. 10% of deaths of adolescents and young children are by suicide.

    C. Many suicides are now occurring in clusters of high school students, often three or four in one class in a week (a recent phenomenon).

    D. Suicide attempts in the United States are estimated to number 300,000–500,000 per year, and an estimated 12,000 suicides occur annually in the United States among children aged 14 years or younger.

    E. 90% of suicides in adolescent girls are by ingestion of drugs; 90% of suicides in adolescent boys are by hanging.

III. Reasons

    A. To get even ("You'll be sorry when I'm gone")

    B. Way out of conflicts with parents; lack of close relationships

    C. Desire to be with someone who died

    D. Impulsiveness

IV. Personality characteristics

    A. Child at risk

        1. Impulsive, acting out

        2. Depressed

        3. Angry

        4. Loner; no social skills, few friends, withdrawn

        5. In crisis due to loss of parent through divorce or death of loved one

        6. Lacks ability to communicate; suicide attempt is cry for help.

    B. Suicide completer

        1. Often very bright intellectually

        2. May go to highly competitive schools

        3. Does not solve problems well

4. Exceedingly demanding of self
5. Sees things as right or wrong
6. Achiever, hard worker
7. Does not respond to therapist in diagnostic interview
8. Loner, socially withdrawn
9. Most importantly, displays termination behaviors: gives important things away and disengages from usual activities

V. **Warning signs and symptoms**

A. Previous attempts: Eight of 10 successful suicides are carried out by persons who have attempted the act before.

B. Threat of suicide

C. Depression: Extreme sadness; feelings of helplessness, hopelessness, and worthlessness; low self-esteem

D. Changes in school behavior that last for more than 2–3 weeks: Emotional outbursts, failing grades, falling asleep in class, inability to communicate, problems with drugs or alcohol

E. Changes in appetite, usually decreasing but sometimes increasing

F. Changes in sleep patterns; too much or too little sleep may indicate depression.

G. Increase in substance abuse (drugs or alcohol)

H. Changes in peer group or peer relationships

I. Stresses

1. Parent–child conflict
2. Physical or sexual abuse by parents
3. Dysfunctional family unit (due to recent divorce, death, or substance abuse, for instance)
4. Rejection or neglect by others; feeling that nobody cares

VI. **Management**

A. Immediate response and rapid intervention are critical.

B. Reassure child he or she does have someone to turn to.

C. Don't lecture. Point out all the reasons a person has to live, but listen and reassure child that he or she can be treated. Take the child seriously and show you care. Do not show shock or disapproval.

D. If a child is depressed, do not be afraid to ask, "Do you feel like killing or harming yourself?"

E. Assess safety of child; get him or her to agree not to act on suicidal impulses. Refer to mental health professional.

F. Be ready to intervene against any suicide attempt.

G. Psychotherapy should include family (in group therapy as well as initial interview), school personnel, and peers. Child may be hospitalized to provide protective, comprehensive therapeutic setting.

H. Record in writing all events, information given, and plan of referral.

NOTES

NOTES

THRUSH

Oral candidiasis is characterized by white plaques on inflamed oral mucosa. It is often associated with cutaneous candidiasis in the diaper or intertriginous areas.

I.   **Etiology**

    A. *Candida albicans*

II.   **Incidence**

    A. Seen primarily in newborns and infants up to 6 months of age, who have less immunity than older children to *C albicans*

    B. Newborns can be infected during passage through the vagina; infants can contract it from mother with breast infection.

III.   **Incubation period**

    A. Highly variable

IV.   **Subjective data**

    A. Fussy, irritable infant

    B. Difficulty feeding or refusal to nurse

    C. White spots on tongue and inside of mouth

    D. Mother may have history of vaginal candidiasis.

    E. Nursing mother may have concomitant infection of nipples and areola.

    F. Infant may have history of concurrent or previous antibiotic therapy.

V.   **Objective data**

    A. White, curdlike plaques on inflamed oral mucosa

    B. Located on tongue, buccal mucosa, gingivae, and throat

    C. Plaques cannot be easily removed. If they are wiped away, bleeding occurs.

    D. Early lesions start as pinpoint in size and grow.

    E. Cracks or fissures may appear in corners of mouth.

    F. Lesions may extend to esophagus.

    G. Inspect skin for concomitant candidiasis of diaper area or intertriginous areas.

VI.   **Assessment**

    A. Diagnosis is readily made by the clinical picture.

    B. Differential diagnosis

        1. Milk deposits: May resemble thrush but are easily removed by wiping with a gauze pad

VII.   **Plan**

    A. Nystatin (Mycostatin) oral suspension

        1. Infants: 1 ml in each side of mouth four times a day

        2. Premature or low-birthweight infants: 0.5 ml in each side of mouth four times a day

        3. Continue for 48 hours after symptoms disappear
        or

    B. Fungizone (amphotericin B) oral suspension

        1. 1 ml (100 mg) four times a day between feedings

        2. Continue treatment for 2 weeks

  C. Candidiasis in diaper area: See Candidiasis (Diaper Rash).

VIII. Education

  A. Give infant small amount of water before medication to rinse inside of mouth.

  B. Try to remove large plaques with cotton swab moistened with water.

  C. Call immediately if infant refuses liquids.

  D. Try infant feeder if infant refuses bottle or breast.

  E. Diaper rash may occur concomitantly. Leave diaper area exposed as much as possible to help eliminate the warmth and moisture that *C albicans* thrives on; see Candidiasis (Diaper Rash).

  F. Sterilize nipples and pacifiers.

  G. Wash toys well to prevent reinfection.

  H. If breast-feeding, wash nipples well with warm water before and after feeding. Allow to air dry.

  I. Observe careful hand-washing technique.

  J. Call if infant does not improve or seems worse.

  K. If mother has symptoms of vaginal candidiasis, she should be referred for treatment.

  L. Newborns can be infected during passage through the vagina of a mother with candidiasis; infants can contract it from mothers with breast infection.

IX. Follow-up

  A. Telephone contact in 3–4 days to assess progress. If no improvement noted, return visit is indicated.

X. Complications

  A. Persistent or recurrent thrush

  B. Systemic candidiasis in debilitated infants or those on immunosuppressive therapy

XI. Consultation/Referral

  A. Persistent or recurrent thrush, for evaluation of immunologic status

  B. No improvement in 5 days

  C. Mother with vaginal candidiasis

NOTES

| TINEA CORPORIS

Ringworm of the body, a superficial fungal infection of the nonhairy skin

I. **Etiology**
   A. *Trichophyton* and *Microsporum* dermatophyte fungi
II. **Incidence**
   A. Most prevalent in hot, humid climates
   B. Children are the most susceptible.
III. **Incubation period**
   A. 4–10 days
IV. **Subjective data**
   A. Pruritic or asymptomatic lesions
   B. Complaint of rash, round sores, or ringworm
   C. History of exposure to infected person or animal
V. **Objective data**
   A. Lesions
      1. Flat, erythematous papules
      2. Spread peripherally
      3. Clear centrally
      4. Develop into circinate or oval lesions with scaling papular or vesicular advancing borders
   B. Distribution: Most commonly seen on face, neck, and arms but may affect any part of the body
   C. Check feet and scalp for tinea pedis (interdigital scaling, maceration, and fissures) and tinea capitis (patchy hair loss with broken stumps in oval or circinate lesions with central clearing).
VI. **Assessment**
   A. Diagnosis
      1. Scrapings from borders of lesions in potassium hydroxide fungal preparation demonstrate hyphae.
      2. History and physical findings may be adequate for diagnosis.
   B. Differential diagnosis
      1. Pityriasis rosea: Herald patch may resemble tinea corporis.
      2. Candidiasis: Lesions more inflamed; no central clearing; satellite lesions present
      3. Psoriasis: Lesions erythematous, circumscribed, and covered with silvery scales
VII. **Plan**
   A. Use one of the following topical creams:
      1. Ketoconazole (Nizoral) 2% cream: Apply once daily for 2 weeks.
      2. Oxiconazole (Oxistat) 1% cream: Apply once daily for 2 weeks.
      3. Clotrimazole (Lotrimin): Apply three times a day for 2 weeks.
   B. Systemic treatment for severe or unresponsive cases: griseofulvin (Grifulvin V), 125–250 mg/day for a child 30–50 lb; 250–500 mg/day for a child over 50 lb; continue treatment for 2–4 weeks.

VIII. **Education**
  A. Transmitted by direct and indirect contact
  B. Communicable as long as lesions are present
  C. Observe for involvement of other family members or sexual contacts.
  D. Ringworm lives on humans and animals; avoid contact with pets.
  E. Check dog or cat for *Microsporum canis*.
  F. Do not lend or borrow clothing.
  G. Bathe or shower daily.
  H. Use talcum or antifungal powder (Caldesene, Tinactin) in intertriginous areas.
  I. Keep skin dry; ringworm thrives in moist areas.
  J. Do not wear tight, constricting clothing; absorbent cotton is preferable.
  K. Launder clothing and linens in hot water.
  L. May see no improvement for 5–6 days; generally takes 1–3 weeks for effective cure
  M. Continue treatment for 1 week after disappearance of symptoms.
  N. Use of corticosteroids will exacerbate lesions.
IX. **Follow-up**
  A. Telephone call in 4–5 days to report progress
  B. Recheck in 7–9 days if no significant improvement.
  C. Return sooner if lesions appear worse or become inflamed.
X. **Complications**
  A. Secondary bacterial infection
  B. Sensitivity to topical antifungal cream
XI. **Consultation/Referral**
  A. If severe or extensive, may require treatment with griseofulvin
  B. If tinea capitis is present

NOTES

| TINEA CRURIS

Ringworm of the groin or "jock itch," a superficial fungal infection of the groin

I. **Etiology**
   A. *Epidermophyton floccosum* and *Trichophyton* dermatophyte fungi

II. **Incidence**
   A. Seen most often in athletes and obese children
   B. Incidence increases in hot, humid weather
   C. More common in males

III. **Subjective data**
   A. Groin and upper inner thighs are red, raw, and sore.
   B. Pruritic when healing
   C. Hurts with activity
   D. Complaint of jock itch
   E. History of exposure to tinea cruris

IV. **Objective data**
   A. Symmetric rash with butterfly appearance on groin and inner aspects of thighs; scrotum, gluteal folds, and buttocks may also be involved.
   B. Rash erythematous with a sharp, raised border with tiny vesicles, central clearing, and peripheral spreading
   C. Check entire body.
      1. Tinea pedis often present
      2. Intertriginous areas susceptible to infection

V. **Assessment**
   A. Diagnosis
      1. Scrapings from active borders of lesions in potassium hydroxide fungal preparation reveal hyphae and spores.
      2. Diagnosis may also be made from history and typical appearance of rash.
   B. Differential diagnosis
      1. Intertrigo: Rash is erythematous with oozing, exudation, and crusting; borders not sharply defined; no central clearing.
      2. Seborrheic dermatitis: Lesions are semiconfluent, yellow, and thick with greasy scaling.
      3. Candidiasis: Lesions are moist and intensely erythematous with sharply defined borders and satellite lesions; more common in females.
      4. Contact dermatitis: Distribution and configuration are the distinguishing features; rash is erythematous with vesicles, oozing, erosion, and eventually ulceration; often coexistent.
      5. Psoriasis: Usually unilateral; other psoriatic lesions on body; plaques with silvery scales

VI. **Plan**
   A. For lesions with erythema and pruritus, order one of the following:
      1. Ketoconazole (Nizoral) 2% cream once daily (also effective against *Candida albicans*)

2. Clotrimazole (Lotrimin, Micatin) cream three times daily (also effective against *C albicans*)

3. Tolnaftate (Tinactin) cream three times daily (over-the-counter preparation; ineffective against *C albicans*)

B. For acute inflammatory lesions

1. Domeboro (Burow's solution) compresses: Apply 30 minutes three times daily for 3 days. Dissolve one powder packet in 1 pt of warm water. Or, vinegar wet packs: Half-cup vinegar to 1 qt warm water; apply 15 minutes twice daily.

2. Antifungal cream as above

VII. Education

A. Expect gradual improvement once treatment is instituted.

B. Continue treatment for 1 week after lesions have cleared.

C. Domeboro solution becomes concentrated on exposure to air; keep in covered container.

D. Use a soft cloth for soaks.

E. Eliminate sources of heat and friction.

F. Hygiene

1. Bathe daily; dry thoroughly after bathing.

2. Use cotton underwear.

3. Change clothing daily.

4. Use clean athletic supporter daily.

5. Use fresh towels daily.

6. Launder linens and clothing in hot water.

G. Tinea is highly communicable and is transmitted by both direct and indirect contact.

H. Check siblings carefully for signs of infection.

I. Alert child and parents to signs and symptoms of secondary infection.

J. *Note:* Prevention is of primary importance. Athletes in particular should be educated about the need for clean, dry clothing and the importance of avoiding direct contact with someone who has jock itch. Athletic supporters, shorts, and socks should not be loaned or borrowed. Daily showers should be encouraged, as well as the prophylactic use of antifungal powders such as Caldesene or Tinactin daily or twice daily.

VIII. Follow-up

A. Telephone call in 3–4 days

B. If severe, with oozing, consider rechecking in 5 days.

IX. Complications

A. Secondary infection

B. Chronic infection (80% of patients acquire immunity; 20% may develop chronic infection)

C. Allergic response to topical antifungal cream (erythema, stinging, blistering, peeling, pruritus)

X. Consultation/Referral

A. If no clinical improvement after 2 weeks, griseofulvin may be indicated.

NOTES

TINEA PEDIS

Ringworm of the foot, or "athlete's foot," a superficial fungal infection of the foot

I. **Etiology**

   A. *Trichophyton mentagrophytes* and *Trichophyton rubrum*, dermatophyte fungi, invade the skin after trauma.

II. **Incidence**

   A. Most common in adolescents and adults, but is found with increasing frequency in preadolescent children, probably because of the use of occlusive footwear

   B. Studies have shown that a susceptibility factor must be present for infection to occur. Males are more susceptible than females.

III. **Subjective data**

   A. One or both feet may be involved.

   B. Pruritus

   C. Cracks between toes

   D. Scaling of feet

   E. Blisters on soles

   F. Pain with deep fissures

   G. History of exposure to predisposing factors (eg, communal showers, prolonged use of sneakers); often seen after trauma or in conjunction with atopic dermatitis

IV. **Objective data**

   A. Interdigital fissures

   B. Widespread fine scaling; extension onto sides of foot and heel is frequent.

   C. Maceration

   D. Vesicular eruption on plantar surface

   E. Secondary infection may be present.

   F. Regional adenopathy

   G. Involvement of nails may occur.

   H. Vesicular eruption of the hands—an "id" reaction—may occur.

   I. Unilateral tinea pedis is common.

V. **Assessment**

   A. Diagnosis

      1. Scrapings from lesions in potassium hydroxide fungal preparation reveal hyphae and spores.

      2. Unilateral involvement is a significant positive clinical finding.

   B. Differential diagnosis

      1. Interdigital candidiasis: Interdigital lesions are moist and erythematous, with well-defined borders and satellite lesions.

      2. Hyperhidrosis: Macerated, tender, peeling, erythematous; usually malodorous; diagnosis made by history and appearance

   3. Contact dermatitis: Reaction to shoes, sneakers, dye, soap, nylon socks. Diagnosis is generally made by history, distribution of rash, and appearance of rash (erythematous, vesicular, and oozing).

VI. Plan

   A. Domeboro (Burow's solution) soaks four times daily for acute lesions with blistering and oozing; one tablet or powder packet to 1 pt of water

   B. Use one of the following antifungal creams:
      1. Oxiconazole (Oxistat) cream 1%, once daily for 4 weeks
      2. Clotrimazole (Lotrimin) or haloprogin (Halotex) cream, three times daily for 4 weeks (also effective against *Candida albicans*)
      3. Tolnaftate (Tinactin) cream, three times daily (over-the-counter preparation; ineffective against *C albicans*)

   C. For severe or unresponsive cases in children over 50 lb: Griseofulvin (Grifulvin V), 250–500 mg daily for 4 to 8 weeks

   D. *Note:* For fungal infection of nails, use flurazepam (Diflucan) 200 mg once a week until nail grows out.

VII. Education

   A. Expect gradual improvement once treatment is instituted.

   B. Continue treatment for several days after lesions have cleared.

   C. Soak feet two to four times a day in a small basin.

   D. Domeboro solution concentrates when left exposed; store in covered container.

   E. Hygiene
      1. Dry interdigital areas thoroughly after bathing.
      2. Use white cotton socks; no colored tights or nylons.
      3. Change socks at least daily.
      4. Wear sandals if possible.
      5. Avoid sneakers and plastic footwear.

   F. Communicable as long as lesions are present

   G. Causative organisms are long-lived, surviving more than 5 months.

   H. Transmitted to traumatized skin by both direct and indirect contact

   I. Alert child and parents to signs and symptoms of secondary infection.

   J. Prevention
      1. Use Tinactin or clotrimazole (Micatin) powder daily.
      2. Use clogs for showers.
      3. Do not lend or borrow shoes.

VIII. Follow-up

   A. Telephone call in 3–4 days

   B. If severe, with deep fissures and oozing, recheck in 5 days; recheck sooner if no improvement is noted.

IX. Complications

   A. Secondary infection

   B. Allergic response to topical antifungal cream (erythema, stinging, blistering, peeling, pruritus)

    C. Untreated or improperly treated tinea presents with scaling and erythema of the sides and dorsum of the foot as well as interdigital areas and plantar surface. The tinea may be distributed in a shoe or sneaker pattern.

X. Consultation/Referral

    A. No clinical improvement after 2 weeks

    B. Severe involvement or secondary infection

NOTES

TINEA VERSICOLOR

A chronic, superficial fungal infection characterized by fine scaling and decreased or increased pigmentation, mainly on the trunk

I. **Etiology**
   A. A superficial fungal infection caused by *Malassezia furfur*, a yeastlike fungus
II. **Incidence**
   A. Seen most often in young adults in temperate zones
   B. Uncommon before puberty
III. **Subjective data**
   A. Slight pruritus or asymptomatic
   B. Chief complaint is cosmetic; patient complains of white, pink, or tan somewhat scaly spots on normal skin.
   C. Often no complaints but found on routine physical examination
IV. **Objective data**
   A. Lesions
      1. Maculosquamous or papulosquamous, irregularly shaped and circinate lesions that can be demonstrated by light scratching
      2. Characteristically tan or reddish-brown, but may vary from white to brown
      3. On skin exposed to the sun, lesions appear hypopigmented because they do not tan. Lesions may be darker than surrounding skin in winter and lighter than surrounding skin in summer.
      4. Areas may coalesce.
   B. Distribution
      1. Primarily on the trunk
      2. Less commonly on the neck and face
V. **Assessment**
   A. Diagnosis
      1. Microscopic examination of scales in potassium hydroxide fungal preparation reveals hyphae and budding yeasts.
      2. On examination by Wood's light, lesions may show gold to orange fluorescence.
   B. Differential diagnosis
      1. Vitiligo: By family history; lesions pure white
      2. Postinflammatory or posttraumatic hypopigmentation: By history
      3. Pityriasis rosea: Lesions oval with definite border; herald patch; acute onset
VI. **Plan**
   A. Ketoconazole (Nizoral) 2% cream: Apply once daily for 2 weeks.
   B. Imidazole (Exelderm) cream or solution 1%: Apply gently once daily for 3 weeks.
   C. Selenium sulfide (Selsun) lotion 2.5%; order 8 oz.
      1. Daily for 7 days:
         a. Bathe.
         b. Rub lesions with a coarse towel.

      c. Apply Selsun to entire trunk and other affected areas.

      d. Lather with a small amount of water.

      e. Leave on skin for 10–20 minutes.

      f. Rinse thoroughly.

  D. For frequent recurrences, ketoconazole, 200 mg/day orally for 2 weeks. Do not order for adolescent females who may become pregnant.

VII. Education

  A. Rub lesions with a coarse towel before applying medication.

  B. Launder clothing, towels, and sheets in hot water.

  C. Scaling should disappear within several days.

  D. Continue treatment for several weeks.

  E. Pigment changes resolve slowly. On sun-exposed skin, lesions will not appear normal until they acquire a tan or until existing tan fades; this may take 6 months.

  F. Recurrence is common but can easily be treated.

  G. Selsun may irritate skin.

  H. Do not use Selsun on genitalia.

  I. Ketoconazole is for use in adolescents and adults.

VIII. Follow-up

  A. Recheck in 2 weeks; scaling should not be present, but pigment changes will still be evident.

  B. Recurrences should be re-treated. If resistant to treatment, give oral ketoconazole by mouth for 1 week.

IX. Complications

  A. None; of cosmetic significance only

X. Consultation/Referral

  A. No improvement after skin color has had an opportunity to return to normal; repigmentation may take 3–6 months.

NOTES

UMBILICAL CORD CARE

Cord care begins in the newborn nursery and is continued until the stump falls off and the area is totally healed. Complete healing may take several weeks.

I. **Subjective data**
   A. Cord clamped; drying begins within hours.
   B. Clamp removed on first or second day of life.
   C. Black, hard stump remains attached for about 6–12 days.

II. **Objective data**
   A. Stump clean and dry
   B. No inflammation surrounding umbilicus
   C. No bleeding, discharge, or odor

III. **Assessment**
   A. Normal healing of umbilical cord

IV. **Plan**
   A. Wash with soap and water and dry thoroughly twice a day.
   B. Apply antibiotic ointment (Neosporin) to umbilicus two or three times a day.
   C. Clean with alcohol once a day.
   D. Clean depression with a cotton swab after stump falls off.

V. **Education**
   A. Keep diapers folded below umbilicus.
   B. With disposable diapers, fold plastic to the outside.
   C. Keep rubber pants below umbilicus.
   D. Watch for oozing, odor, bleeding, or inflammation.
   E. A small amount of discharge is normal for 1–2 days after the cord drops off.
   F. Keep depression clean and dry. It can become a site for the collection of dead skin, powder, and so forth, leading to infection.

VI. **Follow-up**
   A. None necessary unless bleeding, discharge, odor, swelling, or inflammation occurs.

VII. **Complications**
   A. Infection

VIII. **Consultation/Referral**
   A. Bleeding
   B. Discharge
   C. Foul odor
   D. Edema
   E. Inflammation
   F. Moistness at base of cord (may be urachus)

NOTES

NOTES

| UMBILICAL GRANULOMA

A small pink lesion that forms at the base of the umbilical cord

I. **Etiology**
   A. Believed to be the result of a mild infection
II. **Subjective data**
   A. Umbilicus moist, oozing
   B. Pink mass on umbilicus
   C. Foul odor may be present.
   D. History of mild infection with mucopurulent drainage or delayed drying of cord
III. **Objective data**
   A. Soft, pink granulation tissue on umbilicus
   B. Seropurulent discharge
   C. Examine for bleeding, erythema, purulent discharge, edema of stump.
IV. **Assessment**
   A. Diagnosis is made by typical appearance of granulation tissue.
   B. Differential diagnosis
      1. Umbilical polyp: Larger (7–10 mm), firmer mass
      2. Patent urachus: Fistula between bladder and umbilicus that discharges urine when infant voids
V. **Plan**
   A. Cauterize with silver nitrate stick. Do not touch surrounding skin with silver nitrate.
   B. Wash umbilicus 3–5 minutes after cauterizing.
VI. **Education**
   A. Keep diapers and rubber pants below umbilicus.
   B. Clean with alcohol sponge at least three times a day.
   C. Watch for oozing, odor, bleeding.
VII. **Follow-up**
   A. Recheck in 5–7 days to check healing. Repeat cauterization if granuloma is still present.
VIII. **Complications**
   A. Secondary infection
IX. **Consultation/Referral**
   A. Persistence of granuloma after repeat treatment with silver nitrate

NOTES

NOTES

| URINARY TRACT INFECTION

A bacterial infection of any portion of the urinary tract. It may be limited to asymptomatic bacteriuria or may progress to involve the renal pelvis and parenchyma, causing pyelonephritis.

I. **Etiology**
   A. *Escherichia coli* is the most common causative organism (up to 80% of cases).
   B. Other organisms include Klebsiella, Proteus, Pseudomonas, Enterobacteriaceae, and less commonly *Staphylococcus aureus.*

II. **Incidence**
   A. Most common between 2 months and 2 years of age
   B. More frequent in girls than in boys
   C. Recurrence rate after the first infection is estimated at about 40%.
   D. Urinary tract infection is seen in the neonate in 1%–2% of both females and males (generally uncircumcised).
   E. In infancy and childhood, it is more common in females. About 1% of school-age girls have symptomatic infections per year.
   F. Often related to sexual activity in adolescent females; the incidence increases as females become sexually active.

III. **Subjective data**
   A. Classic signs
      1. Fever: May be as high as 104.5°F (40°C)
      2. Chills
      3. Anorexia
      4. Urinary frequency and urgency
      5. Dysuria
      6. Incontinence
      7. Enuresis (nocturnal and diurnal)
      8. Costovertebral angle tenderness (flank pain)
      9. Suprapubic pain
      10. Back pain
   B. Typical symptoms
      1. Infants
         a. Failure to thrive
         b. Fever of unknown origin
         c. Irritability
         d. Strong odor to urine
         e. Hematuria
         f. Gastrointestinal symptoms (vomiting, diarrhea)
      2. Preschoolers
         a. Abdominal pain
         b. Vomiting
         c. Fever
         d. Strong-smelling urine

        e. Enuresis

        f. Urinary frequency and urgency

        g. Dysuria

        h. Vaginal discharge

        i. Hematuria

        j. Dysuria

    3. School-age and older children

        a. Symptoms as for preschool children

        b. Costovertebral angle tenderness

C. Pertinent subjective data to obtain

    1. Character of urinary stream

    2. History of previous urinary tract infection or symptoms

    3. History of possible causes of urethral irritation

        a. Use of bubble bath or feminine sprays

        b. Vaginitis

        c. Pinworms

        d. Masturbation

        e. Sexual activity

    4. Personal hygiene practices

    5. Change in urinary habits

    6. History of constipation

D. *Note:* Urinary tract infection should be suspected in all children who present with failure to thrive, fever of unknown origin, or recurrent abdominal pain.

IV. Objective data

A. Obtain weight and blood pressure.

B. Poor growth rate

C. Fever of up to 104.5°F

D. Abdominal examination may reveal suprapubic or costovertebral angle tenderness.

E. Child may appear toxic with acute infection.

F. Laboratory tests: Urinalysis and urine culture

    1. Because infection may be completely asymptomatic, routine urinalysis should be done yearly on all children to detect asymptomatic bacteriuria. About 2% of females screened are found to have significant bacteriuria.

    2. Proteinuria may be present.

    3. Criteria for diagnosis by urine culture in a symptomatic child

        a. More than 10 white blood cells per high-power field in centrifuged sediment

        b. More than 50,000 bacteria/ml (of the same type of microorganism) in a culture of a clean-voided specimen. Growth of more than one organism usually indicates contamination, not infection.

        c. Any pathogens in a suprapubic aspirate or from a catheter specimen (if first 10 ml is excluded) indicate infection.

    4. Order sensitivity studies as well as urine culture if specimen is to be taken to the laboratory (results will take 24–48 hours).

5. Ideally, two or more urine cultures should be done unless the specimen is obtained by suprapubic aspiration (by physician) or sterile catheterization.

6. If child is not toxic or does not have severe symptoms, postpone treatment and request a first morning clean-voided specimen the next day.

7. Repeat any culture with a count of 10,000–50,000/ml.

V. Assessment

A. Diagnosis is established by positive urine culture.

B. Differential diagnosis

1. Vaginitis: Pyuria of more than 10 white cells per high-power field; urine culture nonspecific. Symptoms may be those of cystitis (frequency, burning, urgency).

2. Urethritis: Normal urine culture. Symptoms may be those of cystitis (frequency, burning, urgency).

3. Gonococcal urethritis: Urethral culture positive; urine culture negative

VI. Plan

A. Pharmacologic therapy: Culture results may necessitate a change in antibiotic therapy.

1. Trimethoprim (TMP)–sulfamethoxazole (SMX) (Bactrim, Septra), 8 mg/kg TMP and 40 mg/kg SMX in 24 hours in two divided doses (10 kg, 5 ml every 12 hours; more than 40 kg, one DS tablet every 12 hours) for 10 days, or

2. Amoxicillin, 40 mg/kg/24 hours in three divided doses (more than 20 kg, 250 mg three times a day) for 10 days, or

3. Cefixime (Suprax) (100 mg/5 ml), 4–8 mg/kg once daily for 10 days

4. Acetaminophen for fever and discomfort, 10–15 mg/kg every 4 hours

B. Repeat urine culture in 48 hours.

C. Encourage fluids.

D. Plan should include attempts to determine mechanism causing infection; consult physician for referral for urologic evaluation.

E. Indications for voiding cystourethrogram (VCUG) and ultrasound

1. Child under 5 years

2. First infection in male

3. Child over 5 years with upper urinary tract infection, or more than one urinary tract infection

F. Radionuclide cystogram may be considered instead of VCUG in females.

1. Lower radiation dose (1% that of VCUG)

2. More sensitive in grades II to V vesicoureteric reflux, but more difficult to see grade I

3. In males, there is poorer definition of structural abnormalities of bladder and urethra (urethral valves); therefore, this is not the primary test for males.

G. Vesicoureteral reflux generally resolves with time, as 20%–30% reflux resolves every 2 years. (As the child grows, the longitudinal muscle develops.) Grades I and II reflux (nondilated ureters) resolve spontaneously. Use prophylactic antibiotic therapy until reflux proved normal by repeat VCUG (done every 6–12 months). Refer grades III to V to urologist.

VII. Education

A. Urine collection

1. Do not force fluids before collecting specimen.

2. Collection of clean-voided, midstream specimen

   a. Use sterile container; boil thoroughly washed jar and cover for 10 minutes.

   b. Female: Clean labia from front to back, using a fresh, soft, clean cloth or gauze sponge for each wipe. Cleanse each side with lightly soaped sponges; then spread labia and cleanse from clitoris to anus. Use fresh sponges to rinse.

   c. Male: Retract foreskin and cleanse glans, first with a lightly soaped cloth or sponge, then with water.

   d. Have child initiate voiding and then stop. Obtain specimen when child begins voiding again.

   e. Take specimen to the office immediately; if a delay of more than a few minutes is expected, refrigerate specimen at 4°C.

3. U-bag collection (difficult to obtain an uncontaminated specimen using this method)

   a. Female: Clean genitalia as above and dry thoroughly. Remove protective covering from bag; apply first to perineum, pressing firmly to ensure adherence; then apply pressure from perineum forward. Be sure seal is tight.

   b. Male: Clean genitalia and dry thoroughly. Apply bag with firm pressure to ensure a tight seal.

   c. Seal edges of bag once infant has voided and take to the office or laboratory immediately.

B. Encourage fluids during treatment.

C. Try to give medication every 6 hours. Give all medication.

D. Call back immediately if child develops a rash or has nausea, vomiting, diarrhea, or headache.

E. Expect child to improve within 24–48 hours.

F. Teach parent and child to be alert to signs and symptoms of urinary tract infection.

G. Do not use bubble baths or feminine sprays.

H. Use showers instead of baths if child is old enough.

I. Do not use deep water for baths.

J. Stress perineal hygiene—wiping from front to back after toileting.

K. Encourage child to void at regular intervals and not to delay voiding.

L. For sexually active adolescents, encourage voiding after intercourse.

M. Minimize constipation (see protocol, p. 268).

VIII. Follow-up

A. Repeat urine culture in 48 hours.

B. Repeat urine culture 48 hours after treatment is discontinued and every month for 3 months, then every 3 months for 1 year.

IX. Complications

A. Recurrent urinary tract infection

    B. Pyelonephritis

    C. Failure to thrive in undiagnosed or untreated cases

X. **Consultation/Referral**

    A. Infants

    B. Males with first urinary tract infection

    C. Females with second urinary tract infection

    D. If patient is symptomatic 2–3 days after initiation of therapy

    E. Vesicoureteral reflux, for administration of long-term prophylaxis. Dosage should be half the standard treatment dose, given at night to ensure concentration in urine.

NOTES

VARICELLA (CHICKENPOX)

A benign, highly contagious viral disease characterized by a mild constitutional prodrome followed by a pruritic rash consisting of macules, papules, vesicles, and crusted lesions, which appear in crops and rapidly progress through various stages

I. **Etiology**

    A. Varicella zoster virus (VZV: primary infection)

II. **Incidence**

    A. Peak incidence: 2–8 years of age

    B. Epidemics are seen in 3–4-year cycles, mainly from January to May.

III. **Incubation period**

    A. 10–21 days; average period is 14–16 days.

IV. **Communicability**

    A. 1 day before appearance of rash to 6 days after

    B. Transmitted by droplet infection and by direct contact

    C. Dried crusts are not infectious.

    D. Chickenpox can be contracted from patients with herpes zoster.

    E. *Note:* Varicella vaccine is now licensed and available in the United States. States have the option of purchasing it under the Vaccines for Children Contract. In Massachusetts, the vaccine is available for children ages 12–18 months and ages 11–12 years with no previous history of varicella.

    F. The VZV vaccine was developed in Japan, where it is licensed for administration and has been used since the 1970s. In Japan, nearly all vaccinees seroconverted in 1 month and were seropositive 5 years later. The protective effect was about 83%, and those that had the disease had a mild clinical course with few lesions.

V. **Subjective data**

    A. History of exposure about 2 weeks before appearance of lesions, or a history of chickenpox in the community

    B. Lesions appear in crops.

    C. Lesions in various stages of development at one time

    D. Prodrome

        1. Child may have low-grade fever, upper respiratory infection, anorexia, headache, and malaise for 24–48 hours before appearance of lesions, or constitutional symptoms may appear simultaneously with exanthem.

        2. Prodrome may be recognized in retrospect only.

    E. Lesions

        1. A few spots on trunk or face initially; then a 3–4-day period during which successive crops erupt on trunk, face, scalp, extremities, and mucous membranes.

        2. Lesions are seen in greatest concentration centrally and on proximal portions of the extremities. They tend to be more abundant on clothed areas and in areas of local inflammation (eg, diaper area in a child with diaper rash).

        3. Lesions are found on the scalp, the mucous membranes, and the conjunctiva.

VI. **Objective data**

  A. Skin

   1. Lesions appear as small red macules and rapidly progress to papules to clear vesicles on an erythematous base to umbilicated to cloudy vesicles to crusted lesions. (Drying occurs in the center of the vesicle, producing an umbilicated appearance before crusting.)

   2. Lesions are seen in various stages in one area. They progress through the stages in 6–8 hours, with crusts forming in 2–4 days.

   3. Total number of lesions is generally 200 to 400.

  B. Mucous membranes

   1. Vesicles rupture rapidly, so are most commonly seen as shallow white ulcers 2–3 mm in diameter.

   2. Lesions may be present on genital mucosa, palpebral conjunctiva, ear canals, and mouth.

  C. Lymphadenopathy may be generalized.

  D. Severity

   1. Varies from mild cases with a few lesions and no systemic symptoms to severe toxicity with hundreds of lesions and fever (104°F).

   2. Systemic manifestations subside after the first 3 days as new crops of lesions cease to appear.

VII. **Assessment**

  A. Diagnosis is usually made by history of contact and development of an exanthem that rapidly progresses through stages (macule to papule to vesicle to crusting); various stages are found in one area.

  B. Differential diagnosis

   1. Smallpox: Severe prodrome; lesions are seen in the same stage, are more prominent peripherally, and progress more slowly (5–6 days) through stages. *Note:* Variola has been virtually eradicated throughout the world and is not a diagnostic consideration in the United States at this time.

   2. Impetigo: Lesions do not appear in crops, differ in appearance and distribution, and do not involve mucous membranes of the mouth. There are no constitutional symptoms.

   3. Insect bites: Lesions do not have vesicular appearance and are not present on mucous membranes. Constitutional symptoms are not present.

   4. Scabies: Lesions do not have characteristic appearance and are not present on mucous membranes, but are characteristically present in the interdigital spaces.

   5. Herpes zoster: Lesions are painful and usually confined to dermatome.

VIII. **Plan**

  A. Symptomatic treatment to alleviate itching

   1. Baking soda or Aveeno oatmeal baths

   2. Calamine lotion as needed to skin

   3. Antihistamines for pruritus

    a. Diphenhydramine (Benadryl), more than 10 kg: 5 mg/kg/day in three or four doses, or

    b. Hydroxyzine (Atarax), more than 6 years of age: 50–100 mg/day in divided doses; less than 6 years: 50 mg/day in divided doses

    B. Acetaminophen as indicated for fever, 10–15 mg/kg every 4 hours

    C. Oral lesions: Warm saline or hydrogen peroxide mouth rinses

    D. Genital lesions: Warm saline or hydrogen peroxide compresses

    E. Infected lesions

        1. One or two lesions: Wash lesions well and apply Neosporin or bacitracin ointment four times daily.

        2. Many lesions: See Impetigo.

    F. Acyclovir (Zovirax): Infectious disease experts do not recommend routine use of acyclovir in varicella. In some instances, however, administration may be indicated because if given within 24 hours of onset of rash, it results in a milder illness. Indications for use should be defined and included in guidelines for individual health centers.

IX. Education

    A. Transmitted by direct contact or inhalation from nose and throat secretions

    B. Communicable 24–48 hours before first lesion appears and until all lesions have crusted

    C. Crusts do not contain active virus.

    D. Second attacks are rare; lifelong immunity is generally conferred.

    E. In mild cases, crusting occurs within 5 days. In severe cases, crusting occurs in 10 days.

    F. Keep child home from school until all vesicles are crusted; this generally takes 7 days.

    G. Do not expose to pregnant women or infants.

    H. Do not expose to children with eczema or malignancies or those on immunosuppressive therapy.

    I. Call immediately if cough, dyspnea, or chest pain occurs within 2–5 days of onset of exanthem.

    J. Call immediately if child develops high fever, stiff neck, headache, listlessness, or hyperirritability.

    K. Keep nails trimmed. Put gloves on child if scratching is a problem.

    L. Use careful hygiene to prevent superimposed infection; keep nails clean, bathe child daily, and change clothing daily.

    M. Encourage fluids.

    N. If genital lesions cause dysuria, encourage child to void in tub.

    O. Crusts fall off in 5–20 days.

    P. When scabs fall off, a shallow pink depression remains. This eventually becomes white, and repigmentation occurs later.

    Q. Scarring is caused by premature removal of scabs or secondarily infected lesions.

    R. Do not use aspirin.

    S. Aveeno baths: Mix 1 cup Aveeno with 2 cups cold water. Shake until well mixed, then pour in tub of tepid water.

X. Follow-up

    A. Generally not indicated in uncomplicated cases

    B. Return to office if:

        1. Any question of secondary infection

    2. Cough, dyspnea, chest pain

    3. Persistent vomiting, abdominal pain

    4. Headache, fever, stiff neck, lethargy, irritability

    5. Fever over 104°F, or any fever after 1 week

    6. Lesions continue to develop after 1 week

XI. Complications

    A. Most common: Secondary bacterial infection

    B. Rare: Encephalitis, pneumonia, Guillain-Barré syndrome, hemorrhagic varicella, Reye's syndrome

    C. Disseminated varicella

XII. Consultation/Referral

    A. Suspected complications

    B. Infants and children with debilitating conditions or those on prednisone, for prophylaxis if exposed to varicella or for antiviral therapy if infected by varicella

        1. Varicella zoster immune globulin (VZIG) should be given within 96 hours of exposure to:

            a. Newborns whose mothers had varicella less than 5 days before delivery or 48 hours after delivery

            b. Premature infants

            c. Children with cancer or collagen vascular disease

            d. Recipients of organ or bone marrow transplants

            e. Children being treated with steroids, cytotoxic chemotherapy, or radiation

            f. Immunodeficient children

            g. Children with severe burns or eczema

            h. Pregnant women

        2. Acyclovir is given to VZV-susceptible high-risk children if they are beyond the fourth day postexposure, when there would be no beneficial effect of passive immunization with VZIG. It is generally given intravenously to children with an immunodeficiency syndrome and children with cancer who are undergoing chemotherapy.

NOTES

VIRAL CROUP

Laryngotracheobronchitis characterized by inspiratory stridor. Inflammation of the respiratory mucosa of all airways is generally present. The classic symptoms are caused by inflammation and edema in the larynx and subglottic area.

I. **Etiology**
   A. Generally caused by the parainfluenza virus; less commonly caused by the respiratory syncytial virus, influenza virus, and adenoviruses

II. **Incidence**
   A. Most common in children ages 3 months to 3 years
   B. Peak incidence, age 1–2 years
   C. Occurs predominantly in late fall or early winter

III. **Subjective data**
   A. History of gradual onset
   B. Symptoms of upper respiratory infection for several days before onset
   C. Low-grade or moderate fever
   D. Harsh, barking cough
   E. Wheezing, with lower respiratory tract involvement
   F. Hoarseness
   G. High-pitched sound on inspiration; often occurs at night
   H. Child does not appear toxic.
   I. The following are important questions to ask in history to rule out epiglottitis. If the answer is affirmative for any or the child appears toxic, do not attempt to examine child but refer to physician immediately.
      1. Acute onset?
      2. Dysphagia?
      3. Drooling?
      4. Apprehension and air hunger?

IV. **Objective data**
   A. Fever
   B. Slight hyperemia and edema of nasopharynx
   C. Inspiratory stridor, usually of abrupt onset
   D. Harsh, barking cough
   E. Hoarseness
   F. Dyspnea
   G. Wheezing, with lower respiratory tract involvement
   H. Prolonged expiratory phase
   I. With increased obstruction, breath sounds decrease and anxiety increases.
   J. Laboratory test: White cell count normal or low
   K. Lateral neck x-ray to rule out epiglottitis

V. **Assessment: Differential diagnosis**
   A. Bacterial croup (epiglottitis): Toxic, drooling, dysphagic, high fever, acute onset, anxious; age range generally 3–7 years

    B. Foreign body: Fever absent; dysphagia, visualization of foreign body, sudden onset of coughing and wheezing; careful history may reveal episode of choking just before onset of wheezing.

    C. Congenital laryngeal stridor: Stridor present from birth.

    D. Bronchiolitis, pneumonia, bronchitis: See Table 2-1, Differential Diagnosis of Viral Croup, Bronchiolitis, Pneumonia, and Bronchitis.

VI. Plan

    A. Home management if:

        1. Child is well hydrated and pink

        2. Little or no retraction

        3. Normal air exchange on auscultation

        4. Respirations and pulse within normal range

        5. Absence of stridor at rest

    B. Cool-mist vaporizer: Use continuously.

    C. Force fluids, especially clear liquids.

    D. Monitor respiratory rate.

    E. Refer to physician for hospitalization if moderate to severe respiratory distress.

VII. Education

    A. Cool-mist vaporizers are preferred over steam vaporizers. Warm steam may have a partial drying effect and may raise the temperature of a febrile child. Also, steam vaporizers are more dangerous to use around small children.

    B. Fluids, especially clear liquids, are important in the acute phase because they help keep secretions thin.

    C. Croup is generally self-limited.

    D. Inspiratory obstruction is at a maximum for the first 24–48 hours. Respiratory symptoms persist for 1 week.

    E. Recurrences are common until 5–6 years of age.

    F. Do not use antihistamines; they tend to cause inspissation of laryngeal and tracheal secretions.

    G. Restlessness and anxiety are indications of hypoxemia.

    H. Monitor respiratory rate; teach parent how to count respirations.

    I. Symptoms generally increase at night.

    J. For immediate relief of acute symptoms, take child into bathroom and turn on hot water. Symptoms also improve when child is taken outside. If no improvement after 5 minutes, take child to hospital.

    K. Signs and symptoms of airway obstruction are tachypnea, cyanosis, increased retractions, and increased anxiety or restlessness. Should any of these occur, call physician immediately.

VIII. Follow-up

    A. Call immediately if child becomes restless or anxious.

    B. Call immediately if respiratory rate or retractions increase.

IX. Complications

    A. Principal complication is asphyxia secondary to laryngeal obstruction.

X. Consultation/Referral

    A. Any child with an acute onset of inspiratory stridor, tachypnea, retractions, or diminished breath sounds

Table 2-1. Differential diagnosis of viral croup, bronchiolitis, pneumonia, and bronchitis

Criteria	Viral Croup (Laryngotracheobronchitis)	Bronchiolitis	Pneumonia	Bronchitis
Etiology	Viral Parainfluenza viruses (most common) Influenza viruses Adenoviruses Rhinoviruses Respiratory syncytial virus	Viral Respiratory syncytial virus (most common) Parainfluenza viruses Adenoviruses Influenza viruses Allergy Inflammation of small and terminal bronchioles Occasionally, secondary bacterial infection	Bacterial Pneumococci Hemolytic streptococci *Haemophilus influenzae* Staphylococci Viral Respiratory syncytial virus Parainfluenza viruses Adenoviruses Influenza viruses Mycoplasmal	Viral, bacterial (including mycoplasmal and fungal)
Incidence	Most common ages: 3 months–3 years Generally seen during late fall or early winter	Most commonly seen under 2 years; spans ages 3 months–3 years Most common in winter	All age groups Most common in winter	Uncommon in childhood as an isolated entity
Subjective findings	History of upper respiratory infection Low-grade or moderate fever Gradual onset of cough and dyspnea Sudden onset of stridor; usually at night	Mild rhinitis for 1–2 days Low-grade or no fever Abrupt onset of dyspnea Wheezing Cough	History of upper respiratory infection Abrupt rise in temperature Cough Tachypnea Chills Chest or abdominal pain Bacterial pneumonia presents with acute onset Viral pneumonia presents with insidious onset	Low-grade fever Dry, hacking, nonproductive cough for 4–6 days Productive cough after 4–6 days Chest pain with coughing

(continued)

Table 2-1 (Continued)

Criteria	Viral Croup (Laryngotracheobronchitis)	Bronchiolitis	Pneumonia	Bronchitis
Objective findings	Variable fever Harsh, barking cough Nasopharynx slightly hyperemic with mild edema Inspiratory stridor Supraclavicular and intercostal retractions Diminished breath sounds	Marked respiratory distress Rapid, shallow respirations Flaring of alae nasi Intermittent cyanosis Rales (diffuse) Expiratory wheezes/grunts Decreased breath sounds Prolonged expiratory phase Displacement of liver edge below costal margin (hyperinflation of lungs leads to depression of the diaphragm, resulting in liver displacement) Tachycardia Hyperresonance on percussion Bilateral involvement	Elevated temperature: 39.5°–40.5°C (103.1°–104.9°F) Respiratory distress varies from mild to marked Tachypnea Decreased breath sounds Inspiratory rales; rales may not be heard until infection is resolving Retractions Hyperresonance over areas of consolidation Unilateral or bilateral involvement	Fever mild or absent Coarse inspiratory rhonchi, which disappear with coughing
Laboratory	WBCs normal or low	WBCs normal Eosinophilia (nasal and peripheral) in allergic infants	WBCs elevated to 18,000–40,000/mm^3 (mainly polys)	WBCs normal or slightly elevated
X-ray		Hyperinflation Increased bronchovascular markings Mild infiltrates	Patchy infiltrates Increased bronchovascular markings Lobar consolidation	Normal or increased bronchovascular markings

Duration of illness	5–7 days	Acute symptoms 2–7 days Total resolution 7–10 days	7–10 days	7–14 days
Diagnosis	Generally apparent from inspiratory stridor and harsh, barking cough	Generally made by history of abrupt onset of dyspnea and wheezing in infant; hyperinflation of lungs and retractions support the diagnosis	Usually made by x-ray studies and physical signs of consolidation; etiology established by culture and clinical features Mycoplasmal (school-age children and adolescents) Insidious onset Nonproductive cough Fever Staphylococcal (children under 3 years) High fever Abdominal distention Respiratory distress Toxic Unilateral involvement Viral Upper respiratory infection often precedes pneumonia Insidious onset WBCs slightly elevated *H influenzae* (infants and young children) Symptoms similar to any of above Failure to respond to penicillin therapy	Diagnosis may by signs and symptoms

(continued)

Table 2-1 (Continued)

Criteria	Viral Croup (Laryngotracheobronchitis)	Bronchiolitis	Pneumonia	Bronchitis
Treatment	Outpatient management Cool-mist vaporizer Parents to monitor respirations and to watch for tachypnea, cyanosis, retractions, anxiety Increase liquid intake Refer for physician management children with acute onset of inspiratory stridor; respiratory distress; signs of acute epiglottitis (sudden onset, elevated temperature, toxic, drooling, anxious)	Refer to physician for airway maintenance and oxygenation; probable hospitalization Cool humidified oxygen Increase liquid intake Antibiotics indicated only with secondary bacterial infection	Penicillin G Streptococcal Staphylococcal Pneumococcal Ampicillin *H influenzae* Erythromycin Mycoplasma Viral Antibiotic therapy only if secondary bacterial infection is suspected Cool-mist vaporizer Increase liquid intake	Symptomatic Postural drainage Chest percussion Avoid inhalants Cool-mist vaporizer Antibiotic therapy with elevated WBCs or production of purulent sputum; amoxicillin is generally the drug of choice

B. Any child with cyanosis, restlessness, anxiety, or flaring of the alae nasi

C. Child under 1 year of age

NOTES

VIRAL GASTROENTERITIS

An acute, generally self-limited inflammation of the gastrointestinal tract, manifested by a sudden onset of vomiting and diarrhea

I. **Etiology**

    A. Most common causative agents: Reovirus, echovirus, Coxsackie virus, adenoviruses, polioviruses, parvovirus

II. **Incidence**

    A. Seen sporadically in day care centers, schools, and communities in epidemic proportions

    B. Common in all age groups

    C. Seen most frequently in winter

III. **Incubation period**

    A. 24–48 hours

IV. **Communicability**

    A. Transmissible during acute stage via fecal–oral route

V. **Subjective data**

    A. Vomiting: Assess duration, frequency, character, amount.

    B. Diarrhea

        1. Assess duration, frequency, consistency of stools, presence of blood or mucus.

        2. Stools are loose with unpleasant odor.

        3. Blood or mucus is rarely present.

    C. Pertinent subjective data to obtain

        1. History of exposure to others with similar symptoms

        2. History of illness in the community

        3. Urinary output: Frequency and amount

        4. Fever

        5. Abdominal pain

        6. Weight loss

        7. Type and amount of feedings before and since onset

    D. Pertinent subjective data to rule out other causes

        1. Exposure to turtles

        2. Exposure to food source outside of home

        3. Ingestion of drugs or toxic substances: If history is positive, refer immediately to physician.

        4. Exposure to stressful situation

        5. Ingestion of home-canned foods: If history is positive, refer immediately to physician.

VI. **Objective data**

    A. Physical examination should include other systems to rule out other infections.

        1. Ears

        2. Throat

        3. Adenopathy

4. Chest

5. Central nervous system for signs of meningeal irritation

   a. Nuchal rigidity

   b. Fontanelle

   c. Kernig's sign

   d. Brudzinski's sign

   e. Irritability, especially paradoxical

   f. Level of sensorium

6. Abdomen for distention, visible peristalsis, bowel sounds, tenderness, spasm, organomegaly, masses

7. Assess state of hydration (see Appendix D, Clinical Signs of Dehydration).

8. Weight, pulse, blood pressure, temperature

B. Laboratory tests

1. Urinalysis; include specific gravity to assess state of dehydration.

2. Stool culture not necessary for all children seen with acute gastroenteritis; indications for culture are diarrhea persisting over 4 days, infants, blood in stool.

VII. Assessment

A. Diagnosis is made by history of exposure, clinical course, and clinical picture. It is generally a diagnosis of exclusion if the history is not suggestive of other bacterial or parasitic etiologies and (if done) the stool culture is negative and there are no leukocytes on stool examination.

B. Differential diagnosis

1. *Escherichia coli* gastroenteritis: Common in children under 2 years of age. Gradual onset of diarrheal stools, which are loose, slimy green, and foul-smelling; vomiting and fever are not usually prominent symptoms.

2. *Salmonella* gastroenteritis (including food poisoning): Incubation period is usually 12–24 hours but can range from 6–72 hours. Severe abdominal cramps and loose, slimy, green stools with odor of rotten eggs are characteristic; vomiting is common. Diagnosis is confirmed by stool culture.

3. Staphylococcal food poisoning: Explosive onset 2–6 hours after ingestion of food contaminated with staphylococci; other persons who ingested the same food have a similar illness. Not transmitted from person to person.

VIII. Plan

A. If concurrent infection is found in addition to gastroenteritis (eg, pneumonia, otitis media, pharyngitis), treat according to protocol. Initially, antibiotics may have to be given parenterally.

B. Dietary management is directed primarily toward fluid and electrolyte management.

1. First 4 hours

   a. Oral rehydration solutions (Ricelyte, Lytren, Pedialyte) for mild to moderate dehydration. Mild: Give 50–60 ml/kg over 4-hour period. Moderate: Give 80–100 ml/kg over 4-hour period.

   b. To control vomiting, begin with 1 tsp/minute; continue even if vomiting persists initially.

   c. When tolerated, gradually increase the amount and decrease the frequency as vomiting subsides. If vomiting recurs, resume giving 1 tsp/minute and again gradually increase amounts.

    d. Repeat phase until rehydration occurs. Refer for intravenous fluids if dehydration worsens or rehydration not accomplished in 8 hours.

    e. Toddlers and older children refusing to take oral rehydration solutions may be given saltines and half-strength apple juice.

  2. Maintenance phase

    a. Breast-feeding on demand

    b. Lactose-free formula

    c. Add the following bland solids in small amounts. Avoid foods high in lactose.

      (1) Infant rice cereal

      (2) Banana flakes or mashed ripe banana

      (3) Saltines

      (4) Dry cereal

      (5) Toast with jelly

      (6) Jell-O

    d. Give 10 ml/kg oral rehydration solution after each watery stool.

  3. Third day

    a. If bland solids have not been added, start with small amounts of the foods listed above.

    b. If bland solids have been started and diarrhea has improved, continue as above and add baked potato and chicken, or similar bland foods.

    c. Gradually return to normal diet, avoiding whole milk, juices, and foods with roughage until diarrhea has completely subsided.

IX. Education

  A. Explain that the disease is self-limited. The usual duration of illness is 5–7 days. Medications such as paregoric, Kaopectate, and diphenoxylate (Lomotil) are not indicated.

  B. If toddler or child refuses oral rehydration solution, try Pedialyte freezer pops (2.1 oz per pop).

  C. Aim of treatment is to rehydrate and keep child well hydrated.

    1. Vomiting generally resolves as fluid repletion occurs.

    2. Clear liquids should be at room temperature. If given, cola or ginger ale is preferable if "flat."

    3. Do not give large amounts. One teaspoon every 1–5 minutes is tolerated best.

    4. If large amounts of cola are given, the caffeine may cause stimulation and increase the severity of diarrhea.

    5. Do not give whole milk for at least 48 hours.

    6. Do not use boiled skim milk; it has a high solute load.

  D. Once vomiting is under control, increase amount of clear liquids and decrease frequency to avoid too-frequent stimulation of the gastrocolic reflex, which might aggravate diarrhea.

  E. Stress the importance of strict adherence to the dietary regime so as not to prolong the course of the illness.

F. If clear liquids only are given for more than 48 hours, reactive loose stools may occur.

G. Starvation stools (scanty, mucoid, loose, green-brown) may be mistaken for diarrheal stools.

H. Monitor temperature and urinary output.

I. Use petroleum jelly on perianal area to prevent excoriation.

J. Support and encourage parent; treatment is time-consuming.

K. Gastroenteritis may occur in the entire family. It is highly communicable by the fecal–oral or fecal–respiratory route.

    1. Careful hand-washing technique must be followed to control spread.

    2. Do not let other children drink from the sick child's glass or use the same utensils.

X. Follow-up

A. Close telephone follow-up every 2 hours if vomiting and diarrhea are frequent.

B. Daily weight measurement until weight is stabilized.

C. Daily or twice-daily telephone contact until all gastrointestinal symptoms have stopped.

XI. Complications

A. The most important complication is dehydration.

XII. Consultation/Referral

A. Infants under 3 months of age

B. Vomiting persisting over 12 hours

C. Diarrhea persisting over 3 days

D. Signs or symptoms of dehydration

E. Abdominal pain or tenderness on examination

NOTES

| VOMITING, ACUTE

The forceful ejection of stomach contents through the esophagus and mouth; a common symptom throughout infancy and childhood

I. **Etiology**
   A. Associated with a variety of illnesses, infections, and emotional stress
   B. Often indicates an abnormality or infection of the gastrointestinal tract, urinary tract, or central nervous system
   C. Etiology varies with age.

II. **Incidence**
   A. One of the most common symptoms throughout infancy and childhood

III. **Subjective data**
   A. Is nausea associated with vomiting?
   B. Does child appear ill?
   C. Duration of vomiting (acute or chronic)
   D. Frequency of vomiting
   E. Character of vomitus (undigested food, bile, fecal material, blood)
   F. Relation to intake
   G. Projectile vomiting or "spitting up"?
   H. Associated fever
   I. Diarrhea or constipation
   J. Exposure to similar illness
   K. Weight loss, or last accurate weight
   L. Decrease in urinary output
   M. Detailed dietary history
   N. Ingestion of drugs or other substances
   O. Stress or changes (family, school)
   P. Associated symptoms
      1. Pulling at ears or complaints of ear pain
      2. Sore throat or distress when swallowing
      3. Stiff neck
      4. Cough
      5. Abdominal pain
      6. Headache
      7. Changes in vision
      8. High-pitched cry
      9. Convulsions
   Q. History of injury (eg, fall on head)

IV. **Objective data**
   A. Physical examination should encompass other systems to rule out other infectious processes.
      1. Ears
      2. Throat

3. Adenopathy
4. Chest
5. Central nervous system for signs of meningeal irritation
   a. Nuchal rigidity
   b. Fontanelle
   c. Kernig's sign
   d. Brudzinski's sign
   e. Irritability, especially paradoxical
   f. Level of sensorium
6. Abdomen for distention, visible peristalsis, bowel sounds, tenderness, spasm, organomegaly, masses
7. Assess state of hydration (see Appendix D, Clinical Signs of Dehydration).
8. Weight, head circumference, pulse, blood pressure, temperature

B. Urinalysis; include specific gravity to assess state of hydration.

V. **Assessment**

A. Type of vomiting
   1. Projectile
      a. Etiology: Upper gastrointestinal tract or increased intracranial pressure
      b. Refer to physician.
   2. Vomiting without nausea
      a. Etiology: Probable increased intracranial pressure
      b. Refer to physician.
   3. Vomiting with nausea
      a. Etiology: Infection or toxicity

B. Vomiting in infants (neonates to toddlers 2 years of age)
   1. Most acute vomiting in this age group is in conjunction with infection. The following causes must also be considered:
      a. Overfeeding
      b. Poor feeding technique (eg, failure to burp baby, propping of bottle)
      c. Congenital anomalies
         (1) Gastrointestinal lesions
            (a) Pyloric stenosis: Onset of vomiting at 2–3 weeks of age; progresses to projectile vomiting
            (b) Chalasia: Vomiting or regurgitation after feedings
            (c) Intussusception: Currant jelly stools, distention, visible peristalsis, bile-stained vomitus
            (d) Volvulus
         (2) Hydrocephalus: Increased head circumference, bulging fontanelle
   2. Infections: Almost any disease with fever at onset
      a. Gastroenteritis
      b. Urinary tract infection
      c. Meningitis
      d. Pneumonia
      e. Otitis media

3. Poisoning

C. Vomiting in children (2 years of age and older). Infection is also the most common etiology in acute vomiting in children over the age of 2 years, but ingestion of toxic substances becomes of increasing importance in this age group. The following are important causes to be considered in this age group:
   1. Acute infection
      a. Gastroenteritis
      b. Urinary tract infection
      c. Meningitis
      d. Pneumonia
      e. Pharyngitis
      f. Otitis media
      g. Acute glomerulonephritis
      h. Hepatitis
   2. Appendicitis
   3. Central nervous system
      a. Increased intracranial pressure due to brain tumor, hydrocephalus
      b. Migraine headaches
   4. Poisoning
      a. Lead
      b. Medications, drugs, salicylates
      c. Poisons

VI. **Plan**

A. Acute vomiting due to infectious cause
   1. First 4 hours
      a. Oral rehydration solution (Ricelyte, Pedialyte, Lytren), 1 tsp every 1–5 minutes
      b. After cessation of vomiting, increase amounts and decrease frequency to avoid overstimulating gastrocolic reflex and causing diarrhea. Give 1–2 oz every 15–30 minutes.
      c. If vomiting recurs, resume 1 tsp every 1–5 minutes until tolerated, and again gradually increase amounts.
      d. Intractable vomiting after 4 hours of therapy: Refer.
   2. Second day
      a. Add infant rice cereal mixed with water, banana, saltines, toast with jelly, Jell-O.
   3. Third day
      a. Gradually resume regular diet, avoiding foods high in lactose, strong-flavored foods, and fried foods until child is completely well.

B. Treatment for concurrent infectious processes must be instituted. Initially, antibiotics may have to be given parenterally.

VII. **Education**

A. Set timer and give 1 tsp of clear liquids every 1–5 minutes.
   1. Some children do not take oral rehydration solutions readily; try half-strength apple juice.

2. Vomiting resolves as fluid repletion occurs.

3. If 5 ml (1 tsp) of oral rehydration is given every minute, rehydration generally occurs with the total 300 ml delivered in 1 hour.

B. Monitor temperature and intake and output.

C. Support and encourage parent; this treatment is time-consuming but is the most effective way to treat vomiting and prevent dehydration.

D. Give parent specific dietary instructions, in writing if possible, and stress the importance of strict adherence to regimen.

E. If clear liquids are used for more than 48 hours, child may have reactive loose stools or starvation stools.

F. Stress hygiene and proper hand-washing technique to prevent spread if vomiting is due to infectious process.

G. Use tepid baths for temperature control if indicated.

VIII. Follow-up

A. Telephone contact at least every 3–4 hours while child is vomiting. Call immediately if any symptoms of dehydration.

B. Check weight in 24 hours.

C. Follow-up for other infectious process per protocol

IX. Complications

A. The most important complication of acute vomiting due to infection is dehydration.

X. Consultation/Referral

A. Infant under 6 months of age

B. Child of any age who appears toxic

C. Signs or symptoms of dehydration

D. Projectile vomiting

E. Blood, fecal material, or bile in vomitus

F. Vomiting persisting over 12 hours

G. Positive findings on abdominal examination

NOTES

VULVOVAGINITIS IN THE PREPUBERTAL CHILD

Inflammation of the vulva and vaginal introitus characterized by dysuria, pruritus, and vaginal discharge

I. **Etiology**

  A. Often a contact reaction to irritants such as bath soaps, bubble bath, laundry products, deodorants, perfumed powders, nylon underpants, panty hose, or tights

  B. Anal scratching (secondary to pinworm infestation), poor perineal hygiene, and masturbation may cause contamination of the vaginal area.

  C. Lack of estrogen makes the immature vaginal mucosa susceptible to infection.

II. **Incidence**

  A. Common in prepubertal females

III. **Subjective data**

  A. Vaginal discharge

  B. Dysuria

  C. Pruritus

  D. Inflammation

  E. Pertinent subjective data to obtain

   1. Use of bubble bath

   2. Use of harsh soaps

   3. Recent change in laundry products

   4. Use of nylon underpants, tights, tight jeans

   5. Improper toileting hygiene (have child demonstrate toileting technique)

   6. Symptoms of pinworm infestation (see Pinworms)

   7. Exposure to infection (eg, streptococcal upper respiratory infection)

   8. Recent infection (eg, group A beta-hemolytic streptococcus)

   9. Recent course of antibiotics

   10. Determine duration, amount, and type of discharge (bloody, purulent, mucoid).

   11. Masturbation

   12. Detailed history to determine possibility of sexual abuse. Include any behavioral changes that may suggest abuse.

IV. **Objective data**

  A. Vaginal discharge: Thin and mucoid, but may be copious and purulent

  B. Erythema of vulva and vaginal introitus

  C. Check hymenal opening; a minute high hymenal opening can impair vaginal drainage.

  D. If symptoms are severe, examine vagina with child in the knee–chest position using an otoscope with a nasal speculum or veterinary otoscope.

  E. Check for anal excoriation.

  F. Rectal exam, to detect foreign body or mass

  G. Laboratory tests

   1. Urinalysis, to rule out urinary tract infection and diabetes

    2. Hematocrit, to rule out anemia

    3. Culture of purulent discharge, both aerobically and on Thayer-Martin medium

V. Assessment

  A. Diagnosis: 80% of cases in prepubertal children are nonspecific vulvovaginitis.

  B. Differential diagnosis

    1. Physiologic leukorrhea

    2. Foreign body: Foreign body visualized; foul-smelling drainage

    3. Gonorrhea: Culture positive for *Neisseria gonorrhoeae*

    4. Herpes simplex: Vesicular eruptions; may be ulcerations; painful. Herpes simplex type 1 can cause simultaneous lesions in the mouth and vulva of young girls.

    5. Moniliasis: Vulvar and vaginal erythema; white, cheesy vaginal discharge; presence of *Candida* in potassium hydroxide wet preparation

    6. *Trichomonas* vaginitis: Vaginal erythema; profuse frothy discharge that is gray or green and malodorous. *Trichomonas* is seen as a motile, pear-shaped, flagellated protozoan on microscopic examination of wet preparation. Trichomoniasis may also be detected by Pap smear.

    7. Pinworms: Pinworm eggs visualized microscopically on Scotch tape slide

    8. Sexual abuse: Rule out by careful history. If high index of suspicion and history negative, refer to mental health worker with expertise in the field.

VI. Plan

  A. Sitz baths three times a day

  B. Proper perineal hygiene

  C. White cotton underpants

  D. Use mild soap (Dove or Johnson's Baby Bath).

  E. Scotch tape slide for pinworms if infestation suspected

  F. Neosporin ointment or 1% hydrocortisone cream applied locally three or four times a day

  G. Antibiotics as indicated by culture

    1. Group A beta-hemolytic streptococcus or pneumococcus: Penicillin 125–250 mg four times a day for 10 days, or erythromycin 50 mg/kg/day in four divided doses (more than 40 kg, 250 mg four times a day) for 10 days

    2. *Haemophilus influenzae*: Amoxicillin 40 mg/kg/day in three divided doses (more than 25 kg, 250 mg three times a day) for 10 days

    3. *N gonorrhoeae*: Consult physician for parenteral penicillin and order serology for syphilis.

VII. Education

  A. Teach careful perineal hygiene.

    1. Use cool, wet tissue, cotton balls, or Tucks (witch hazel) pads.

    2. Wipe from front to back.

  B. Sitz baths

    1. Warm water

    2. May add baking soda

    3. Duration of 15–20 minutes

4. Pat dry or air dry after bathing; do not rub. May use hair dryer on cool setting.

C. Avoid shampooing hair in bathtub.

D. Do not use bubble bath.

E. Use Dove or other bland soap in bath.

F. Change underpants frequently. White cotton underpants should be used; they are more absorbent than synthetic materials and free of dyes.

G. Use Ivory Snow for laundry.

H. Discontinue use of bleach and fabric softeners.

I. Avoid perfumed powders.

J. Avoid nylon underpants, tight jeans or slacks, pantyhose, and tights; they lead to maceration of the vulva.

K. Encourage child to void in tub if dysuria is a problem.

L. Wash all new items of clothing before child wears them.

M. Avoid long periods of time in wet bathing suits or spandex.

N. Overweight girls are particularly prone to recurrences.

VIII. Follow-up

A. Mild symptoms: Have parent call back in 5 days.

B. Moderate to severe symptoms
1. Have parent call back in 24–48 hours.
2. If pruritus is still a problem, use 1% hydrocortisone cream three times daily on vulva, or give diphenhydramine (Benadryl), 5 mg/kg/day orally in four doses.

C. Most cases of nonspecific vulvovaginitis improve within 2 weeks. If symptoms have not improved, vaginal examination and cultures must be done. If no specific causative organism is found, give amoxicillin three times daily (dosage according to age and weight) and use sulfanilamide (Vagitrol) or Sultrin cream locally.

IX. Consultation/Referral

A. Any question of sexual abuse

B. No improvement within 2 weeks using plan outlined above

C. Culture positive for *N gonorrhoeae*

NOTES

NOTES

|WARTS, COMMON AND PLANTAR

Benign intraepidermal tumors of the skin

I. **Etiology**
   A. Human papilloma virus, a papovavirus that grows within the nucleus of the epithelial cells and causes hyperplasia

II. **Incidence**
   A. Worldwide
   B. Plantar and common warts are most frequently seen in children 12–16 years of age. Both are more common in females.

III. **Subjective data**
   A. Common warts (verruca vulgaris)
      1. Complaints of warts that started as small papules and grew over a period of weeks or months
      2. May be no presenting complaints; warts may be found on physical examination.
      3. Complaint is generally prompted by cosmetic appearance, but some large warts may be irritated by pressure (eg, use of a pencil may cause pain in wart on finger).
   B. Plantar warts (verruca plantaris)
      1. Pain on sole of foot on weight bearing or walking
      2. Corn or callus on sole of foot
      3. Complaint of plantar wart
      4. May be history of trauma

IV. **Objective data**
   A. Common warts
      1. Lesions begin as tiny, translucent papules and progress to sharply circumscribed, circinate, firm lesions. Surface is roughened and pitted with papillary protuberances. Black pinpoint spots are often seen on the surface (thrombosed capillaries). Color of lesions ranges from skin-colored to gray-brown.
      2. Found most often in multiple distribution on the hands, but may occur anywhere on epidermis, usually on sites subject to trauma
   B. Plantar warts
      1. Lesions are flat (because of weight bearing) or slightly elevated.
      2. Resemble a callus, with pinpoint depressions on the surface
      3. Capillary dots may be seen.
      4. Interrupt natural skin lines; calluses do not.
      5. May be a single wart or a multiple distribution

V. **Assessment**
   A. Diagnosis is usually made by appearance.
   B. Differential diagnosis
      1. Molluscum contagiosum: umbilicated waxy papules; molluscum body can be expressed.
      2. Foreign body reaction: By history and surrounding erythema

    3. Callus: Does not interrupt skin lines, as does a plantar wart

VI. Plan

  A. Many treatments available, including benign neglect

  B. Vigorous treatment, which may cause pain and scarring, is not generally recommended.

  C. Treatment is not always successful; rate of recurrence is high.

  D. Many warts resolve spontaneously (66% within 2 years).

  E. Treatment modality selected must be individualized according to child and location of wart.

  F. Common warts

    1. Occlusive therapy: Periungual and subungual warts, which tend to be painful, may respond well to this therapy.

      a. Completely occlude wart with adhesive tape.

      b. Leave tape undisturbed for 1 week.

      c. After 1 week, soak wart thoroughly in warm water.

      d. Scrape surface of wart with emery board or fingernail.

      e. Reapply adhesive tape, and repeat process.

      f. May take several weeks for wart to disappear.

    2. Duofilm (salicylic and lactic acid in collodion)

      a. Soak wart for 10 minutes.

      b. Scrape surface with emery board.

      c. Apply Duofilm to wart only, using a toothpick.

      d. Allow to dry.

      e. Repeat every 24 hours.

    3. Trans-Ver-Sal patch (salicylic acid 15%), 6- or 12-mm size

      a. Cut patch to size of wart.

      b. Clean skin and smooth wart surface with emery board.

      c. Moisten wart with drop of water.

      d. Apply patch and secure with tape.

      e. Apply at bedtime and remove in morning, about 8 hours later.

      f. Use nightly until wart is gone.

    4. Tretinoin (Retin-A) gel, 0.01%: Use once daily.

    5. Cryosurgery (Histofreezer)

  G. Plantar warts

    1. Duofilm

      a. Soak foot in warm water for 10 minutes.

      b. Scrape surface of wart with emery board.

      c. Apply Duofilm to wart with toothpick; allow to dry and apply more if necessary to cover wart.

      d. Apply adhesive tape to wart once Duofilm is dry, and leave on for 24 hours.

      e. Repeat process daily.

    2. Trans-plantar patch (salicylic acid 21%), 20-mm size: Follow directions for Trans-Ver-Sal patch.

    3. Hyperthermia

        a. Hot water (113°F) immersion for 30–45 minutes two or three times a week for 10 treatments

        b. Wart virus is thermolabile.

    4. Fluorinated corticosteroid cream with occlusive dressing

        a. Diprosone cream 0.05% (middle potency), Maxivate cream 0.05% (middle to high potency), or Temovate cream 0.05% (high potency)

        b. Apply small amount at night.

        c. Cover with Saran wrap.

        d. Leave on for 12–48 hours.

        e. Reapply.

    5. Cryosurgery (Histofreezer)

VII. Education

  A. Warts are a virus.

  B. Warts generally occur after trauma to the skin.

  C. Warts are transmitted by direct contact, but plantar warts can be transmitted by fomites and floors.

  D. Virus concentration is greatest in warts of 6–12 months' duration.

  E. Most warts eventually disappear without treatment. About 66% resolve spontaneously within 2 years.

  F. Recurrences occur in 20%–30% of all cases.

  G. Duofilm

    1. Do not use applicator with Duofilm; drops are large and apt to get on surrounding skin.

    2. Do not apply to surrounding skin; causes desquamation and tissue destruction.

    3. Keep Duofilm bottle tightly closed.

    4. With erythema or tenderness, discontinue treatment until inflammation subsides.

    5. Do not use on infected or recently treated areas.

    6. Overtreatment causes scarring.

  H. Trans-plantar or Trans-Ver-Sal

    1. Do not apply to surrounding skin.

    2. Do not use on any other lesions. Use only on warts that have been diagnosed as such.

    3. Directions and emery board are included in package.

  I. Wear correctly fitting shoes to avoid pressure and trauma to the feet.

  J. Treatment may require several weeks.

  K. With occlusive therapy, if skin is sensitive to tape, use Micropore or Dermicel.

  L. Visible clinical improvement should be noted in 2–4 weeks. Complete resolution may take 6–12 weeks.

VIII. Follow-up

  A. Return in 1 week if using Duofilm.

  B. Phone in 2 weeks with occlusive therapy.

    C. Recheck periungual or subungual warts treated with occlusive therapy every 10–14 days.

IX. **Complications**

    A. Secondary infection

    B. Trauma to surrounding skin

X. **Consultation/Referral**

    A. For more vigorous treatment: Electrodesiccation for common warts or laser surgery for plantar warts

    B. Diabetics

    C. Venereal warts (condyloma acuminatum): Soft, friable, vegetative clusters on the foreskin, penis, labia, vaginal mucosa, or perianal area

NOTES

| BIBLIOGRAPHY

AIDS/HIV Infection Policies for Early Childhood and School Settings. Massachusetts Department of Public Health & Massachusetts Board of Education, 1993.

Annunziato P, Gershon A. Herpes simplex virus infections. *Pediatrics in Review,* 17:12, December 1996.

Behrman RE, Kliegman R. *Nelson Textbook of Pediatrics,* 14th ed. Philadelphia: WB Saunders, 1992.

Biddle C. *Adolescents, AIDS and HIV.* Washington DC: Center for Population Options, 1991.

Carlson LH. Otitis media in children. *Advance for Nurse Practitioners,* 2:2, February 1996.

Ceftriaxone: Associated biliary complications of treatment of suspected disseminated Lyme disease, New Jersey, 1990–1992. *Morbidity and Mortality Weekly Report,* 42:2, January 1993.

Connor E. Pediatric HIV infection: What you can do. *The Journal of Respiratory Diseases,* 14:1, January 1993.

Cranston K. Notes from the VIII International Conference on AIDS. Amsterdam, July 1992.

Cunningham AS. Antibiotics for otitis media: Restraint, not routine. *Contemporary Pediatrics,* 11:3, March 1994.

Eigen H. Asthma diagnosis: Getting back to the basics. *Journal of Respiratory Diseases,* 13:10 Supplement, October 1992.

Fireman P. Diagnosis of allergic disorders. *Pediatrics in Review,* 16:4, April 1995.

Fischbach F. *A Manual of Laboratory & Diagnostic Tests,* 5th ed. Philadelphia: JB Lippincott, 1996.

Gerber M, Markowitz M. Streptococcal pharyngitis: Clearing up the controversies. *Contemporary Pediatrics,* 9:10, October 1992.

Gigliotti F. Acute conjunctivitis. *Pediatrics in Review,* 16:6, June 1995.

Guidelines for the Diagnosis and Management of Asthma. Bethesda, MD: National Asthma Education Program, U.S. Department of Health and Human Services, August 1991.

Hatcher RA et al. *Contraceptive Technology,* 16th ed. New York: Irvington Publishers, Inc., 1994.

Healy GB. Consultation with the specialist: Otitis media. *Pediatrics in Review,* 13:1, January 1992.

HIV/AIDS Surveillance. Atlanta: U.S. Department of Health and Human Services, December 1996.

HIV/HBV in health care settings. *AIDS Newsletter.* Boston: Massachusetts Department of Public Health, December 1992.

Hoeprich PD, Jordan M, Ronald AR. *Infectious Diseases,* 5th ed. Philadelphia: JB Lippincott, 1994.

Hoole AJ, Greenberg RA, Pickard CG Jr. *Patient Care Guidelines for Nurse Practitioners,* 4th ed. Philadelphia: JB Lippincott, 1995.

Hoth DF Jr, Myers MW, Stein DS. Current status of HIV therapy: Antiretroviral agents. *Hospital Practice,* 27:9, September 1992.

Kaplan EL, ed. Group A streptococcal infections. *Pediatrics,* 87:6 Supplement, June 1996.

Karch AM. *Lippincott's Nursing Drug Guide.* Philadelphia: JB Lippincott, 1997.

Katcher ML. Cold, cough, and allergy medications: Uses and abuses. *Pediatrics in Review,* 17:1, January 1996.

Kemper K. Chronic asthma: An update. *Pediatrics in Review,* 17:4, April 1996.

Konig P. A step-wise approach to the changing drug therapy of Asthma. *Pediatric Annals,* 21:9, September 1992.

Kreipe RE. Eating disorders among children and adolescents. *Pediatrics in Review,* 16:10, October 1995.

Kruks G. Gay and lesbian homeless/street youth: Special issues and concerns. *Journal of Adolescent Health,* 12:7, November 1991.

Managing Otitis Media with Effusion in Young Children. Otitis Media Guideline Panel, U.S. Department of Health and Human Services, October 1994.

Mansfield MJ, Eliot AO. *Eating Disorders: Obesity, Anorexia and Bulimia Nervosa.* Syllabus, Postgraduate Course, Adolescent Medicine, Children's Hospital, Boston, May 1992.

Maxson S, Yamauche T. Acute otitis media. *Pediatrics in Review,* 17:6, June 1996.

Merenstein GB, Kaplan DW, Rosenberg AA. *Handbook of Pediatrics,* 17th ed. Norwalk: Appleton & Lange, 1994.

Meyers BR. *Antimicrobial Therapy Guide.* Newtown, PA: Antimicrobial Prescribing, 1992.

Middleton AD. Managing asthma: It takes teamwork. *American Journal of Nursing,* 97:1, January 1997.

Milgrom H, Bender B. Behavioral side effects of medications used to treat asthma and allergic rhinitis. *Pediatrics in Review,* 16:9, September 1995.

Murphy SJ. Treatment of acute asthma: What's new? *Audio Digest Foundation,* 42:15, August 1996.

Murphy SJ, Kelly HW. Advances in the management of acute asthma in children. *Pediatrics in Review,* 17:7, July 1996.

Nelson JD. *Pocket Book of Pediatric Antimicrobial Therapy,* 12th ed. Philadelphia: Williams & Wilkins, 1996.

Oski FA. *Principles and Practice of Pediatrics,* 2d ed. Philadelphia: JB Lippincott, 1994.

Pediatric spectrum of HIV disease in Massachusetts. *AIDS Newsletter.* Boston: Massachusetts Department of Public Health, January 1993.

Physicians Desk Reference, 50th ed. Montvale, NJ: Medical Economics, 1996.

Platts-Mills TAE. Controlling indoor allergens in patients with asthma. *Journal of Respiratory Diseases,* 13:10 Supplement, October 1992.

Rachelefsky GS. Guidelines for effective long-term use of theophylline. *Journal of Respiratory Diseases,* 13:10 Supplement, October 1992.

Report of the Committee on Infectious Diseases, 23d ed. Elk Grove Village, IL.: American Academy of Pediatrics, 1994.

Richards W. Asthma, allergies, and school. *Pediatric Annals,* 21:9, September 1992.

Rudolph C, Benaroch L. Hirschsprung disease. *Pediatrics in Review,* 16:1, January 1995

Saryan JA, O'Loughlin JM. Anaphylaxis in children. *Pediatric Annals,* 21:9, September 1992.

Sauer GC, Hall JC. *Manual of Skin Diseases,* 7th ed. Philadelphia: Lippincott-Raven, 1996.

Schidlow DV, Callahan CW. Pneumonia. *Pediatrics in Review,* 17:9, September 1996.

Schmitt BD. When your child has a fever. *Contemporary Pediatrics,* 10:6, June 1993.

Schotte, DE, Stunkard, AJ. Bulimia vs. bulimic behaviors on a college campus. *Journal of the American Medical Association,* 258:9, September, 1987.

Schuster CS, Ashburn SS. *The Process of Human Development*, 3rd ed. Philadelphia: JB Lippincott, 1992.

Shadick NA, Liang MH. Management of Lyme disease. *Brigham and Women's Hospital Medical Update*, 5:1, January 1993.

Shapiro ED. Bacterial respiratory infections and otitis media. *Pediatric Annals*, 20:8, August 1991.

Shapiro GG. Childhood asthma: Update. *Pediatrics in Review*, 13:11, November 1992.

Sheffer AL. Where beta$_2$-adrenergics fit into step care for asthma. *Journal of Respiratory Diseases*, 13:10 Supplement, October 1992.

Siedfried EC. Warts on children: An approach to therapy. *Pediatric Annals*, 25:2, February 1996.

Singalavanija S, Frieden I. Diaper Dermatitis. *Pediatrics in Review*, 16:4, April 1995.

Sonnenblick HC. Abstract: Erythema infectiosum. *Pediatrics in Review*, 13:6, June 1992.

Strasburger VC, Brown RT. *Adolescent Medicine*, 1st ed. Boston: Little, Brown, 1991.

Survival with AIDS in Massachusetts. *AIDS Newsletter*. Massachusetts Department of Public Health, November 1992.

Tierney LM, McPhee SJ, Papadakis MA. *Current Medical Diagnosis and Treatment*, 33rd ed. Norwalk: Appleton & Lange, 1994.

Wilson MH. Update of urinary tract infections. *Audio Digest Foundation*, 42:19, October 1996.

III

Drug Index

Rose W. Boynton

The Drug Index provides a quick reference to help medical professionals confirm their knowledge of medications. It contains a list of the most common drugs used in ambulatory pediatric practice. This part of the manual provides a comprehensive outline of each medication, including the generic name and composition, pediatric dosage, action of the drug, and the facts parents should know about the drug.

ACLOVATE (Topical Cream, Ointment)

I. **Generic name.** Aclometasone dipropionate cream, 0.05%; ointment, 0.05%

II. **Manufacturer/How supplied.** Glaxo Wellcome; 15-, 45-, or 60-g tubes (both cream and ointment)

III. **Route.** Topical cream or ointment

IV. **Uses.** Synthetic corticosteroid used to treat symptoms of inflammatory and pruritic rashes when corticosteroid activity is required

V. **Dosage and administration**

    A. Apply a small amount of cream or ointment to the affected area two or three times a day; massage gently into skin until absorbed.

    B. Use of an occlusive dressing may be more beneficial with psoriasis or lichen simplex chronicus. Cover lesion with medication and light gauze dressing, and then cover the area with pliable plastic film. Seal the edges with tape. Leave dressing in place for 1–4 days.

    C. Discontinue use if signs of infection occur.

VI. **Side effects.** Burning, itching, dryness, hypopigmentation, allergic contact dermatitis

VII. **Contraindications.** Hypersensitivity to any ingredients in this preparation or to other corticosteroids

VIII. **Precautions**

    A. Children may have a greater sensitivity to topical corticosteroid-induced HPA axis suppression and Cushing's syndrome than do older people because of a larger ratio of skin surface to body weight. Manifestations of adrenal suppression in children include mental retardation, retardation of linear growth, poor weight gain, low plasma cortisol levels, absence of ACTH stimulation, bulging fontanelles, headache, and bilateral papilledema.

    B. Use the lowest dose compatible with effective therapeutic regimen.

    C. Do not use over an extended period of time in children.

    D. Not suggested for use in pregnant patients

    E. Medication is excreted in breast milk, so use with caution during lactation.

IX. **Education**

    A. Keep all medication out of children's reach.

    B. Children may absorb proportionately more topical corticosteroids and therefore may be more susceptible to toxicity.

    C. If irritation, side effects, or infections develop, discontinue use immediately and call the office.

    D. Do not use medication near or in the eyes.

    E. Do not use medication over a prolonged period of time or over large surface areas.

    F. Do not bandage or cover skin area unless advised to do so by medical provider.

    G. Do not use in the diaper area.

    H. Do not use on the face, groin, or underarm area.

    I. Store medication at 36°–86°F.

ACTIFED (ANTIHISTAMINE-DECONGESTANT)

I. **Composition.** Triprolidine hydrochloride 2.5 mg, pseudoephedrine hydrochloride 60 mg

II. **Manufacturer/How supplied.** Warner-Wellcome; tablets (bottles of 100 and 1,000; boxes of 12, 24, and 48)

III. **Route.** Oral

IV. **Action and uses.** Antihistamine and decongestant used in seasonal and perennial rhinitis, allergic rhinitis, mild upper respiratory symptoms, and sinus congestion.

V. **Dosage.** Ages 6–12, one-half tablet every 4–6 hours; ages 12 and older, 1 tablet every 4–6 hours

VI. **Contraindications.** High blood pressure, heart disease, diabetes, thyroid disease, asthma, glaucoma

VII. **Precautions.** Reacts with monoamine oxidase inhibitors and tricyclic antidepressants

VIII. **Education**

    A. Keep all medication out of children's reach.

    B. May cause excitability in some children

    C. May cause drowsiness

    D. Do not exceed four doses in 24 hours.

    E. Store tablets at 59°–77°F in a dry dark place.

ADRENALIN CHLORIDE SOLUTION (EPINEPHRINE HYDROCHLORIDE)

I. **Composition.** Sterile solution contains 1 mg adrenaline (epinephrine as a hydrochloride) in each 1-ml ampule (1:1,000).

II. **Manufacturer/How supplied.** Parke-Davis; ampules, packages of 10; solution, 30-ml vial

III. **Route.** Subcutaneous or intramuscular

IV. **Action.** Epinephrine is a sympathomimetic drug. It stimulates an adrenergic receptive mechanism on effector cells and imitates all actions of the sympathetic nervous system, except those on the arteries of the face and on the sweat glands.

V. **Uses.** Most commonly used to relieve respiratory distress due to bronchospasm, especially bronchial asthmatic paroxysms. Also used to relieve hypersensitivity to drugs and other allergens and to control rhinitis, urticaria, and acute sinusitis.

VI. **Dosage.** 0.2–1 ml (mg) subcutaneously; use small dose to start and increase if required. Pediatric dose is 0.01 mg/kg, to a maximum of 0.5 mg subcutaneously every 4 hours.

VII. **Side effects.** Anxiety, headache, fever, palpitations

VIII. **Contraindications**

    A. Patients with congestive glaucoma or organic brain disease

    B. Patients receiving local anesthesia of certain areas (eg, toes or fingers); it may cause vasoconstriction and sloughing of tissue.

C. Patients taking digitalis, mercurial diuretics, or other drugs that sensitize the heart to arrhythmias

IX. Education

A. Keep all medication out of children's reach.

B. Protect from light.

C. Do not remove from carton until ready to use.

D. Do not use if medication is brown or a precipitant is evident.

E. Action of epinephrine may be affected by tricyclic antidepressants and certain antihistamines.

F. Repeated local injections of epinephrine may result in necrosis at injection sites.

G. "Epinephrine-fastness" can occur with prolonged use.

H. Use in pregnancy only if the benefit outweighs the risk to the fetus.

I. Use with caution in patients with long-standing bronchial asthma and emphysema who have developed degenerative heart disease.

J. Use with caution in persons with cardiovascular disease, hypertension, diabetes, or hyperthyroidism, and in psychoneurotic persons.

K. Overdose or inadvertent intravenous injection of epinephrine may cause cerebrovascular hemorrhage due to the sudden increase in blood pressure.

L. Epinephrine may cause pulmonary edema due to peripheral constriction and cardiac stimulation.

M. Rapid-acting vasodilators such as nitrates or alpha-blocking agents may counteract the marked pressure effects of epinephrine.

AMOXICILLIN (SYNTHETIC ANTIBIOTIC)

I. **Manufacturer/How supplied.** SmithKline Beecham; pediatric drops: 50 mg/ml; oral suspension: 125 or 250 mg/5 ml; chewables: 250 mg (Amoxil); capsules: 250 or 500 mg

II. **Route.** Oral

III. **Uses.** Upper and lower respiratory tract infections caused by gram-negative and gram-positive organisms. Effective in infections of the ears, nose, throat, soft tissues, skin, and genitourinary tract. Also used before oral surgical procedures.

IV. **Dosage**

A. For infections other than of lower respiratory tract, 20 mg/kg/day in divided doses every 8 hours

1. Under 13 lb: 0.75 ml pediatric drops every 8 hours

2. 13–15 lb: 1 ml every 8 hours

3. 16–18 lb: 125 ml every 8 hours

4. 18 lb or more: 250 mg every 9 hours

B. For infections of lower respiratory tract, 40 mg/kg/day in divided doses every 8 hours

1. Under 13 lb: 1.25 ml pediatric drops every 8 hours

2. 13–15 lb: 2 ml every 8 hours

3. 16–18 lb: 125 or 250 mg every 8 hours

4. 20 kg and over: 500 mg every 8 hours

C. Oral prophylaxis before dental surgery or dental procedures: Adults 2g, Children, 50 mg orally 1 hour before procedure.

V. **Side effects.** Nausea, vomiting, diarrhea, urticaria, maculopapular rash

VI. **Contraindications.** Allergy to penicillin; renal or hepatic malfunction

VII. **Precautions.** Safety of use in pregnancy has not been established.

VIII. **Education**

A. Keep all medication out of children's reach.

B. Take medication for 10 full days even though symptoms disappear.

C. Medication may be given with meals.

D. Suspension may be placed directly in mouth for swallowing or may be mixed with juice, formula, or soft drinks.

E. Shake oral suspension and pediatric drops well before using.

F. Keep bottle tightly capped.

G. Discard unused portion of medication after 14 days.

H. Refrigeration preferred but not required

I. Diabetics using Clinitest will get a falsely high sugar reading.

J. If side effects occur, discontinue use and call the office.

Ampicillin (Antibiotic)

I. **Generic name.** Ampicillin trihydrate

II. **Composition.** Oral suspension: 125 or 250 mg/5 ml; capsules: 250 or 500 mg

III. **Route.** Oral, intramuscular, or intravenous

IV. **Action and uses**

A. Inhibition of cell wall synthesis; broad-spectrum activity against gram-negative and gram-positive bacteria

B. Used for treatment of genitourinary, respiratory, and gastrointestinal infections caused by *Escherichia coli, Haemophilus influenzae, Neisseria gonorrhoeae,* salmonella, shigella, and *Proteus mirabilis,* septicemia, and bacterial meningitis

C. Also effective against gram-positive pneumococcal staphylococci, groups A and B beta-hemolytic streptococci, and *Bacillus anthracis.*

V. **Dosage**

A. 25–50 mg/kg/day in divided doses every 8 hours

B. For septicemia and bacterial meningitis: 50–200 mg/kg/day in divided doses every 4 hours

C. 11–22 lb: 125 mg by mouth every 6 hours

D. Over 25 lb: 250 mg by mouth every 6 hours

VI. **Side effects.** Nausea, vomiting, stomatitis, diarrhea, urticaria, rash (maculopapular or erythema multiforme), and black, hairy tongue. Hematologic side effects include anemia, thrombocytopenia, purpura, eosinophilia, agranulocytosis.

VII. **Contraindications.** History of hypersensitivity to any penicillins

VIII. Precautions

A. Not suggested for, or to be used with caution in, children with asthma, severe hay fever, or allergies.

B. Treatment may cause overgrowth of nonsusceptible organisms.

C. Smaller dosages are suggested for premature infants and neonates; use with caution in this age group because of poor renal clearance.

D. Oral contraceptives may be less effective; breakthrough bleeding may occur. Clinitest may produce false-positive results.

IX. Education

A. Keep all medication out of children's reach.

B. Discontinue drug if signs of allergy appear; call the office.

C. Take medication on an empty stomach 1 hour before or 2 hours after eating; absorption may be affected by food.

D. Shake liquid well before using.

E. Take for 10 full days as instructed.

F. Store liquid form in refrigerator.

ANAPROX (NONSTEROIDAL ANTI-INFLAMMATORY)

I. Generic name. Naproxen sodium

II. Composition. 275 mg naproxen sodium equivalent of 250 mg; 250 mg naproxen sodium with 25 mg (1 mEq) sodium

III. Manufacturer/How supplied. Roche; bottles of 100 film-coated tablets or cartons of 100 blister-pack tablets

IV. Route. Oral

V. Uses. Mild to moderate pain associated with primary dysmenorrhea, acute tendinitis, bursitis, juvenile arthritis, rheumatoid arthritis, osteoarthritis, ankylosing spondylitis, and acute gout

VI. Dosage

A. Mild to moderate pain in primary dysmenorrhea, acute tendinitis, and bursitis: Starting dose two tablets (550 mg) followed by one tablet (275 mg) in 6–8 hours. Total daily dose not to exceed 1,375 mg.

B. Children age 2 and older with juvenile arthritis: Single dose of 2.5–5 mg/kg; total dose not to exceed 15 mg/kg/day. Anaprox 275-mg tablet is not well suited for younger children; use Naprosyn 250-mg scored tablet or suspension (125 mg/5 ml) for juvenile arthritis in younger children.

C. Adult rheumatoid arthritis, osteoarthritis, and ankylosing spondylitis: One tablet (275 or 500 mg) twice daily; lower dose may suffice. For long-term administration, do not treat more than twice daily.

VII. Side effects. Gastrointestinal discomfort, drowsiness, dizziness, vertigo, or depression. Serious side effect of gastrointestinal bleeding may require hospitalization or might be fatal.

VIII. Contraindications

A. Allergy to ingredients in medication or sensitivity to aspirin or other nonsteroidal anti-inflammatory medications that induce asthma, rhinitis or nasal polyps, or hypertension

   B. History of peptic ulcer disease, alcoholism, gastrointestinal bleeding disorders, renal dysfunction, hypertension, or heart disease

   C. Pregnancy or lactation

IX. Precautions

   A. Do not use concomitantly with Naprosyn.

   B. Long-term use of Anaprox can result in acute interstitial nephritis with hematuria, proteinuria, and occasionally nephrotic syndrome.

X. Education

   A. Keep all medication out of children's reach.

   B. If side effects occur, discontinue use and call the office.

   C. If overdose occurs, call the office immediately.

   D. Safety in use in children under age 2 is not established.

   E. Do not exceed daily recommended dose. Do not use medication longer than necessary.

   F. Single daily dose is recommended in children with juvenile arthritis.

   G. When treating primary dysmenorrhea, prescribe only eight tablets at a time and do not treat longer than 3 days. Have the patient call the office after her next menstrual period regarding effectiveness. Reevaluate patient every 3–4 months with follow-up visit.

ARISTOCORT A (TOPICAL CREAM)

I. Generic name. Triamcinolone acetonide

II. Composition. Each gram of 0.025% topical cream contains 0.25 mg of the highly active steroid triamcinolone acetonide. Each gram of 1% topical cream contains 0.1 mg triamcinolone acetonide.

III. How supplied. 15- or 60-g tubes

IV. Route. Topical

V. Uses. Inflammatory and pruritic rashes, minor skin irritations, allergic contact dermatitis

VI. Dosage and administration. Apply a light film sparingly to the affected area three times daily.

VII. Contraindications

   A. Sensitivity to ingredients of medication

   B. Safety during pregnancy has not been established. Not suggested for use by nursing mothers.

VIII. Precautions. Children may absorb proportionally larger amounts of topical corticosteroids and therefore may be more susceptible to systemic toxicity than more mature patients because of larger ratio of skin surface area to body weight.

IX. Education

   A. Keep all medication out of children's reach.

   B. Administration of topical corticosteroids to children should be limited to the least amount compatible with an effective therapeutic regimen.

C. Chronic corticosteroid therapy may interfere with growth and development in children.

D. If skin does not respond to medication, immediately discontinue use.

E. Do not use in management of extensive area, particularly in small children.

F. Occlusive dressings may be used rarely for the management of psoriasis or recalcitrant conditions. If infection develops, the use of occlusive dressings should be discontinued and appropriate antimicrobial therapy instituted.

G. Use medication as directed.

H. Avoid contact with face and eyes.

I. Do not use medication for any other rash.

J. Do not use medication under tight-fitting diapers or plastic pants in children.

ASPIRIN (ANALGESIC)

I. **Generic name.** Acetylsalicylic acid

II. **Composition.** Orange-flavored chewable tablets, 1.25 grains

III. **Route.** Oral

IV. **Action and uses.** Antipyretic, anti-inflammatory, analgesic. Used to treat headache, simple upper respiratory infection, teething discomfort, immunization discomfort, otitis media, pharyngitis, juvenile rheumatoid arthritis, acute rheumatic fever, Kawasaki disease.

V. **Dosage**

A. 65 mg/kg/day in divided doses every 6 hours, not to exceed 3.6 g/day

B. Administer every 4 hours, no more than five times a day.

   1. 2–4 years: Two tablets
   2. 4–6 years: Three tablets
   3. 6–9 years: Four tablets
   4. 9–11 years: Five tablets

VI. **Contraindications**

A. Sensitivity to salicylates

B. Not recommended for influenza symptoms or chickenpox because of risk of Reye's syndrome

VII. **Precautions**

A. Use cautiously in patients with peptic ulcer or asthma or those on anticoagulant therapy.

B. Use of aspirin during pregnancy and lactation is usually not advised. Do not use aspirin during the last 3 months of pregnancy, as it may cause fetal problems or complications during delivery.

VIII. **Education**

A. Do not use over a prolonged period of time.

B. If intense itching and general rash occur, discontinue medication and call the office.

C. Tinnitus is an early sign of toxicity; discontinue use or decrease dosage.

D. Prolonged high doses of aspirin can lead to iron-deficiency anemia, especially in young women.

E. High levels of salicylates can cause gastric irritation and gastric bleeding.

F. *Warning:* Keep out of children's reach. One of the most common causes of poisoning in children is accidental ingestion of aspirin, and this drug is often used in teenage suicides, particularly by females.

ATARAX (ANTIANXIETY, ANTIHISTAMINE)

I. **Generic name.** Hydroxyzine hydrochloride

II. **Composition.** Syrup: 10 mg/5 ml in pint bottles; tablets: 10, 25, 50, or 100 mg

III. **Route.** Oral

IV. **Action.** Suppression of activity in certain regions of subcortical area of central nervous system; primary skeletal muscle relaxant, bronchodilator activity with antihistamine and analgesic effects. May have an antiemetic effect.

V. **Uses**

A. Pruritus due to allergic conditions (chronic urticaria, atopic and contact dermatitis) and in histamine-mediated pruritus

B. Symptomatic relief of anxiety and tension

C. For sedation in premedication and after general anesthesia

VI. **Dosage**

A. Under age 6: 50 mg daily in divided doses four times a day

B. Over age 6: 50–100 mg daily in divided doses three or four times a day

VII. **Side effects.** Dry mouth, drowsiness, rare instances of trauma and convulsions

VIII. **Contraindications**

A. Safety during pregnancy has not been established.

B. Previous hypersensitivity to Atarax

C. Not suggested for use by nursing mothers; unknown whether this drug is excreted in human milk

IX. **Precautions.** Potentiating action of hydroxyzine must be considered when drug is used in conjunction with central nervous system depressants. Atarax potentiates the effects of meperidine (Demerol) and barbiturates, so their use in preanesthetic adjunctive therapy should be modified. Atropine and other belladonna alkaloids are not affected. Digitalis may be used with Atarax successfully.

X. **Education**

A. Keep all medication out of children's reach.

B. Patients should be advised against simultaneous use of central nervous system depressants; the effect of alcohol may be increased.

C. Overdose causes hypersedation. If overdose occurs, call the office immediately. No specific antidote; if vomiting has not occurred spontaneously it should be induced immediately. Gastric lavage is also recommended.

D. Effectiveness as an antianxiety agent (more than 4 months) has not been established by clinical studies.

AUGMENTIN (ORAL ANTIBIOTIC)

I.   **Generic name.** Amoxicillin and clavulanate potassium

II. **Manufacturer/How supplied.** SmithKline Beecham; 250- or 500-mg white coated tablets; 125- or 250-mg chewable tablets; 125- or 250-mg orange- or banana-flavored suspension

III. **Route.** Oral

IV. **Uses.** Lower respiratory tract infections (especially beta-lactamase–producing strains of *Haemophilus influenzae*), otitis media, sinusitis, skin and skin structure infections, urinary tract infections caused by *Escherichia coli, Klebsiella,* and *Enterobacter* species

V.   **Dosage**
   A. 20 mg/kg/day (based on amoxicillin component)
   B. 18 lb and over: 125 or 250 mg every 8 hours
   C. 20 kg and over: 500 mg every 8 hours

VI. **Side effects.** Loose stools or diarrhea, vomiting, skin rash, urticaria, vaginitis, flatulence, headache, abdominal discomfort

VII. **Contraindications**
   A. Allergy to penicillin
   B. Lactation (Augmentin secreted in breast milk)

VIII. **Education**
   A. Keep all medication out of children's reach.
   B. Take medication for 10 full days even though symptoms disappear.
   C. Shake oral suspension well before using.
   D. Refrigerate suspension.
   E. Discard medication after 10 days.
   F. May be administered with meals.
   G. Discontinue drug if signs of allergy appear.
   H. 250- and 500-mg tablets contain the same amount of clavulanic acid; therefore, two 250-mg tablets are not equivalent to one 500-mg tablet.

AURALGAN OTIC SOLUTION (TOPICAL OTIC ANALGESIC)

I.   **Composition.** Antipyrine, benzocaine, dehydrated glycerin

II. **Manufacturer/How supplied.** Wyeth-Ayerst; 10-ml bottle

III. **Route.** External canal of ear

IV. **Action and uses.** Topical analgesic to reduce inflammation and pain associated with acute otitis media

V.   **Dosage and administration.** Instill drops until ear canal is filled. Do not touch ear with dropper. Insert a wick of cotton into the meatus; moisten cotton with Auralgan. Repeat procedure every 1–2 hours until pain is relieved.

VI. **Contraindications**

A. Hypersensitivity to any of the components or substances related to them

B. Effect on fetus unknown; use not recommended in pregnancy or by nursing mothers

VII. **Education**

A. Keep all medication out of children's reach.

B. Warm bottle by holding in palm of hand; do not heat in hot water.

C. Keep bottle tightly closed.

D. Do not rinse dropper after use; water reduces strength of medication.

E. Discard remaining medication after treatment has been completed.

F. Protect solution from light and heat.

G. Do not use solution if it is brown or contains precipitate.

H. Discard product 6 months after dropper is first placed in drug solution.

A ZMACORT (ORAL INHALER)

I. **Generic name.** Triamcinolone acetonide

II. **Composition.** Each inhalation contains about 200 mcg triamcinolone acetonide.

III. **Manufacturer/How supplied.** Rhone-Poulenc Rorer; metered aerosol unit with 240 actuations. Instructions and an oral adapter are supplied.

IV. **Route.** Oral inhalation in aerosol

V. **Action and uses.** Chronic treatment with corticosteroids for symptoms of bronchial asthma. This is not a bronchodilator and is not indicated for rapid response to bronchospasm.

VI. **Dosage.** Ages 6–12 years: One or two inhalations four times a day, not to exceed 12 inhalations a day

VII. **Side effects.** Dry throat, hoarseness, dry mouth, increased cough or wheezing

VIII. **Contraindications**

A. Primary treatment of status asthmaticus or acute attacks of asthma where intensive treatment is required

B. Hypersensitivity to ingredients in preparation

C. Not indicated for asthma that can be controlled by bronchodilators or other nonsteroidal medications

D. Not indicated for patients who require systemic corticosteroid treatments infrequently

E. Not indicated in the treatment of nonasthmatic bronchitis

F. Not indicated for patients with positive mouth and throat cultures for *Candida albicans*

G. Not recommended for children on immunosuppressant drugs

H. Not recommended for children with measles or chickenpox

I. Not indicated for use during pregnancy

IX. **Precautions.** Use with caution in persons already receiving alternate-day prednisone treatment for any disease.

X. Education

A. Keep all medication out of children's reach.

B. Monitor children's growth and development carefully while on medication, especially suppression of growth.

C. Not recommended for children under age 6 years

D. Patients receiving a bronchodilator by inhalation should use the bronchodilator before using the Azmacort inhaler.

E. Practice good oral hygiene; rinse the mouth after using the inhaler.

F. Best used on a regular schedule rather than as needed

G. Do not give live vaccines with immunosuppressive doses of corticosteroids.

H. Do not increase dose; follow directions carefully.

I. If side effects occur, discontinue medication and call the office.

BACTRIM OR SEPTRA (SYNTHETIC ANTIBACTERIAL)

I. **Generic name.** Trimethoprim–sulfamethoxazole

II. **Composition.** Cherry-flavored suspension: Trimethoprim 40 mg/5 ml, sulfamethoxazole 200 mg/5 ml; tablets: trimethoprim 80 mg, sulfamethoxazole 400 mg; double-strength tablets: trimethoprim 160 mg, sulfamethoxazole 800 mg

III. **Route.** Oral

IV. **Uses.** Urinary tract infection, otitis media, *Pneumocystis carinii* pneumonitis. The organisms most affected in urinary tract infections are *Escherichia coli*, *Klebsiella–Enterobacter*, *Proteus mirabilis*, *Proteus vulgaris*, and *Proteus morganii*. Also traveler's diarrhea in adults.

V. **Dosage.** Administer twice daily for 10 days.

Body Weight (kg)	(lbs)	Suspension		Tablets
10	22	1 tsp (5 ml)	or	$1/2$ tablet
20	44	2 tsp (10 ml)	or	1 tablet
30	66	3 tsp (15 ml)	or	$1^1/_2$ tablets
40	88	4 tsp (20 ml)	or	2 tablets or 1 double-strength tablet

VI. **Side effects**

A. Blood dyscrasia, allergic manifestations (eg, urticaria, erythema multiforme, pruritus, periorbital edema, photosensitivity, gastrointestinal complaints, nausea, vomiting, diarrhea, headaches, tinnitus, vertigo, insomnia)

B. Minor side effects: Mild fluid retention, itching of skin, ringing of ears

VII. **Contraindications**

A. Sensitivity to sulfonamides

B. Infants less than 2 months of age

C. Renal insufficiency

D. Severe allergy or asthma

    E. Pregnant women and nursing mothers (drug passes the placental barrier and is excreted in breast milk)

    F. Not to be used in treatment of streptococcal pharyngitis

    G. Not to be used by AIDS patients; they may not tolerate or respond to Bactrim in the same manner as patients without AIDS.

    H. Not indicated for prophylactic or prolonged treatment of otitis media at any age

VIII. Precautions

    A. Discontinue at first appearance of skin rash or any adverse reaction.

    B. *Warning:* Fatalities associated with administration of sulfonamides have occurred due to severe adverse reactions (Stevens-Johnson syndrome, toxic epidermal necrolysis, agranulocytosis, aplastic anemia, fulminant hepatic necrosis).

IX. Education

    A. Keep all medication out of children's reach.

    B. Increase fluid intake by several glasses of water a day.

    C. Discontinue drug if any signs of allergy occur, and call the office immediately.

    D. Take medication for 10 full days as directed.

    E. Store tablets and liquid medicine at 59°–86°F, away from light.

BACTROBAN 2% OINTMENT (TOPICAL OINTMENT, DERMATOLOGIC USE)

I. **Generic name.** Mupirocin

II. **Composition.** Each gram contains 20 mg mupirocin in a bland, water-miscible ointment base.

III. **Manufacturer/How supplied.** SmithKline Beecham; 15- or 30-g tubes or 1-g single-unit packages

IV. **Route.** Topical; not for ophthalmic use

V. **Action and uses.** Inhibits bacterial protein synthesis by reversibly and specifically binding to bacterial isoleucyl transfer-RNA synthetase. Used for treatment of impetigo due to *Streptococcus pyogenes, Staphylococcus aureus,* and beta-hemolytic streptococcus.

VI. **Dosage and administration.** Apply a small amount of ointment to the affected area three times a day for 3–5 days.

VII. **Side effects.** Itching, burning, stinging, rash, nausea, dry skin, tenderness, swelling, increased exudate

VIII. Contraindications

    A. History of sensitivity reactions to any components of the drug

    B. Safety of use in pregnancy has not been established.

IX. Precautions

    A. If a reaction suggesting sensitivity or chemical irritation occurs, discontinue treatment.

    B. Nursing should be temporarily discontinued while using Bactroban. It is unknown whether Bactroban is present in breast milk.

X. Education

A. Keep all medication out of children's reach.

B. Reevaluate patients who do not show a clinical response within 3–5 days.

C. Store medication at 59°–86°F (controlled room temperature).

D. The area treated may be covered with a gauze dressing if desired.

E. Prolonged use may result in overgrowth of nonsusceptible organisms, including fungi.

F. Due to the mode of action, Bactroban shows no cross resistance with chloramphenicol, erythromycin, fusidic acid, gentamicin, lincomycin, methicillin, neomycin, novobiocin, penicillin, streptomycin, and tetracycline.

BIAXIN (SEMISYNTHETIC MACROLIDE ANTIBIOTIC)

I. Generic name. Clarithromycin

II. Manufacturer/How supplied. Abbott; 250- or 500-mg tablets; granules for oral suspension, 100 mg after suspension (125 or 250 mg/5 ml)

III. Route. Oral

IV. Action and uses. An antibacterial medication that binds the 50S ribosomal subunit of susceptible microorganisms, resulting in inhibition of protein synthesis. It is used in acute maxillary sinusitis, uncomplicated skin infections due to *Staphylococcus aureus* or *Streptococcus pyogenes*, or pneumonia due to streptococcus.

V. Dosage

Body Weight (kg)	(lbs)	Dose q12h	125/5 ml	250 mg/5 ml
9	20	62.5 mg	2.5 ml q12h	1.25 ml q12h
17	37	125 mg	5 ml q12h	2.5 ml q12h
25	55	187.5 mg	7.5 ml q12h	3.75 ml q12h
33	73	250 mg	10 ml q12h	5 ml q12h

VI. Contraindications

A. Known hypersensitivity to clarithromycin, erythromycin, or any of the macrolide antibiotics

B. Patients receiving tertenadine therapy who have preexisting cardiac abnormalities or electrolyte disturbances

C. Do not use in pregnant women due to potential hazard to the fetus.

D. Safety and effectiveness in children under 6 months of age are unknown.

VII. Education

A. Keep all medication out of children's reach.

B. Can be taken with or without food; can be taken with milk.

C. Do not refrigerate the suspension.

D. Keep at 59°–86°F.

E. Most strains of methicillin- and oxacillin-resistant staphylococci are resistant to clarithromycin.

F. Patients receiving theophylline may show an increase in serum theophylline concentration. Monitoring of these levels should be considered for patients receiving high doses of theophylline.

G. Unknown if clarithromycin is excreted in breast milk

H. Follow instructions carefully. Add half the volume of water to the bottle and shake vigorously. Add rest of water to the bottle and shake well before use.

I. Keep bottle tightly closed.

J. Use medication within 14 days.

K. Discontinue use of medication if severe diarrhea, vomiting, nausea, or rash occurs; call the office immediately.

BROMFED DM (COUGH SYRUP)

I. **Composition.** Each teaspoon of syrup contains 2 mg brompheniramine maleate, 30 mg pseudoephedrine hydrochloride, and 10 mg dextromethorphan hydrobromide. Tablets contain 4 mg brompheniramine maleate and 60 mg pseudoephedrine hydrochloride.

II. **Manufacturer/How supplied.** Muro; syrup or tablets

III. **Route.** Oral

IV. **Uses.** Seasonal and allergic rhinitis, vascular rhinitis, nasal congestion

V. **Dosage**

A. Syrup: 6–12 years: 1 tsp every 4–6 hours; 12 years to adult: 2 tsp every 4–6 hours

B. Tablets (not to exceed 6 doses in 24 hours): 6–12 years: 1/2 tablet every four hours; 12 years to adult: 1 tablet every four hours

VI. **Contraindications**

A. Hypersensitivity to any of the ingredients

B. Persons who have severe hypertension, coronary disease, narrow-angle glaucoma, urinary retention, or peptic ulcer

C. Persons taking monoamine oxidase inhibitors

D. Anyone during an asthma attack

E. Safety in pregnancy has not been established.

F. Do not use in nursing mothers. Pseudoephedrine is excreted in breast milk.

G. Do not give medication to children under age 6 except on the advice of a physician.

VII. **Precautions.** Use caution in patients with diabetes, hyperthyroidism, and mitral ocular pressure.

VIII. **Adverse reactions.** Drowsiness, nausea, dry mouth, blurred vision, cardiac palpitations, flushing, increased irritability or excitement, especially in children

IX. **Education**

A. Keep all medication out of children's reach.

B. Antihistamines may cause irritability and excitability in children. At dosages higher than recommended, dizziness, sleeplessness, and nervousness may occur.

C. Keep tablets in an airtight container.

D. Store at controlled temperature (59°–86°F).

E. Dispense in child-resistant container.

BROMFED PD (ANTIHISTAMINE, DECONGESTANT)

I. **Composition.** Pseudoephedrine hydrochloride 60 mg, brompheniramine maleate 6 mg

II. **Manufacturer/How supplied.** Muro; bottles of 50, 100, 500

III. **Uses.** Antihistamine and nasal decongestant

IV. **Dosage**

A. Ages 6–12 years: One capsule every 12 hours

B. Ages 12 years and older: One or two capsules every 12 hours

V. **Side effects.** Increased irritability, dryness of the mouth, nausea, blurred vision, drowsiness

VI. **Contraindications**

A. Sensitivity to any of the ingredients of the medication

B. Patients taking monoamine oxidase inhibitors

C. Patients having an asthma attack

D. Patients with severe hypertension

E. Pregnancy

F. Children under age 6

VII. **Education**

A. Keep all medication out of children's reach.

B. Keep medication tightly sealed in child-resistant containers.

C. Store at room temperature.

D. Medication may cause drowsiness; caution those driving or using machinery.

E. Take medication as directed. Do not increase dosage.

F. If symptoms persist, discontinue medication and call the office.

CEFACLOR (SEMISYNTHETIC CEPHALOSPORIN ANTIBIOTIC)

I. **Manufacturer/How supplied.** Eli Lilly & Co.; oral suspension: 125, 187, 250, or 375 mg/5 cc; pulvules: 250 or 500 mg

II. **Route.** Oral

III. **Actions and uses.** Semisynthetic cephalosporin antibiotic used for treatment of clinical infections caused by staphylococci, group A beta-hemolytic streptococci, *Streptococcus pneumoniae, Escherichia coli, Proteus mirabilis, Klebsiella* species, *Haemophilus influenzae,* and some beta-lactamase–producing ampicillin-resistant strains. Also used to treat otitis media, urinary tract infections, lower and upper respiratory infections, and skin and skin structure infections. It is not known whether cefaclor is effective in preventing rheumatic fever.

IV. **Dosage**

    A. Usual dosage for children: 20 mg/kg/day in divided doses every 8 hours

    B. For serious infections: 40 mg/kg/day; maximum dosage, 1 g/day

Body Weight	125 mg/5 ml	250 mg/5 ml
9 kg (20 lbs)	$^1/_2$ tsp tid	$^1/_2$ tsp tid
18 kg (40 lbs)	1 tsp tid	
Ceclor suspension 20 mg/kg/day		
9 kg (20 lbs)	1 tsp tid	$^1/_2$ tsp tid
18 kg (40 lbs)		— 1 tsp tid

    C. For otitis media and pharyngitis, the total daily dosage may be divided and administered every 12 hours.

V. **Contraindications**

    A. Allergy to cephalosporins

    B. Safety in infants less than 1 month old is unknown.

    C. In penicillin-sensitive children, cephalosporin antibiotics should be administered cautiously. Some cross allergenicity between the cephalosporins and penicillin has been shown, including anaphylaxis.

    D. Use caution in administering to nursing mothers; use in pregnancy only if needed.

VI. **Education**

    A. Keep all medication out of children's reach.

    B. Some serum sickness–like reactions can occur in children (erythema multiforme, signs of arthritis, arthralgia with or without fever).

    C. Toxic signs may include severe epigastric distress or diarrhea. More severe signs of toxicity include Stevens-Johnson syndrome.

    D. Hepatic effects may include elevated SGOT, SGPT, and alkaline phosphatase values.

    E. If side effects occur, discontinue use and call the office immediately.

    F. After mixing medication, shake vigorously before using. Store in tightly capped bottle in the refrigerator.

CEFTIN (SECOND-GENERATION CEPHALOSPORIN ANTIBIOTIC)

I.   **Generic name.** Cefuroxime axetil

II. **Manufacturer/How supplied.** Glaxo Wellcome; tablets: 250 or 500 mg; oral suspension: 125 or 250 mg/5 ml

III. **Route.** Oral

IV. **Uses.** Second-generation cephalosporin for treatment of:

    A. Pharyngitis, tonsillitis, and nasopharynx infections caused by *Streptococcus pyogenes*

    B. Otitis media caused by *Streptococcus pneumoniae, Haemophilus influenzae, Moraxella (Branhamella) catarrhalis*

C. Uncomplicated urinary tract infections caused by *Escherichia coli* or *Klebsiella pneumoniae*

D. Uncomplicated gonorrhea (urethral and endocervical caused by non-penicillinase-producing *Neisseria gonorrhoeae*)

E. Lower respiratory tract infections secondary to bacterial infection of acute bacterial exacerbation of chronic bronchitis caused by *S pneumoniae*, *H influenzae* (beta-lactamase positive and negative strains), and *M catarrhalis*

F. Skin and skin structure of infections

G. Uncomplicated skin infections caused by *Staphylococcus aureus* or *S pyogenes*

H. Culture and sensitivity tests should be taken before treatment whenever necessary.

V. Dosage

Age	Total Daily Dose	Duration
6 months–12 years	15 mg/kg q12h	10 days
13 years–older	250 mg q12h	10 days
	or 500 mg q24h	10 days
	or 500 mg q12h	10 days

VI. Side effects. Diarrhea, nausea, vomiting, rash, diaper rash, superinfection, anaphylaxis, Stevens-Johnson syndrome, erythema multiforme

VII. Contraindications

A. Allergies to cephalosporin; determine any allergy to penicillin and other drugs.

B. Safety and efficacy in children under age 6 is unknown.

C. Pregnancy and lactation

VIII. Education

A. Keep all medication out of children's reach.

B. Give liquid medication to children who cannot swallow tablets whole (crushed tablet has a bitter taste).

C. Follow directions on box for mixing Ceftin for oral suspension.

D. May be given with food to lessen gastric symptoms

E. Shake oral suspension well before each administration.

F. Replace cap tightly after each opening.

G. Suspension may be stored in the refrigerator or at room temperature.

H. Discard unused medication after 10 days.

I. Discontinue medication and immediately call the office if any side effects occur.

CEFZIL (SECOND-GENERATION CEPHALOSPORIN ANTIBIOTIC)

I. Generic name. Cefprozil

II. Manufacturer/How supplied. Bristol-Myers Squibb; film-coated tablets, 250 or 500 mg (bottle of 100 tablets); bubble gum–flavored oral suspension, 125 or 250 mg/5 ml in 50-, 75-, or 100-ml bottles

III. Route. Oral

IV. Action and uses. Cefzil is a broad-spectrum cephalosporin antibiotic used for the treatment of:

  A. Upper respiratory tract infections caused by *Streptococcus pyogenes*

  B. Otitis media caused by *Haemophilus influenzae*, *Streptococcus pneumoniae*, and *Moraxella catarrhalis*

  C. Lower respiratory tract infections of acute bronchitis, acute bacterial exacerbation of chronic bronchitis

  D. Uncomplicated skin and skin structure infections caused by *Staphylococcus aureus* or *S pyogenes*

V. Dosage

Age	Type of Infection	Total Daily Dose	Duration
6 months–12 years	Otitis media and upper respiratory infection	15 mg/kg q12h	10 days
2–12 years	Upper respiratory tract, pharyngitis/tonsillitis	7.5 mg/kg q12h	10 days
13 years–to adult	Upper respiratory tract, pharyngitis/tonsillitis, lower respiratory tract, secondary bronchitis, chronic bronchitis	500 q24h	10 days
	Skin and skin structure infections	250 mg q12h	10 days
		or 500 mg q24h	10 days
		or 500 mg q12h	10 days

VI. Contraindications

  A. Allergies to cephalosporins; use with caution in patients with a known penicillin allergy.

  B. Safety and effectiveness in children under age 6 months are not known.

  C. Safety in lactation is unknown.

VII. Side effects. Diarrhea, rash, dizziness, diaper rash, genital pruritus, vaginitis

VIII. Education

  A. Keep all medication out of children's reach.

  B. Culture and sensitivity tests must be performed before treatment of skin and skin structure infections.

  C. May be given with food or drinks

  D. Refrigerate suspension; discard unused medication after 14 days.

  E. Complete full course of medication as directed.

  F. Discontinue medication if hypersensitivity (rash, hives, difficulty breathing, severe diarrhea) or bleeding occurs; call the office.

CLARITIN (ANTIHISTAMINE)

I. Generic name. Loratidine

II. **Manufacturer/How supplied.** Schering; 10-mg tablets

III. **Route.** Oral

IV. **Uses.** Long-acting antihistamine for the relief of symptoms of seasonal allergic rhinitis

V. **Dosage.** Children age 12 and older: One 10-mg tablet daily

VI. **Side effects.** Blurred vision, nausea, vomiting, itchy dry skin, agitation, irritability

VII. **Contraindications**
   A. Allergy to any of the ingredients
   B. Pregnancy and lactation
   C. Children under age 12

VIII. **Education**
   A. Keep all medication out of children's reach.
   B. Do not exceed the recommended dose.
   C. Store medication at 36°–86°F.

COLACE (STOOL SOFTENER)

I. **Generic name.** Docusate sodium

II. **Composition.** Syrup: 20 mg/5 ml (1 tsp); liquid drops (1% solution) 10 mg/ml; capsules: 50 or 100 mg

III. **Manufacturer/How supplied.** Roberts; syrup: bottles of 8 or 16 fluid oz; liquid drops: 1% solution with calibrated dropper, 16 or 30 fluid oz; capsules: bottles of 30, 60, 250, or 1,000, or 100 single-unit packs

IV. **Route.** Oral

V. **Action and uses.** A stool softener, not a laxative; used in chronic constipation and in children with anal fissures

VI. **Dosage**
   A. Under 3 years: 10–40 mg/day or 10 mg three times a day (0.5 tsp syrup three times a day)
   B. Ages 3–6 years: 60 mg/day or 20 mg three times a day (1 tsp syrup three times a day)
   C. Ages 6–12 years: 40–120 mg/day (2 tsp syrup three times a day)
   D. Older children: 50–200 mg/day (one 50-mg capsule three times a day)
   E. Higher doses are suggested for initial therapy.

VII. **Side effects.** Throat irritation, nausea, rash, bitter taste in mouth

VIII. **Education**
   A. Keep all medication out of children's reach.
   B. No contraindications to use
   C. During pregnancy and in nursing mothers, ask physician's advice before prescribing.
   D. Not habit-forming
   E. Give in formula, juice, or milk to mask the flavor.
   F. Store capsules at room temperature.

G. Medication takes effect in 1–3 days.

H. Adjust dosage to patient.

I. Keep child on medication for 1 week; call office regarding results.

J. Gradually taper off medication.

DOMEBORO POWDER PACKETS (TOPICAL SOLUTION)

I. **Generic name.** Aluminum sulfate and calcium acetate

II. **Composition**

A. One packet with 1 pt water = Burow's solution 1:40 dilution

B. Two packets with 1 pt water = Burow's solution 1:20 dilution

III. **Manufacturer/How supplied.** Bayer; powder packets, boxes of 12 and 100; each packet contains 2.2 g.

IV. **Route.** Topical solution for external use

V. **Uses.** Severe inflammatory dermatitis, poison ivy, insect bites, diaper rash, athlete's foot

VI. **Dosage and administration.** Apply wet soaks to skin for 15–30 minutes every 4–8 hours.

VII. **Education**

A. Keep all medication out of children's reach.

B. Dissolve one or two packets in 1 pt water. Stir until mixture is dissolved. Shake well and apply as wet dressing.

C. Do not use plastic or rubber pants or occlusive bandages.

D. For external use only

E. May be stored for 7 days at room temperature

F. Keep away from eyes.

G. May treat for symptomatic relief for 1 week; if condition is worse or not relieved in 1 week, discontinue use and seek medical advice.

DONNAGEL (ANTIDIARRHEAL)

I. **Composition.** Each tablespoon (15 ml) or chewable tablet contains 600 mg attapulgite.

II. **Manufacturer/How supplied.** Wyeth-Ayerst; bottles of 4 or 16 fluid oz; packages of 18 tablets

III. **Route.** Oral

IV. **Uses.** Symptomatic relief of diarrhea; relieves cramping, reduces the number of loose stools, and improves the consistency of the stool

V. **Dosage**

A. Ages 3–6 years: 0.5 tablespoon or half a tablet after loose bowel movement

B. Ages 6–12 years: 1 tablespoon or one tablet after loose bowel movement

    C. Age 12 years or older: 2 tablespoons or two tablets after loose bowel movement

    D. Do not exceed seven doses in a 24-hour period.

VI. Contraindications

    A. Hypersensitivity to any of the ingredients in the medication

    B. Not recommended for use in children age 3 or under unless under care and consultation of a physician

    C. Not recommended for pregnant women or nursing mothers unless directed by physician

VII. Education

    A. Keep all medication out of children's reach.

    B. Chew tablets well, then swallow.

    C. Shake liquid medication well before using.

    D. Store medication at controlled room temperature (59°–86°F).

    E. Discontinue use of medication and call office if any signs of dehydration—sunken fontanelle, dry mouth, decreased urination, or sunken eyes.

    F. Call office if symptoms persist beyond 2 days.

    G. Call office if temperature is above 100°F or child is vomiting.

    H. Do not exceed recommended dosage.

    I. Call Poison Control Center if overdose occurs.

DONNATAL (ANTICHOLINERGIC/ANTISPASMODIC, MILD SEDATION)

I. **Composition.** Each tablet, capsule, or teaspoon contains phenobarbital (0.25 grain) 16.2 mg, hyoscyamine sulfate 0.1037 mg, atropine sulfate 0.0194 mg, and hyoscine hydrobromide 0.0065 mg.

II. **Manufacturer/How supplied.** A.H. Robins; green citrus-flavored elixir in bottle of 4 fluid oz; tablets: bottle of 100 or 1,000 or dose package of 100; capsules: bottle of 100 or 1,000

III. **Route.** Oral

IV. **Action and uses.** Anticholinergic and antispasmodic with mild sedation; used in colic and irritable bowel syndrome

V. **Dosage.** Children (elixir). May have every 4–6 hours

Body Weight			
(kg)	(lbs)	**q4h**	**q6h**
4.5	10	0.5 ml	0.75 ml
9.1	20	1.0 ml	1.5 ml
13.6	30	1.5 ml	2.0 ml
22.7	50	$^1/_2$ tsp	$^3/_4$ tsp
34.0	75	$^3/_4$ tsp	1 tsp
45.4	100	1 tsp	$1^1/_2$ tsp

Older children and adults: One or two tablets or capsules three or four times a day

VI. **Side effects.** Headache, blurred vision, drowsiness, constipation, suppression of lactation, nervousness, hyperactivity

VII. **Contraindications**

    A. Bleeding disorder, cardiac disease, question of pyloric stenosis or hepatic dysfunction

    B. Pregnancy and lactation; suppresses lactation

VIII. **Education**

    A. Keep all medication out of children's reach.

    B. May be habit-forming

    C. Do not use in patients with history of drug dependency.

    D. Return call in 1 week regarding progress of colic.

    E. Use with caution in a very warm climate because of association with increased heat prostration and heat stroke due to increased sweating.

    F. Symptoms of overdose: Severe headache, nausea, vomiting, hot and dry skin, dilated pupils, dry mouth, difficulty swallowing, central nervous system stimulation

    G. If overdose occurs, call the office immediately. Overdose is treated by gastric lavage, emetics, activated charcoal.

DORCOL PEDIATRIC COUGH SYRUP

I. **Composition.** Pseudoephedrine hydrochloride 15 mg, guaifenesin 50 mg, dextromethorphan hydrobromide 5 mg in each 5 ml

II. **Manufacturer/How supplied.** Sandoz; grape-flavored syrup in bottles of 4 or 8 fluid oz with tamper-proof, child-resistant cap

III. **Route.** Oral

IV. **Actions and uses.** Temporary relief of common cold; prompt relief of upper respiratory infection; helps in excretion of mucous secretions. Contains a decongestant, expectorant, and antitussive. Antihistamine-free formula.

V. **Dosage**

    A. Ages 3–12 months: 3 gtt/kg every 4 hours (on physician's advice only)

    B. Ages 12–24 months: 7 gtt (0.2 ml)/kg every 4 hours (on physician's advice only)

    C. Ages 2–6 years: 1 tsp every 4 hours

    D. Ages 6–12 years: 2 tsp every 4 hours

    E. By weight: 24–47 lb, 1 tsp every 4 hours; 48–95 lb, 2 tsp every 4 hours

    F. Do not exceed four doses in 24 hours.

VI. **Side effects.** Dizziness, gastrointestinal upset, insomnia, hyperactivity

VII. **Contraindications**

    A. Ongoing chronic cough due to bronchitis, bronchial asthma, or emphysema

    B. Diabetes mellitus, high blood pressure, heart disease, or thyroid disease

    C. Patients taking antidepressants or antihypertensive medication

VIII. **Education**

A. Keep all medication out of children's reach.

B. Do not exceed recommended dose.

C. If overdose occurs, call Poison Control Center immediately.

D. If cough persists longer than 1 week, call office.

E. Return to office or call if rash appears or if persistent headache, vomiting, or high fever occurs.

DURICEF (FIRST-GENERATION CEPHALOSPORIN ANTIBIOTIC)

I. **Generic name.** Cefadroxil monohydrate

II. **Manufacturer/How supplied.** Bristol-Meyers Squibb; capsules: 500 mg; film-coated tablets, 1 g; orange-and-pineapple-flavored oral suspension, 125, 250, or 500 mg/5 ml

III. **Route.** Oral

IV. **Actions and uses**

A. Urinary tract infections caused by *Escherichia coli*, *Proteus mirabilis*, and *Klebsiella* species

B. Skin and suture infections caused by staphylococci or streptococci

C. Pharyngitis and tonsillitis caused by beta-hemolytic streptococci; penicillin is still the drug of choice in the treatment and prevention of streptococcal infections.

D. Efficacy in preventing rheumatic fever is unknown.

V. **Dosage**

Body Weight

(kg)	(lbs)	125 mg/5 ml	250 mg/5 ml	500 mg/5 ml
4.5	10	1 tsp		
9.1	20	2 tsp	1 tsp	—
13.6	30	3 tsp	1¹/₂ tsp	—
18.2	40	4 tsp	2 tsp	1 tsp
22.7	50	5 tsp	2¹/₂ tsp	1¹/₄ tsp
27.3	60	6 tsp	3 tsp	1¹/₂ tsp
31.8+	70+	—	—	2 tsp

Adult Dose: 1–2 g/day in divided doses or single dose, ie:

A. Uncomplicated urinary tract infection 30 mg/kg/day in divided doses every 12 hours

B. Skin and skin structure infections 30 g/kg/day in equally divided doses every 12 hours

C. Group A beta-hemolytic striptococcus pharyngitis and tonsillitis 30 g/kg/day in divided doses every 12 hours

VI. **Side effects.** Pseudomembranous colitis, diarrhea, rashes, urticaria and angioedema, genital pruritus, genital moniliasis, vaginitis, neutropenia

VII. **Contraindications**

A. Not known to be safe in pregnancy or lactation

    B. Impaired renal function

    C. *Warning:* Use with caution in penicillin-allergic patients; there is evidence that they may also be allergic to cephalosporins. It is safer not to use in patients with a known penicillin allergy.

VIII. Precautions

    A. Prolonged use may result in overgrowth of nonsusceptible organisms.

    B. Coombs' test may be positive while patient is on Duricef.

    C. Use with caution in patients with gastrointestinal disease, particularly colitis.

IX. Education

    A. Keep all medication out of children's reach.

    B. Culture and sensitivity tests should be done before and during therapy.

    C. Do not use medication if packaging or seal on the cap is broken.

    D. If side effects occur, discontinue medication and call the office immediately.

    E. Medication may be given with or without food but is better tolerated if given with meals.

    F. Shake suspension well before administration.

    G. Keep cap tightly closed.

    H. Keep medication in the refrigerator.

    I. Discontinue use after 14 days.

ERYCETTE TOPICAL SOLUTION

I.   **Generic name.** 2% erythromycin topical solution

II.   **Manufacturer/How supplied.** Ortho; 20 mg of erythromycin base in a vehicle of alcohol (66%) and propylene glycol; boxes of 60 swabs

III.   **Actions and uses.** Acne vulgaris on face, neck, shoulders, back, and chest; reduces inflammatory acne vulgaris, presumably by its antibiotic action

IV.   **Dosage and administration.** Apply topically to affected area twice daily after skin is thoroughly washed and dried.

V.   **Side effects.** Tenderness, dryness, erythema, desquamation, pruritus of affected areas

VI.   **Contraindications**

    A. Sensitivity to ingredients

    B. Safety of use during pregnancy is unknown.

VII.   **Precautions**

    A. Discontinue use immediately if urticaria or side effects occur.

    B. Safety of use in nursing mothers is unknown; use cautiously.

VIII.   **Education**

    A. Keep all medication out of children's reach.

    B. Store at controlled room temperature (59°–86°F).

    C. Not intended for ophthalmic use or use in mouth or nose

    D. If overgrowth of bacterial organisms occurs, discontinue use and call the office.

    E. Use each swab only once; discard after use.

ERYTHROMYCIN (ANTIBIOTIC)

I. **How supplied.** Tablets, capsules, liquid, chewable tablets, drops, granules

II. **Route.** Oral

III. **Action and uses**

    A. A macrolide group of antibiotics used to inhibit protein synthesis without changing nucleic acid synthesis

    B. Used for upper and lower respiratory tract infections (eg, bronchitis, pneumonia, pertussis), intestinal infections, soft-tissue and nasal infections, pharyngitis, primary syphilis, Legionnaire's disease

    C. Long-term prophylaxis against rheumatic fever

    D. Urologic and gynecologic infections due to *Chlamydia trachomatis*

    E. Prevention of bacterial endocarditis

    F. Oral prophylaxis before oral surgery and surgical procedures

IV. **Dosage**

    A. Dosage determined by severity of infection, weight, and age

    B. For mild to moderate infections (total daily dose)

        1. 10–15 lb: 200 mg

        2. 16–25 lb: 400 mg

        3. 26–50 lb: 800 mg

        4. 51–100 lb: 1,200 mg

        5. Over 100 lb: 1,600 mg

    C. 30–50 mg/kg/day in divided doses every 6 hours, or 15–25 mg/kg twice a day

    D. For pertussis: 40–50 mg/kg/day for 14 days

    E. For *Chlamydia trachomatis* infection: 50 mg/kg/day in divided doses for 14 days

    F. Oral prophylaxis before oral surgery or procedure: 800 mg or 1 g 2 hours before procedure, then half dose 6 hours after surgery or procedure

V. **Side effects**

    A. Nausea, vomiting, abdominal pain

    B. Symptoms of hepatic dysfunction may occur, with or without abnormal liver function.

    C. Rash may appear with pruritus (urticaria, eczema, or bullae).

    D. Severe anaphylaxis and transient deafness can occur.

VI. **Contraindications**

    A. Hypersensitivity to the medication

    B. Safety during pregnancy has not been established.

    C. Effect during labor and delivery is unknown.

    D. Excreted in breast milk

    E. Concomitant use with Seldane (terfenadine) can be toxic; not recommended.

    F. Children receiving high levels of theophylline may show an increase of serum theophylline and potential theophylline toxicity if erythromycin is taken concomitantly.

VII. **Education**

    A. Prolonged use may cause overgrowth of bacteria or a fungal infection. If so, discontinue use.

    B. Some organisms are resistant to erythromycin. Whenever possible, obtain specimens for culture and sensitivity. When indicated, incision and drainage or another surgical procedure is best done, as well as antibiotic therapy.

    C. Medication is best given without food, but suspension and tablets may be given with meals if gastrointestinal symptoms occur.

    D. Mix pellets with applesauce before administering.

    E. Store liquid medication in the refrigerator.

    F. Chewable tablets should be chewed or crushed, never swallowed.

    G. Suspensions are stable for 14 days at room temperature, but palatability increases if they are kept refrigerated.

    H. Order generic form to minimize cost. Best ordered in coated tablets or caplet form to reduce side effects.

EURAX (SCABICIDE/ANTIPRURITIC)

I.   **Generic name.** Crotamiton

II.   **Manufacturer/How supplied.** Westwood Squibb; lotion and cream are available in 60-g tubes containing 10% synthetic crotamiton.

III.   **Route.** Topical use

IV.   **Action and uses.** Antipruritic and antiscabies medication used to eradicate scabies and provide symptomatic treatment for pruritus

V.   **Dosage and administration.** Apply lotion or cream to skin from neck down. Massage into skin, leave cream on overnight, and wash off in the morning.

VI.   **Contraindications**

    A. Sensitivity or known allergy to the ingredients

    B. Pregnancy or lactation

    C. Safety in children has not been established.

VII.   **Side effects.** Skin irritation

VIII.   **Education**

    A. Keep all medication out of children's reach.

    B. Shake medication well before using.

    C. For scabies

        1. After bath or shower, pat dry and massage medication into skin, covering all areas from neck down.

        2. A second application may be advisable 24 hours later (60-g tube is sufficient for two applications).

        3. Bed linens and clothing should be washed in hot, soapy water. Other contaminated clothing should be dry cleaned.

        4. A bath is recommended 48 hours after the last treatment.

    D. For pruritus: Apply small amount of medication and massage gently into affected area.

E. Discontinue use if skin becomes severely irritated.

F. Keep medication away from eyes and mouth.

G. If ingested, call Poison Control Center immediately.

H. Do not apply to acutely inflamed skin that has open sores or is weeping or severely red.

FEOSOL ELIXIR (NONPRESCRIPTION IRON SUPPLEMENT)

I. **Generic name.** Ferrous sulfate

II. **Composition.** 200 mg ferrous sulfate (44 mg elemental iron) per 5 ml

III. **How supplied.** Clear orange liquid in 16-oz bottle; also available in tablets and capsules

IV. **Route.** Oral

V. **Uses.** Iron-deficiency anemia or simple iron deficiency

VI. **Dosage**

    A. 6 mg/kg/day

    B. Infants: Begin with 4 gtt, then increase to 0.5 tsp three times a day for 1 month.

    C. Children: 0.5–1 tsp three times a day for 4 weeks, between meals

    D. Adults: 1–2 tsp three times a day

VII. **Education**

    A. Keep all medication out of children's reach.

    B. Do not take iron supplements within 2 hours of tetracycline due to malabsorption.

    C. If gastrointestinal irritation occurs, take iron supplement with meals starting with a lower dose, gradually increasing to recommended dose.

    D. Iron may cause constipation, dark stools, or diarrhea.

    E. Liquid may cause temporary staining of teeth; dilute elixir with water or juice and use a straw.

    F. Do not mix with milk, milk products, or wine-based materials.

    G. Take medication for 3–4 weeks and return for reevaluation.

    H. Request tamper-resistant packing. If seal is broken or missing, do not use product.

    I. If overdose occurs, call the office and the Poison Control Center immediately.

ILOTYCIN OPHTHALMIC OINTMENT (ERYTHROMYCIN)

I. **Composition.** Erythromycin in a sterile ophthalmic base

II. **Manufacturer/How supplied.** Dista; 5 mg/g in 0.125-oz tamper-resistant tube

III. **Route.** Topical ophthalmic ointment

IV. **Uses**

    A. Treatment of ocular infections involving conjunctiva or cornea

    B. Prophylaxis of neonatal ophthalmia

V. **Dosage and administration.** Apply a ribbon of ointment 1 cm long to the lower conjunctival sac of the affected eye two to six times a day, depending on severity of infection.

VI. **Contraindications**

    A. Sensitivity to erythromycin

    B. Safety during pregnancy is unknown.

VII. **Education**

    A. Keep all medication out of children's reach.

    B. Occasionally an overgrowth of antibiotic-resistant organisms occurs; if this happens, stop all medications and call the office.

    C. Do not flush ointment from eyes after application.

    D. Medication may cause temporary blurring of vision shortly after application.

    E. Use a separate tube of medication for each patient.

    F. If eyes seem sensitive to medication, stop medication and call the office.

INTAL INHALER (ANTIASTHMATIC)

I. **Generic name.** Cromolyn sodium

II. **Composition.** Each metered inhalation contains about 800 mcg cromolyn sodium. Each canister contains 112 metered inhalations (56 doses).

III. **Route.** Oral inhalation

IV. **Uses**

    A. Treatment and management of bronchial asthma

    B. Prevention of exercise-induced bronchoconstriction or environmental antigen reactions

V. **Dosage**

    A. For management of bronchial asthma: Two metered inhalations four times a day. Do not exceed this dose.

    B. For exercise-induced asthma or exposure to cold dry air: Two metered inhalations 10–15 minutes (not more than 1 hour) before prolonged exercise or exposure to cold dry air

    C. Decrease dosage in patients with renal or hepatic dysfunction.

VI. **Contraindications**

    A. Hypersensitivity to cromolyn sodium

    B. Eosinophilic pneumonia or pulmonary infiltrates with eosinophilia

    C. Coronary artery disease or history of cardiac arrhythmias

    D. Pregnancy and lactation

    E. Children under 5 years

    F. *Warning:* Do not use to treat acute attack of asthma, especially status asthmaticus.

VII. **Side effects.** Decreased sense of taste, cough, irritated throat, wheeze and dryness, dizziness, dysuria

VIII. Education

   A. Keep all medication out of children's reach.

   B. May take 4 weeks to be effective

   C. Relieves bronchospasm in some, but not all, patients with exercise-induced asthma

   D. Use as directed; do not increase frequency.

   E. If side effects occur, discontinue use and call the office.

   F. Gradually decrease use when withdrawal is desired.

   G. Do not use during an acute asthma attack; begin treatment when the acute episode is controlled.

   H. Do not use on a long-term basis in children.

KEFLEX (CEPHALOSPORIN ANTIBIOTIC)

I.   **Generic name.** Cephalexin

II. **Manufacturer/How supplied.** Dista; oral suspension, 125 or 250 mg/5 ml; pulvule, 250 or 500 mg

III. **Route.** Oral

IV. **Action and uses.** Cephalosporin antibiotic for the treatment of bacterial infections:

   A. Respiratory tract infections caused by pneumonia and group A beta-hemolytic streptococci (not rheumatic fever)

   B. Otitis media due to *Streptococcus pneumoniae, Haemophilus influenzae,* streptococci, staphylococci, and *Moraxella catarrhalis*

   C. Soft-tissue infections caused by staphylococci and streptococci

   D. Bone infections caused by staphylococci or *Proteus mirabilis*

   E. Genitourinary infections caused by *Escherichia coli, P mirabilis,* and *Klebsiella*

V. **Dosage**

   A. Children: 25–50 mg/kg/day; otitis media: 75–100 mg/kg/day in four divided doses

   B. Adult: 1–4 g/day, usually 250 mg orally every 6 hours

   C. Keflex suspension

Body Weight			
(kg)	(lbs)	**125 mg/5 ml**	**250 mg/5 ml**
10	22	½–1 tsp qid	¼–½ tsp qid
20	44	1–2 tsp qid	1–2 tsp qid
40	88	2–4 tsp qid	1–2 tsp qid

VI. **Side effects**

   A. Headache, diarrhea, vomiting, abdominal cramps, dyspepsia; hypersensitivity (urticaria, rash, angioedema)

   B. Genital and anal pruritus

   C. Dizziness, fatigue

VII. **Contraindications**
   A. Allergy to any antibiotics, especially penicillin-sensitive patients
   B. Renal failure
   C. Safety during pregnancy is unknown.
VIII. **Precautions.** Use with caution in nursing mothers and patients with a history of colitis.
IX. **Education**
   A. Keep all medication out of children's reach.
   B. Diabetics taking Keflex will have falsely high readings on Clinitest.
   C. After mixing the medication, store in the refrigerator.
   D. Mixture may be kept for 14 days. Discard unused medication after 14 days.
   E. Shake well before using.
   F. Keep cap tightly closed.
   G. Call the office immediately if side effects occur.
   H. May be given without regard to meals
   I. Medication is rapidly absorbed.
   J. Culture and sensitivity tests are required before and during therapy when indicated.

KWELL LOTION (PEDICULOCIDE, SCABICIDE)

I. **Composition.** Lindane 1%
II. **Manufacturer/How supplied.** Reedoc; bottles of 2 oz, 16 oz, and 1 gallon
III. **Route.** Topical
IV. **Uses.** Treatment of scabies and pediculosis
V. **Dosage and administration.** After bathing and patting dry, apply a thin layer of lotion to skin from neck down all over body; leave lotion on overnight and wash it off in the morning. One application generally is effective.
VI. **Contraindications**
   A. Premature infants
   B. Seizure disorders
   C. Sensitivity to any components in medication
VII. **Precautions**
   A. Safety of lindane use in pregnancy is unknown. Women should not exceed two treatments during pregnancy.
   B. Lindane is excreted in low concentrations in breast milk.
   C. Lindane can cause central nervous system toxicity, especially in the young. Overdose or oral ingestion can cause central nervous system reaction.
VIII. **Education**
   A. Keep all medication out of children's reach.
   B. Do not use on open cuts or abrasions.
   C. Some children continue to have pruritus after treatment; this is not a sign of treatment failure.

   D. Do not re-treat unless live mites are a consideration.

   E. Treat sexual contacts.

   F. Do not use near eyes.

   G. Use only as directed; do not exceed recommended dose.

KWELL SHAMPOO (ANTIPARASITIC)

I. **Composition.** Lindane 1%.

II. **Route.** Topical

III. **Uses.** Treatment of head lice

IV. **Dosage**

   A. Apply 1 oz shampoo to dry hair and leave it on for 4 minutes. Add enough water to make a good lather. Shampoo, rinse thoroughly with water, and towel dry.

   B. Remove nits with a nit comb.

V. **Contraindications**

   A. Premature infants

   B. Seizure disorders

   C. Sensitivity to any component in medication

VI. **Precautions**

   A. Seizures may occur after excessive use or oral ingestion.

   B. Lindane is absorbed through the skin and can cause central nervous system toxicity, especially in children.

   C. Lindane is excreted in low concentrations in breast milk.

   D. Use cautiously in pregnancy. Do not exceed two treatments during pregnancy.

VII. **Education**

   A. Keep all medication out of children's reach.

   B. Do not use on open cuts or abrasions.

   C. Some children continue to have pruritus after treatment; this is not a sign of treatment failure.

   D. Do not re-treat unless live mites are a consideration.

   E. Do not use as prophylaxis for possible infestation.

   F. Treat household contacts.

   G. Hair oils may enhance absorption; medication should be applied onto clean hair.

   H. Avoid contact with eyes.

LORABID (SECOND-GENERATION ANTIBIOTIC)

I. **Generic name.** Loracarbef

II. **Route.** Oral

III. **Uses.** Lorabid, a second-generation antibiotic, is used for the treatment of mild to moderate infections, such as:

A. Secondary bacterial infection of acute bronchitis and acute exacerbation of chronic bronchitis caused by *Streptococcus pneumoniae, Haemophilus influenzae* and of catarrha pneumonia caused by *S pneumoniae* or *H influenzae* (non-beta-lactamase–producing strains only)

B. Otitis media caused by *S pneumoniae* (including beta-lactamase-producing strains) and of catarrhalis (including beta-lactamase–producing strains or *Streptococcus pyogenes*)

C. Acute maxillary sinusitis caused by *S pneumoniae, H influenzae* (non-beta-lactamase-producing strains only), or *Moraxella catarrhalis* (including beta-lactamase-producing strains)

D. Pharyngitis or tonsillitis caused by *S pyogenes*

E. Skin and skin structure infections caused by *Staphylococcus aureus*

F. Uncomplicated urinary tract infections (cystitis) caused by *Escherichia coli* or *Staphylococcus saprophyticus*

G. Uncomplicated pyelonephritis caused by *E coli*

IV. **Dosage**

Age	Type of Infection	Total Daily Dose	Duration
6 months–12 years	Acute otitis media	30 mg/kg/day in divided doses q12h	10 days
	Pharyngitis/tonsillitis	15 mg/kg/day in divided doses q12h	10 days
	Skin and skin structure	15 mg/kg/day in divided doses q17h	7 days
13 years and older	Acute bronchitis	200–400 mg q12h	7 days
	Exacerbation of chronic bronchitis	400 mg q12h	14 days
	Pneumonia	400 mg q12h	10 days
	Sinusitis	400 mg q12h	10 days
	Uncomplicated skin and skin structure	200 mg q12h	10 days
	Uncomplicated cystitis	200 mg q24h	7 days
	Uncomplicated pyelonephritis	400 mg q12h	14 days

V. **Contraindications**

A. Allergy to loracarbef or cephalosporin-class antibiotics

B. Not recommended for nursing mothers

C. Not recommended during labor and delivery

D. Not recommended in children under 6 months

E. Not recommended for patients with renal failure

VI. **Side effects.** Nausea, vomiting, abdominal pain, rash, headache, rhinitis, unusual bleeding or bruising

VII. **Education**

A. Keep all medication out of children's reach.

B. For treatment of otitis media, use oral suspension rather than capsules.

   C. Take medication 1 hour before or 2 hours after eating.

   D. Follow directions carefully when reconstituting the suspension.

   E. Store at room temperature (59°–86°F).

   F. Discard unused medication after 14 days.

   G. Discontinue use if side effects occur, and call the office.

   H. Culture and sensitivity tests should be done before beginning medication whenever prudent.

LOTRIMIN CREAM (ANTIFUNGAL)

   I. **Generic name.** Clotrimazole

   II. **Composition.** 10 mg/g (1%)

  III. **Manufacturer/How supplied.** Schering; 12- or 24-g tubes

  IV. **Route.** Topical; not for ophthalmic use

   V. **Action.** Broad-spectrum antifungal

  VI. **Uses.** Inhibits growth of pathogenic dermatophytes, yeasts, and *Malassezia furfur;* used for tinea pedis, cruris, corporis

 VII. **Dosage and administration.** Gently massage into affected area and surrounding skin twice daily.

VIII. **Side effects.** Erythema, stinging, blistering, peeling, edema, pruritus, urticaria, generalized irritation of the skin

  IX. **Contraindications**

   A. Hypersensitivity to any components of the medication

   B. Use in first trimester of pregnancy only if essential to patient's welfare.

   X. **Education**

   A. Keep all medication out of children's reach.

   B. Clinical improvement usually occurs within the first week of treatment. If no improvement occurs after 4 weeks, review the diagnosis.

   C. Store at 34°–86°F.

   D. Not for ophthalmic use

   E. Do not use for nails or scalp.

   F. Discontinue use if irritation develops, and call the office.

LURIDE (FLOURIDE SUPPLEMENT)

   I. **Generic name.** Sodium fluoride

   II. **Manufacturer/How supplied.** Colgate-Hoyt; drops: About 0.125 mg fluoride per drop in squeeze bottles of 50 ml (peach-flavored); tablets: 1.0, 0.5, or 0.25 mg in bottles of 120

  III. **Uses.** Prevention of dental caries in children, birth up to age 16

  IV. **Dosage**

    A. Drops

        1. Drinking water less than 0.3 ppm

            a. Ages 6 months–2 years: 0.5 ml (0.5 dropperful)

            b. Ages 2–3: 1 ml (one dropperful)

            c. Ages 3–14: 2 ml (two dropperfuls)

        2. Drinking water more than 0.3 ppm

            a. Ages 6 months–2 years: Fluoride supplement not indicated

            b. Ages 2–3: 0.5 ml (0.5 dropperful)

            c. Ages 3–14: 1 ml (one dropperful)

        3. Topical rinse

            a. Ages 6–12: 5–10 ml; swish around teeth and spit out.

            b. Do not swallow rinse.

    B. Tablets

        1. Drinking water less than 0.3 ppm

            a. Ages 6 months–3 years: 0.25 mg

            b. Ages 3–6: 0.5 mg

            c. Ages 6–16: 1 mg

        2. Drinking water 0.3–0.6 ppm

            a. Ages 6 months–3 years: No supplement indicated

            b. Ages 3–6: 0.25 mg

            c. Ages 6–16: 0.5 mg

    C. Adult: up to 60 mg/d with calcium supplements, vitamin D, and estrogen to prevent osteoporosis.

V. **Contraindications.** Contraindicated if drinking water contains more than 0.6 ppm fluoride

VI. **Precautions.** Do not exceed recommended daily dose; excessive fluoride will result in fluorosis.

VII. **Education**

    A. Keep all medication out of children's reach.

    B. If overdose occurs, call office immediately.

    C. Daily dose should be given at bedtime, after brushing teeth.

    D. Medication is poorly absorbed if given with dairy foods.

    E. Prolonged use results in pitting of the teeth (fluorosis).

    F. Dispense only one 15-ml bottle or 120 tablets at a time.

    G. Recommend chewing tablets before swallowing.

    H. Federal law prohibits dispensing without prescription.

    I. Check the amount of fluoride in drinking water before prescribing.

MONISTAT 7 VAGINAL CREAM (ANTIFUNGAL)

I. **Generic name and composition.** Water-miscible white cream containing miconazole nitrate 2%

II. **Manufacturer/How supplied.** Ortho; 1.66-oz (47-g) tubes with applicator

III. **Route.** Intravaginal

IV. **Action.** Exhibits fungicidal activity against *Candida* species; mode of action unknown

V. **Uses.** Treatment of moniliasis (vulvovaginal candidiasis) previously diagnosed by physician and confirmed by KOH smear

VI. **Dosage and administration.** One applicatorful intravaginally once a day at bedtime for 7 days (age 12 and older)

VII. **Side effects.** Vulvovaginal burning, itching, irritation; vaginal burning, pelvic cramps, hives, skin rash, headache

VIII. Contraindications

  A. Hypersensitivity to the drug

  B. Do not use in first trimester of pregnancy unless essential to patient's welfare.

IX. Education

  A. Keep all medication out of children's reach.

  B. Discontinue use if irritation develops.

  C. Do not use tampons while using cream.

  D. Course may be repeated after other pathogens have been ruled out by appropriate smears and cultures.

  E. Discontinue use if infection worsens or does not improve in 3 days (fever 100°F; lower abdominal, back, or shoulder pain; odoriferous vaginal discharge).

  F. Oil from the cream weakens the latex of condoms and diaphragms; therefore, they are not reliable forms of birth control or prophylaxis for sexually transmitted diseases during use of Monistat 7.

  G. If ingested, call office and Poison Control Center immediately.

Monistat 3 Vaginal Suppositories (Antifungal)

I. **Generic name.** Miconazole nitrate, 200 mg

II. **Manufacturer/How supplied.** Ortho; package of three suppositories

III. **Route.** Intravaginal

IV. **Uses.** A broad-spectrum antifungal used for the local treatment of vulvovaginal candidiasis (moniliasis) previously diagnosed by positive KOH smear

V. **Dosage and administration.** One suppository inserted intravaginally at bedtime for 3 consecutive days

VI. **Side effects.** Vulvovaginal burning, itching, irritation

VII. Contraindications

  A. Allergy to medication

  B. Not recommended during pregnancy or lactation

  C. Not recommended for diabetic patients

VIII. Education

  A. Keep all medication out of children's reach.

  B. Do not use with vaginal contraceptive diaphragm.

  C. Before suggesting another course of medication, reconfirm the diagnosis by smears and cultures to rule out other pathogens.

  D. Insert suppository with vaginal applicator per package directions.

  E. Store at 59°–86°F.

  F. Discontinue medication if side effects occur, and call the office.

MOTRIN FOR CHILDREN (NONSTEROIDAL ANTI-INFLAMMATORY ANALGESIC)

I. **Generic name.** Ibuprofen

II. **Composition.** Each 5 ml (teaspoon) contains 100 mg ibuprofen.

III. **Manufacturer/How supplied.** McNeil; bottles of 2 or 4 fluid oz

IV. **Route.** Oral

V. **Uses.** Relief of minor pain and aches due to colds, influenza, sore throat, headache, toothaches; relief of fever; used for children 6 months and older

VI. **Dosage**

Age	Body Weight	Dosage	Time
2–3 y	24–35 lbs	1 tsp	
4–5 y	36–47 lbs	1½ tsp	may repeat
6–8 y	48–59 lbs	2 tsp	6–8 hours
9–10 y	60–71 lbs	2½ tsp	no more
11 y	72–95 lbs	3 tsp	than 4 x day

VII. **Side effects.** Vomiting, rash, stomach upset

VIII. **Contraindications**

    A. Allergy to aspirin

    B. Not recommended for children with stomach pain

    C. Do not give with aspirin, naproxen sodium, or acetaminophen.

    D. Do not give to infants and children with dehydration due to poor liquid intake or prolonged vomiting and diarrhea.

IX. **Education**

    A. Keep all medication out of children's reach.

    B. May be given with food or liquid

    C. Follow directions carefully; do not give more than the recommended dose. One dose lasts 6–8 hours.

    D. If overdose occurs, call Poison Control Center immediately.

    E. Shake bottle well before using.

    F. Keep cap tightly closed.

    G. Store at room temperature.

MOTRIN (ANTIRHEUMATIC, ANALGESIC, FEVER REDUCER)

I. **Generic name.** Ibuprofen

II. **How supplied** 300-, 400-, or 600-mg tablets or caplets in bottles of 24, 50, 100, or 165

III. **Route.** Oral

IV. **Action.** This nonsteroidal, anti-inflammatory, and antiarthritic agent also has analgesic and antipyretic properties. Mode of action is unknown.

V. **Uses.** Relief of signs and symptoms of rheumatoid arthritis and osteoarthritis; relief of mild to moderate pain (especially helpful for menstrual pain)

VI. **Dosage**

    A. Rheumatoid arthritis and osteoarthritis: Dosage tailored to each patient. Do not exceed six tablets in 24 hours.

    B. Menstrual pain: One tablet at start of period or cramping, then one tablet every 6 hours for 1–2 days

VII. **Side effects**

    A. Most frequent: Nausea, epigastric pain, diarrhea, abdominal distress, vomiting, dizziness, headache, edema, tinnitus, maculopapular rash

    B. Infrequent: Gastric or duodenal ulcers, blurred vision, scotomas or changes in color vision, erythema multiforme, leukopenia, circulatory impairment in patients with marginal cardiac function

VIII. **Contraindications**

    A. Children under 12 years

    B. Aspirin-sensitive patients

    C. Hypersensitivity to drug

    D. Patients with symptoms of nasal polyps, angioedema, and bronchospastic reactivity to aspirin or other nonsteroidal anti-inflammatory agents

    E. Not recommended during pregnancy or lactation

IX. **Precautions**

    A. Use with caution in patients with history of cardiac decompensation.

    B. Use with caution in patients with intrinsic coagulation defects and those on anticoagulant therapy.

    C. Motrin can inhibit platelet aggregation and prolong bleeding time.

    D. Patients on prolonged corticosteroid therapy should have their therapy tapered slowly rather than discontinued abruptly when Motrin is added.

    E. Not recommended for pain more than 10 days or fever more than 3 days

    F. Interactions with coumadin-type anticoagulants and aspirin (net decrease in anti-inflammatory activity).

X. **Education**

    A. Keep all medication out of children's reach.

    B. Use smallest dose that yields acceptable control.

    C. Stop use immediately if blurred or diminished vision, scotomas, changes in color vision, black stools, skin rash, weight gain, edema, or fever occurs.

    D. If gastrointestinal disturbances occur, take with meals or milk.

    E. May cause dizziness; use caution with hazardous mechanical operations

    F. Store at room temperature.

MYCELEX-G 500 MG (ANTIFUNGAL VAGINAL TABLET)

I. **Generic name.** Clotrimazole

II. **Manufacturer/How supplied.** Bayer; 500-mg bullet-shaped vaginal tablet with plastic applicator

III. **Route.** Intravaginal

IV. **Uses**

   A. Treatment of vulvovaginal candidiasis when one-time therapy is warranted. In cases of severe vulvovaginitis due to candidiasis, longer antimycotic therapy is recommended.

   B. Diagnosis should be confirmed by KOH smears and cultures.

V. **Dosage.** One tablet intravaginally at bedtime, for not more than 5 days

VI. **Side effects.** Vaginal irritation

VII. **Contraindications**

   A. Allergy to any components of medication

   B. Not recommended during first trimester of pregnancy

VIII. **Education**

   A. Persistence of signs of vaginitis after 5 days of treatment indicates that another pathogen may be causing the condition; return to office.

   B. Store medication below 86°F.

MYCOSTATIN (ANTIFUNGAL)

I. **Generic name.** Nystatin

II. **Composition.** Ointment and cream: 100,000 U/g; oral suspension: 100,000 U/ml in a vehicle containing 50% sucrose

III. **Manufacturer/How supplied.** Squibb; cream and ointment: 15- or 30-g tubes; oral suspension: 60-ml bottles with calibrated dropper

IV. **Route.** Topical or oral

V. **Action**

   A. Nystatin probably acts by binding to sterols in the cell membrane of the fungus with a resultant change in membrane permeability, allowing leakage of intracellular components.

   B. No appreciable activity against bacteria or trichomonads

VI. **Uses**

   A. Topical preparations: Treatment of cutaneous or mucocutaneous mycotic infections caused by *Candida albicans* and other candidal species

   B. Oral suspension: Treatment of candidiasis in the oral cavity

VII. **Dosage and administration**

   A. Cream or ointment: Apply liberally to affected area twice a day until healed.

   B. Oral suspension

      1. Infants: 2 ml four times a day (1 ml in each side of mouth)

      2. Premature and low-birthweight infants: 1 ml four times a day

      3. Continue treatment 48 hours after perioral symptoms have disappeared.

VIII. **Side effects**

   A. Topical preparations: Minor skin irritation

   B. Oral suspension: Diarrhea, gastrointestinal distress, nausea, vomiting

IX. **Contraindications.** Hypersensitivity to the drug

X. Education

    A. Keep all medication out of children's reach.

    B. Preparations do not stain skin or mucous membranes.

    C. Store at room temperature; avoid freezing.

    D. Apply oral suspension after feeding. Keep bottle nipples and pacifiers clean, and use Mycostatin cream on breasts if nursing.

    E. Discontinue use immediately if hypersensitivity reaction occurs.

    F. Return to office for follow-up after 1 week's treatment.

Nasacort Inhaler

I. Generic name. Triamcinolone acetonide, 55 mcg per dose

II. Manufacturer/How supplied. Rhone-Poulenc Rorer; metered-dose inhaler with nasal adapter

III. Route. Intranasal

IV. Uses. Nasal treatment of symptoms of seasonal and perennial allergic rhinitis

V. Dosage. Age over 12 years: Starting dose, two sprays in each nostril once a day

VI. Side effects. Nasal irritation, burning, or stinging, throat discomfort, sneezing, epistaxis

VII. Contraindications

    A. Sensitivity to ingredients of medication

    B. Pregnancy or lactation

    C. Children under 12 years

    D. Measles or chickenpox

VIII. Precautions. Use with caution in patients with active or quiescent tuberculosis infections of the respiratory tract, those with ocular herpes simplex, and those with systemic viral infections.

IX. Education

    A. Keep all medication out of children's reach.

    B. Take medication as directed; do not increase dosage.

    C. Discontinue use if side effects occur, and call the office.

    D. Follow directions provided for administration of medication.

    E. Monitor growth and development of children, particularly growth suppression.

    F. If no improvement occurs in 1–2 weeks, call the office; patient should be re-evaluated.

    G. Most patients improve within a few days.

    H. Do not puncture the container.

    I. Do not throw canister into a fire or incinerator.

    J. Store at room temperature (59°–86°F); do not store above 120°F.

Nix (TOPICAL PEDICULICIDE)

I. **Generic name.** Permethrin 1%

II. **Manufacturer/How supplied.** Warner-Wellcome; plastic squeeze bottles containing 2 fluid oz

III. **Route.** Topical

IV. **Uses.** Treatment of head lice and nits

V. **Dosage and administration**
   A. After shampooing and towel-drying hair, apply 1–2 oz, enough to saturate hair and scalp. Allow to remain on hair for at least 10 minutes before rinsing off with water.
   B. One treatment is sufficient to eliminate head lice infestation.
   C. Combing of nits is not required but may be done for cosmetic reasons.
   D. If live lice are observed at least 1 week after application, a second application may be given. Remove nits with comb.

VI. **Contraindications**
   A. Sensitivity to ingredients, to any synthetic pyrethroid or pyrethrin, or to chrysanthemums
   B. Pregnancy or lactation
   C. Children under 2 years

VII. **Side effects.** Head lice infestation is often accompanied by pruritus, erythema, and edema; treatment may temporarily exacerbate these conditions.

VIII. **Education**
   A. Keep all medication out of children's reach.
   B. Some itching, redness, or swelling of the scalp may occur after application.
   C. Pruritus is the most common problem associated with use, but the pruritus is actually caused by the lice infestation itself.
   D. If symptoms persist, do not use medication again; call the office.
   E. If sensitivity occurs, discontinue use.
   F. If ingested, use gastric lavage and general supportive measures.
   G. Nix is not irritating to the eyes, but avoid contact with eyes during application. If contact occurs, flush eyes immediately with water.
   H. Discard contents after treatment.
   I. Wash all linens and clothes in hot water and dry in hot dryer; dry clean if unable to wash.
   J. Vacuum rooms used by patient; wash combs and brushes in hot soapy water.
   K. All family members should be examined and treated.

Novahistine DMX (ANTITUSSIVE/EXPECTORANT)

I. **Composition.** Each 5 ml contains dextromethorphan hydrobromide 30 mg, pseudoephedrine hydrochloride 30 mg, and guaifenesin 100 mg.

II. **Manufacturer/How supplied.** SmithKline Beecham; bottles containing 4 or 8 fluid oz

III. **Route.** Oral

IV. **Action.** Cough suppressant; affects medulla; nonanalgesic and nonaddictive

V. **Uses.** To control cough spasms or change a dry cough into a productive one. Helpful for cough, especially a dry, nonproductive one, associated with mild upper respiratory infection, influenza, or bronchitis.

VI. **Dosage**
   A. Ages 6–12 years: 1 tsp every 5 hours
   B. Over 12 years: 2 tsp every 4–6 hours
   C. No more than four doses a day, for no longer than 7 days

VII. **Side effects.** Nausea, dizziness, vomiting, mild stimulation

VIII. **Contraindications**
   A. Persistent or chronic cough (eg, asthma) or cough with excessive secretions
   B. Heart problems, diabetes, high blood pressure, or thyroid disease
   C. Patients on monoamine oxidase inhibitor therapy
   D. Pregnancy or lactation

IX. **Precautions**
   A. Refer to physician if cough persists longer than 1 week, recurs, or is associated with high fever, rash, or persistent headache.
   B. Drugs containing dextromethorphan should not be given with monoamine oxidase inhibitors or antidepressants.
   C. Dextromethorphan is incompatible with salicylates, tetracyclines, penicillin, and iodides.
   D. Consult physician for use in children under 6 years.

X. **Education**
   A. Keep all medication out of children's reach.
   B. Do not exceed recommended dose.
   C. If overdose occurs, call Poison Control Center immediately.
   D. Available over the counter
   E. Do not drive a car or operate machinery while on medication.
   F. If cough persists longer than 1 week, call office.

PEDIACARE

I. **Composition**
   A. PediaCare 1 (Children's Cough Relief Liquid): Dextromethorphan hydrobromide 5 mg/5 ml
   B. PediaCare 2 (Children's Cold Relief Liquid): Pseudoephedrine hydrochloride 15 mg, chlorpheniramine maleate 1 mg/5 ml
   C. PediaCare 3 (Children's Cold Relief)
      1. Liquid: Pseudoephedrine hydrochloride 15 mg, chlorpheniramine maleate 1 mg, and dextromethorphan hydrobromide 5 mg

2. Chewable tablets: Pseudoephedrine hydrochloride 7.5 mg, chlorphenira-mine maleate 0.5 mg, and dextromethorphan hydrobromide 2.5 mg

D. PediaCare Drops (Infants' Cold Relief Decongestant): Pseudoephedrine hy-drochloride 7.5 mg/0.8 ml

II. **Manufacturer/How supplied.** McNeil Consumer Products; cherry-flavored liquid: Bottles containing 4 fluid oz; fruit-flavored tablets: Bottles of 24; cherry-flavored drops: Bottles of 0.5 fluid oz with calibrated dropper

III. **Route.** Oral

IV. **Uses**

A. PediaCare 1: Cough due to minor irritation

B. PediaCare 2: Nasal congestion or runny nose due to hay fever or upper respiratory infection

C. PediaCare 3: Nasal congestion, runny nose, hay fever, or cough

V. **Dosage**

A. PediaCare Drops

1. Ages 0–3 months (6–11 lb): 0.5 dropperful (0.4 ml) every 4–6 hours
2. Ages 4–11 months (12–17 lb): One dropperful (0.8 ml) every 4–6 hours
3. Ages 12–23 months (18–23 lb): 1.5 dropperfuls (1.2 ml) every 4–6 hours
4. Ages 2–3 years (24–36 lb): Two dropperfuls every 4–6 hours

B. PediaCare 1, 2, and 3

1. Ages 2–3 years (24–36 lb): 1 tsp liquid or one tablet every 4–6 hours
2. Ages 4–5 years (36–47 lb): 1.5 tsp liquid or 1.5 tablets every 4–6 hours
3. Ages 6–8 years (48–59 lb): 2 tsp liquid or two tablets every 4–6 hours
4. Ages 9–10 years (60–71 lb): 2.5 tsp liquid or 2.5 tablets every 4–6 hours

C. PediaCare Night Rest liquid or tablets

1. Ages 2–3 years: 1 tsp or one tablet every 4–6 hours
2. Ages 4–5 years: 1.5 tsp or 1.5 tablets every 4–6 hours
3. Ages 6–8 years: 2 tsp or two tablets every 4–6 hours
4. Ages 9–10 years: 2.5 tsp or 2.5 tablets every 4–6 hours
5. Age 11 years: 3 tsp or three tablets every 4–6 hours

VI. **Contraindications.** Heart disease, high blood pressure, thyroid disease, diabetes, glaucoma, asthma, depression

VII. **Education**

A. Keep all medication out of children's reach.

B. Discontinue use after 7 days.

C. Call office if cough continues, high fever occurs, or headache or rash appears.

D. May cause irritability and drowsiness

E. Persistent cough is a sign of a serious illness; call the office.

F. Do not exceed six doses in 24 hours.

G. Not for nasal use; administer orally only.

H. Do not exceed the recommended dose.

I. If overdose occurs, call the Poison Control Center immediately.

J. Do not use medication if seal is broken, cap is open, or carton is opened.

K. PediaCare Night Rest may be used every 6–8 hours.

PEDIALYTE (ORAL ELECTROLYTE SOLUTION)

I. **Composition.** Each liter contains sodium 45 mEq, potassium 20 mEq, chloride 35 mEq, citrate 30 mEq, and dextrose 25 g; 100 calories.

II. **Manufacturer/How supplied.** Ross Laboratories; bottles (8 fluid oz) and cans (32 fluid oz)

III. **Route.** Oral

IV. **Action and uses.** To maintain and replace the normal electrolyte balance in infants and children with moderate to mild diarrhea

V. **Dosage**

    A. Carefully calculate the amount needed according to the child's weight.

        1. 7–13 lb: 13–28 fluid oz/day

        2. 17–20 lb: 40–44 fluid oz/day

        3. 23–25 lb: 41–45 fluid oz/day

        4. 28–30 lb: 53–56 fluid oz/day

        5. 32–35 lb: 58–69 fluid oz/day

        6. 38–41 lb: 62–66 fluid oz/day

    B. Divide daily doses into frequent small feedings for rehydration.

VI. **Contraindications.** Do not use for very small infants (ie, 1 week of age).

VII. **Education**

    A. Discontinue all solid foods and follow diarrhea protocol carefully.

    B. Give frequent small feedings of Pedialyte.

    C. Children age 6 years and older may have 2 qt/day.

    D. Ready-to-use liter bottles are available at grocery stores, drugstores, and convenience stores.

PENICILLIN V POTASSIUM (ANTIBIOTIC)

I. **Composition.** Oral suspension: 125 or 250 mg/5 ml; tablets: 250 or 500 mg

II. **Route.** Oral

III. **Uses**

    A. Upper respiratory infections caused by streptococci, including pharyngitis and scarlet fever

    B. Pneumococcal infection of otitis media

    C. Prophylaxis in rheumatic fever and mild staphylococcal infection of soft tissue and skin

    D. Lyme disease

IV. **Dosage**

    A. Under 12 years: 25–50 mg/kg/day in divided doses every 6 or 8 hours for 10 days

    B. Over 12 years: 125–500 mg every 6 or 8 hours for 10 days

V. **Side effects.** Sore mouth, black tongue, nausea, decreased appetite, vomiting, diarrhea, skin eruptions, urticaria

VI. **Contraindications.** Allergy to penicillin or ampicillin

VII. **Precautions**

A. Use cautiously in patients with asthma or a history of allergies.

B. Order culture and sensitivity tests of skin infection before prescribing.

C. Order throat culture before treating in cases of streptococcal pharyngitis.

VIII. **Education**

A. Keep all medication out of children's reach.

B. Discontinue medication if there are any signs of rash, pruritus, or anaphylaxis.

C. May be administered with food, but blood levels are higher if given on an empty stomach

D. Keep medication refrigerated and tightly capped.

E. Shake bottle well before pouring oral solution.

F. Take medication for 10 full days even though symptoms disappear.

G. Order generic form of medication.

H. Discard any unused medication after 10 days.

PHENERGAN EXPECTORANT WITH CODEINE (COUGH FORMULA)

I. **Composition.** Promethazine hydrochloride 6.25 mg/5 ml, codeine phosphate 10 mg

II. **Route.** Oral

III. **Action and uses.** Antihistamine, antiemetic, and sedative qualities useful for persistent cough, perennial and seasonal allergic rhinitis, and allergic conjunctivitis

IV. **Dosage**

A. Ages 2–6 years: 0.25–0.5 tsp every 4–6 hours, not to exceed 15 ml in 24 hours

B. Ages 6–12 years: 0.5–1 tsp every 6 hours, not to exceed 30 ml in 24 hours

V. **Contraindications**

A. Children under 2 years

B. Pregnancy and lactation

C. History of drug dependency

VI. **Precautions.** Doses of 75–125 mg of promethazine hydrochloride may cause paradoxical reaction characterized by hyperexcitability and nightmares.

VII. **Education**

A. Keep all medication out of children's reach.

B. Use only at night to manage persistent cough in sleepless child (no longer than 4 days).

C. Order 4 oz, with no refills.

D. May be habit-forming; carefully monitor medical plan.

E. May have a sedating effect. Do not use medication when driving a vehicle or farm machinery; children should be discouraged from riding bikes when taking medication.

F. Do not use with tranquilizers, alcohol, or central nervous system depressants.

G. Overdose may result in respiratory depression, stupor or coma, cold clammy skin, bradycardia, Cheyne-Stokes respiration, pinpoint pupils, cardiac arrest, and death. Call office immediately if overdose occurs.

H. If cough continues or if fever or course of illness worsens, discontinue medication and call office.

Ponstel (Anti-inflammatory, Non-narcotic Analgesic)

I.   Generic name. Mefenamic acid

II. Manufacturer/How supplied. Parke-Davis; 250-mg Kapseals in bottles of 100

III. Route. Oral

IV. Action. In clinical trials with animals, analgesic, antipyretic, and anti-inflammatory activities were demonstrated.

V.   Uses. Relief of mild to moderate pain of primary dysmenorrhea

VI. Dosage

    A. Over 14 years: 500 mg initially, then 250 mg every 6 hours as needed, not to exceed 1 week

    B. Start at beginning of menses; therapy should not exceed 1 week (usually needed only 2–3 days).

VII. Side effects

    A. Nausea, gastrointestinal discomfort, vomiting, gas, diarrhea

    B. Drowsiness, dizziness, nervousness, headache, blurred vision, insomnia

    C. Urticaria, rash, facial edema, mild renal toxicity, dysuria, hematuria

    D. Severe autoimmune hemolytic anemia if used for prolonged periods of time

    E. Eye irritation, ear pain, perspiration, mild hepatic toxicity; increased need for insulin in diabetics

VIII. Contraindications

    A. Under age 14 years

    B. Hypersensitivity to mefenamic acid

    C. Ulcerations or chronic inflammation of upper or lower gastrointestinal tract

    D. Pregnancy and lactation

IX. Precautions

    A. Use with caution in patients with inflammatory disease of the gastrointestinal tract or a history of kidney or liver disease.

    B. Autoimmune hemolytic anemia may occur with continuous use for 12 months or longer.

X.   Education

    A. Keep all medication out of children's reach.

    B. Take medication with food.

    C. Do not exceed 1 week of therapy.

    D. If overdose occurs, call Poison Control Center immediately.

    E. If rash or diarrhea occurs, reduce dose or discontinue use temporarily and call the office.

F. Blood urea nitrogen values may rise during therapy.

G. May prolong prothrombin time

H. May exacerbate asthma

I. Produces false-positive reaction for urinary bile in diazo tablet test

PROSTAPHILIN (ANTIBIOTIC)

I. Generic name. Oxacillin sodium

II. How supplied. Oral solution, 250 mg/5 ml

III. Route. Oral

IV. Uses

    A. Infections caused by penicillinase-producing staphylococci, beta-hemolytic streptococci, or pneumococci

    B. Useful for therapy in suspected staphylococcal infection pending culture and sensitivity tests

V. Dosage. 50–100 mg/kg/day in four equal doses for 1–2 weeks

VI. Side effects. Diarrhea, nausea, vomiting, pruritus, rash, hives, wheezing; elevated SGOT and SGPT values; transient hematuria and superinfection

VII. Contraindications

    A. Sensitivity to penicillins or cephalosporins

    B. Renal impairment

VIII. Precautions. Use cautiously in children with a history of asthma.

IX. Education

    A. Keep all medication out of children's reach.

    B. Give medication on an empty stomach 1 hour before or 2 hours after eating or drinking.

    C. Keep medication tightly capped.

    D. Keep medication in the refrigerator (solution remains stable for 14 days in the refrigerator).

    E. Take drug for required length of time as prescribed.

    F. If rash or hives develop, discontinue medication and call the office.

PROVENTIL SYRUP (BRONCHODILATOR-ANTIASTHMATIC)

I. Generic name. Albuterol sulfate

II. Manufacturer/How supplied. Schering; bottle (16 fluid oz) containing 2 mg of albuterol as 2.5 mg of albuterol sulfate in each 5 ml (teaspoonful)

III. Route. Oral

IV. Uses. Relief of bronchospasm in reversible airway disease

V. Dosage

    A. Ages 2–6 years: Initial dose 0.1 mg/kg (not to exceed 1 tsp) three times a day

    B. Ages 6–14 years: 1 tsp three or four times a day

    C. Ages 14 and older: 1–2 tsp three or four times a day

    D. For those who do not respond well:

        1. Ages 2–6: Increase dose cautiously to 0.2 mg/kg (not to exceed 2 tsp) three times a day.

        2. Ages 6–14: Increase dose cautiously, not to exceed 24 mg/day in divided doses.

        3. Ages 14 and older: Increase dose cautiously, not to exceed 8 mg four times a day.

VI. **Side effects.** Irritability, anorexia, tremors, rash, cough, nausea, sputum increase, rarely Stevens-Johnson syndrome, erythema multiforme

VII. **Contraindications**

    A. Allergy to ingredients of medication

    B. Under 2 years of age

    C. Pregnancy and lactation

    D. Labor and delivery

VIII. **Precautions.** Use with caution in patients with hypertension, diabetes mellitus, cardiac arrhythmias, convulsive disorders, or coronary insufficiency.

IX. **Education**

    A. Keep all medication out of children's reach.

    B. Take as directed. Do not increase dosage or frequency without medical input.

    C. If symptoms increase, discontinue use and call office immediately.

    D. Keep medication tightly capped.

    E. Store at 36°–86°F.

PYRIDIUM (URINARY ANALGESIC)

I. **Generic name.** Phenazopyridine hydrochloride

II. **Manufacturer/How supplied.** Parke-Davis; tablets of 100 or 200 mg

III. **Route.** Oral

IV. **Uses.** To relieve symptoms of dysuria in adolescents; especially helpful during interval between diagnosis and treatment

V. **Dosage.** 200 mg three times a day after meals for 2 days only

VI. **Side effects.** Mild gastrointestinal symptoms

VII. **Contraindications**

    A. Pregnancy and lactation

    B. Renal insufficiency

    C. Sensitivity to ingredients in medication

VIII. **Precautions.** Yellowish tinge of skin or sclera may indicate decline in renal function.

IX. **Education**

    A. Keep all medication out of children's reach.

    B. Take medication three times a day after meals.

C. Medication will give urine a reddish-orange tint and may stain fabric.

D. Use only as long as symptoms persist; do not use for more than 2 days.

E. Discontinue use if skin or sclera becomes yellow; call the office immediately.

F. Discontinue use if headache, rash, pruritus, or gastrointestinal disturbance occurs.

G. If overdose occurs, call the office immediately.

Rondec-DM (Antihistamine/Decongestant/Antitussive)

I. **Composition.** Drops: Each 1-ml dropperful contains carbinoxamine maleate 2 mg, pseudoephedrine hydrochloride 25 mg, dextromethorphan hydrobromide 4 mg, and less than 0.6% alcohol. Syrup: Each 5 ml (1 tsp) contains carbinoxamine maleate 4 mg, pseudoephedrine hydrochloride 60 mg, dextromethorphan hydrobromide 15 mg, and less than 0.6% alcohol.

II. **Manufacturer/How supplied.** Dura; drops: 30-ml bottles with dropper (grape-flavored); syrup: bottles of 4 or 16 fluid oz (grape-flavored)

III. **Route.** Oral

IV. **Action and uses.** Relief of symptoms of nasopharyngitis, common cold, bronchitis, bronchial cough, and recurrent cough; nonnarcotic, antitussive, decongestive, and antihistaminic

V. **Dosage**

A. Drops

1. Ages 1–3 months: 0.25 dropperful four times a day

2. Ages 3–6 months: 0.5 dropperful four times a day

3. Ages 6–9 months: 0.75 dropperful four times a day

4. Ages 9–18 months: One dropperful four times a day

B. Syrup

1. Ages 18 months–5 years: 0.5 tsp (2.5 ml) four times a day

2. Ages 6 years and over: 1 tsp (5 ml) four times a day

VI. **Side effects.** Sedation, moderate drowsiness, dizziness, vomiting, headache, nausea, dysuria, polyuria, cardiac arrhythmias, respiratory difficulty, tremors, hallucinations, weakness, pallor

VII. **Contraindications**

A. Glaucoma, urinary retention, ulcer, or coronary disease

B. Hypertension or ischemic heart disease

C. Patients taking monoamine oxidase inhibitors

D. During asthma attacks

E. Pregnancy

VIII. **Precautions**

A. Use with caution in patients with a history of asthma, diabetes, or hyperthyroidism.

B. Use with caution in nursing mothers.

IX. **Education**

    A. Keep all medication out of children's reach.

    B. If overdose occurs, call Poison Control Center immediately.

    C. May be given with analgesics and antibiotics

    D. Give three times a day if side effects occur.

    E. Avoid exposing medication to excessive heat.

    F. Keep liquid in a cool and dark place.

    G. Keep tightly capped.

    H. Antihistamine may enhance the effects of barbiturates, alcohol, antidepressants, or other central nervous system depressants.

    I. If cough worsens or fever ensues, call the office immediately.

SUDAFED (ADRENERGIC)

I. **Generic name.** Pseudoephedrine hydrochloride

II. **Manufacturer/How supplied.** Warner-Wellcome; syrup: 4 oz; tablets: Boxes of 24 or 48

III. **Route.** Oral

IV. **Uses**

    A. Nasal congestion, bronchial congestion, acute coryza, rhinitis, and serous otitis media with eustachian tube congestion

    B. May be used in combination with antibiotics, analgesics, antihistamines, or expectorants in cases of allergic rhinitis, sinusitis, acute otitis media, or tracheobronchitis

V. **Dosage.** Do not exceed recommended daily dosage. Do not exceed four doses in 24 hours.

    A. Ages 2–6 years: 0.5 tsp syrup every 4–6 hours

    B. Ages 6–12 years: 1 tsp syrup or one tablet every 4–6 hours

    C. Over 12 years: Two 30-mg tablets four times a day

VI. **Side effects.** Mild stimulation and nausea

VII. **Contraindications.** Hypertension, diabetes, or hyperthyroidism

VIII. **Precautions.** Sudafed interacts with monoamine oxidase inhibitors and guanethidine.

IX. **Education**

    A. Keep all medication out of children's reach.

    B. Sudafed is an over-the-counter drug.

    C. Do not take any other nonprescription drug with Sudafed without approval of physician.

    D. Avoid taking medication at bedtime; it may cause restlessness and sleeplessness.

    E. Discontinue use if extreme restlessness, agitation, tachycardia, or anorexia occurs.

    F. Do not use for more than 7 days.

G. Call office immediately if overdose occurs.

H. If symptoms do not improve, cough is worse, or fever ensues, call office.

I. Store at 59°–77°F; protect from light.

SUPRAX (SEMISYNTHETIC CEPHALOSPORIN ANTIBIOTIC)

I. **Generic name.** Cefixime

II. **Manufacturer/How supplied.** Lederle; oral suspension: 100 mg/5 cc; scored 200- or 400-mg film-coated tablets

III. **Route.** Oral

IV. **Actions and uses.** A semisynthetic cephalosporin antibiotic used for the treatment of:

   A. Uncomplicated urinary tract infections caused by *Escherichia coli* and *Proteus mirabilis*

   B. Otitis media caused by *Haemophilus influenzae*, *Moraxella catarrhalis*, and *Streptococcus pyogenes*

   C. Pharyngitis and tonsillitis caused by *Streptococcus pyogenes*

   D. Active bronchitis and acute exacerbations of chronic bronchitis caused by *Streptococcus pneumoniae* and *H influenzae*

   E. Uncomplicated gonorrhea (culture and sensitivity tests should be obtained before treatment)

V. **Dosage.** Administer for 10 days.

   A. A normal guide:

Body Weight (kg)	Suspension (Dose/d)	Tablets (Dose/d)
6.25	½ tsp (2.5 ml)	50 mg
12.5	1 tsp (5 ml)	100 mg
18.75	1½ tsp (7.5 ml)	150 mg
25.0	2 tsp (10 ml)	200 mg
31.25	2½ tsp (12.5 ml)	250 mg
37.5	3 tsp (15 ml)	300 mg

   B. More than 50 kg: One 400-mg tablet per day or one 200-mg tablet twice a day

   C. For otitis media, use suspension rather than tablets; peak flow is higher on suspension than tablets.

VI. **Side effects**

   A. Gastrointestinal: Diarrhea, abdominal pain, nausea and vomiting

   B. Central nervous system: Headache, dizziness

   C. Hypersensitivity reactions: Rashes, urticaria, pruritus

   D. Hepatic: Elevated SGPT, SGOT, alkaline phosphatase, blood urea nitrogen, creatinine levels

   E. In severe cases, cephalosporins may trigger seizures.

VII. **Contraindications.** Allergy to penicillin or the cephalosporin group of antibiotics (cross hypersensitivity in up to 10% of patients with penicillin allergy)

VIII. Precautions

- **A.** Safety of use in pregnancy has not been established.
- **B.** It is not known if Suprax is excreted in human milk.
- **C.** Safety and effectiveness in children under age 6 months has not been established.
- **D.** Not recommended for prophylaxis of rheumatic fever

IX. Education

- **A.** Keep all medication out of children's reach.
- **B.** Take medication for 10 days, even though symptoms disappear.
- **C.** Carefully follow directions for reconstituting oral suspension.
- **D.** Shake suspension well before using.
- **E.** Suspension may be kept for 14 days at room temperature or may be refrigerated.
- **F.** Keep bottle tightly capped.
- **G.** Discard unused portion of medication after 14 days.
- **H.** Medication may be taken with or without food.
- **I.** With extended use, overgrowth of resistant organisms may occur; call the office immediately.

TAVIST SYRUP (ANTIHISTAMINE)

- **I. Generic name.** Clemastine fumarate
- **II. Composition.** Each tsp (5 ml) contains 0.67 mg clemastine fumarate.
- **III. Manufacturer/How supplied.** Sandoz; bottle containing 4 fluid oz
- **IV. Route.** Oral
- **V. Uses.** Relief of allergic rhinitis and allergic pruritus, urticaria, and angioedema
- **VI. Dosage**
  - **A.** Age 6–12 years: 1 tsp twice a day for symptoms of allergic rhinitis; 2 tsp twice a day (starting dose) for urticaria and angioedema. Do not exceed 6 tsp in 24-hour period.
  - **B.** Ages 12 and over: 2 tsp twice a day for symptoms of allergic rhinitis; 4 tsp twice a day for urticaria and angioedema. Do not exceed 12 tsp in 24-hour period.
- **VII. Side effects.** Dryness of mouth, nose, and throat; drug rash, headache, sleepiness, anorexia
- **VIII. Contraindications**
  - **A.** Lower respiratory disease, especially asthma
  - **B.** Lactation
  - **C.** Hypersensitivity to the drug or other antihistamines
  - **D.** Newborns or premature infants
  - **E.** Concomitant use of hypnotics, sedatives, tranquilizers, or alcohol
  - **F.** Children under 6 years
  - **G.** Safety of medication during pregnancy is unknown.
- **IX. Precautions**
  - **A.** Use with caution in patients with narrow-angle glaucoma, stenosing peptic ulcer, pyloroduodenal obstruction, or bladder neck obstruction.

B. Use with caution in patients with hypertension, bronchial asthma, increased intraocular pressure, hyperthyroidism, or cardiovascular disease.

C. Monoamine oxidase inhibitors prolong and increase the intensity of anticholinergic effects of antihistamines.

D. Before administering, determine if patient has a history of glaucoma, urinary retention, peptic ulcer, or pregnancy.

X. **Education**

A. Keep all medication out of children's reach.

B. Do not exceed recommended dose.

C. Signs of antihistamine toxicity in children include fixed dilated pupils, dry mouth, flushed face, fever, excitation and agitation, hallucinations, ataxia, incoordination, tonic–clonic convulsions, and postictal depression.

D. Overdose of antihistamines can cause hallucinations, convulsions, and death.

E. Store medication in tightly closed, upright container in dry, cool place, away from sunlight and heat.

F. Do not take alcohol, sleeping pills, sedatives, or tranquilizers while taking antihistamines.

G. May cause dizziness, headache, drowsiness, dry mouth, blurred vision, nausea, or nervousness

H. Do not use when operating machinery or driving a car.

TETRACYCLINE CAPSULES (ANTIBIOTIC)

I. **Manufacturer/How supplied.** Lederle; 250- or 500-mg capsules

II. **Route.** Oral

III. **Action and uses**

A. Inhibits protein synthesis

B. Active against a broad range of gram-positive and gram-negative organisms, especially *Mycoplasma pneumoniae, Escherichia coli, Shigella, Haemophilus influenzae, Klebsiella*

C. Also used for intestinal amebiasis and in severe acne

IV. **Dosage.** Ages 9 years and over: 10–20 mg/kg/day in two or four equal doses, or 25–50 mg/kg/day in four equal doses

V. **Side effects.** Nausea, vomiting, diarrhea, glossitis, enteritis, monilial overgrowth, loss of appetite

VI. **Contraindications**

A. Hypersensitivity to tetracycline

B. Renal impairment

C. Children under 9 years of age, in whom it may cause permanent discoloration of teeth

D. Tetracycline is present in the breast milk of lactating women taking the medication and is not recommended during breast feeding.

E. Pregnancy

VII. Education

A. Keep all medication out of children's reach.

B. Take on an empty stomach 1 hour before or 2 hours after eating.

C. Do not take with any milk products or iron preparations.

D. Overexposure to the sun can have adverse effects.

E. Avoid oral antacids and diuretics when taking tetracycline.

F. Take for the prescribed period of time.

G. Order generically to save money.

H. Limit refills when treating acne to ensure follow-up visits.

I. Acne may require at least 1 month of treatment before noticeable effects occur. If acne seems worse, discontinue use and call the office.

TINACTIN (ANTIFUNGAL)

I. **Generic name.** Tolnaftate

II. **Composition.** Cream 1% and powder 1%: 10 mg/g; solution 1%: Each 1 ml contains tolnaftate 10 mg and butylated hydroxytoluene 1 mg.

III. **Manufacturer/How supplied.** Schering; cream: 15-g tubes; powder: 45-g container; solution: 10-ml bottles

IV. **Route.** Topical

V. **Action.** Active ingredient is a highly active synthetic fungicidal agent that is effective in the treatment of superficial fungal infections of the skin. It is inactive systemically, is virtually nonsensitizing, and does not ordinarily sting or irritate intact or broken skin, even in the presence of acute inflammatory reactions.

VI. **Uses.** To treat superficial fungal infections of the skin that cause tinea pedis (athlete's foot), tinea cruris (jock itch), or tinea corporis (body ringworm)

VII. **Dosage and administration**

A. Wash and dry infected area twice a day, then apply.

B. Rub 0.5″ ribbon of cream gently on infected area, massage two or three drops of solution gently to cover infected area, or sprinkle powder liberally on all infected areas and in shoes and socks.

VIII. **Side effects.** None

IX. **Contraindications.** Children under 2 years

X. **Precautions**

A. If burning or itching does not improve within 10 days or becomes worse or if irritation occurs, discontinue use and consult physician.

B. For external use only. Keep out of eyes.

C. Cream and solution are not recommended for nail or scalp infections.

D. Powder is not recommended for use on scalp.

E. Children under age 12 should be supervised while using product.

XI. **Education**

A. Keep all medication out of children's reach.

B. Products are odorless and greaseless and do not stain or discolor the skin, hair, or nails.

   C. All forms begin to relieve burning, itching, and soreness within 24 hours. Symptoms are usually cleared in 2–3 weeks.

   D. Where skin is thickened, treatment may take 4–6 weeks.

   E. To prevent recurrence, continue treatment for 2 weeks after disappearance of all symptoms.

   F. Store at 36°–86°F.

TOFRANIL (ANTIDEPRESSANT)

I.   **Generic name.** Imipramine hydrochloride

II.   **Manufacturer/How supplied.** Geigy; 10- 25-, or 50-mg tablets in bottles of 100, 1,000, or 5,000

III.   **Route.** Oral

IV.   **Uses**

   A. Nocturnal enuresis in children age 6 years and over; given only after appropriate tests have ruled out organic disease

   B. Safety of use in children for indications other than nocturnal enuresis is not established.

V.   **Dosage.** 25–50 mg 1 hour before bedtime; do not exceed 2.5 mg/kg/day.

   A. Ages 6 and over: Start at 25 mg for 1 week. If no response, increase to 50 mg nightly.

   B. Over 12 years: Up to 75 mg

   C. After 3 months, decrease medication, slowly withdrawing over a 3-month period.

   D. If child has a breakthrough, maintain 50-mg level for a full 6 months.

   E. Lower doses are recommended in adolescents.

VI.   **Side effects.** Nervousness, sleep disorders, mild gastrointestinal symptoms, constipation, anxiety, emotional outbursts, skin rash, petechiae, urticaria, itching, dry mouth, black tongue, jaundice

VII.   **Contraindications**

   A. Hyperthyroidism

   B. History of urinary retention, seizure disorder, glaucoma, or cardiovascular disease

VIII.   **Education**

   A. Time is needed for full therapeutic effect.

   B. Store tablets in a tightly closed container.

   C. Return to office for follow-up at 1-month intervals.

   D. Blood and urine levels of imipramine may not correlate with the degree of intoxication and are not dependable indicators in clinical management.

   E. Do not use with alcohol, decongestants, or local anesthetics.

   F. Medication may impair mental or physical abilities required to operate a car or farm machinery.

   G. Write prescription for least amount possible.

   H. Before elective surgery, discontinue medication for as long as possible.

I. Overexposure to sunlight may cause photosensitization.

J. Elevation or lowering of blood sugar may occur.

K. If overdose occurs, call office and Poison Control Center regarding treatment.

Tussi-Organidin DM (Antitussive/Expectorant)

I. **Composition.** Each 5 ml contains guaifenesin 100 mg and dextromethorphan hydrobromide 10 mg.

II. **Manufacturer/How supplied.** Wallace; orange syrup in bottles of 4 fluid oz or 10 or 30 ml

III. **Route.** Oral

IV. **Action and uses.** Antitussive and expectorant formula for the common cold and upper respiratory conditions

V. **Dosage**

    A. Ages 6 months–2 years: 0.125–0.25 tsp every 4 hours, not to exceed 1.5 tsp in 24 hours

    B. Ages 2–6 years: 0.5–1 tsp every 4 hours

    C. Ages 6–12 years: 1 tsp every 4 hours

    D. Age 12 and over: 2 tsp every 4 hours, not to exceed 12 tsp in 24 hours

VI. **Contraindications**

    A. Sensitivity to ingredients

    B. Children under 6 months

    C. Pregnancy or lactation

    D. Patient taking drugs for depression or Parkinson's disease

    E. Patient taking monoamine oxidase inhibitors

VII. **Side effects.** Nausea, vomiting, dizziness, rash, headache

VIII. **Education**

    A. Keep all medication out of children's reach.

    B. Store at 59°–86°F. Do not freeze or expose to heat.

    C. Keep bottle tightly closed and away from light.

    D. Discontinue use if rash appears, and call the office immediately.

    E. Do not use over prolonged period of time.

    F. Do not exceed recommended dose.

    G. If cough worsens, fever ensues, or cold symptoms do not improve in a few days, discontinue use and call the office.

Vantin (Second-Generation Cephalosporin Antibiotic)

I. **Generic name.** Cefpodoxime

II. **Manufacturer/How supplied.** Upjohn; tablets: 100 or 200 mg; oral suspension: 50 or 100 mg/5 ml

III. **Route.** Oral

IV. **Uses.** A cephalosporin antibiotic used for the treatment of:

   A. Acute otitis media caused by *Streptococcus pneumoniae, Haemophilus influenzae,* including beta-lactamase-producing strains or *Moraxella*

   B. Pharyngitis or tonsillitis caused by *Streptococcus pyogenes*

   C. Urinary tract infection caused by *Escherichia coli, Klebsiella, S pneumoniae, Proteus mirabilis,* or *Staphylococcus saprophyticus*

   D. Skin and skin structure infections caused by *Staphylococcus aureus* or *S pyogenes* (abscess should be incised and drained as clinically indicated)

   E. Uncomplicated urethral and cervical gonorrhea caused by *Neisseria gonorrhoeae*

   F. Acute community-acquired pneumonia caused by *S pneumoniae* or *H influenzae* (non-beta-lactamase–producing strains only)

   G. Acute bacterial exacerbation of chronic bronchitis caused by *S pneumoniae* or *H influenzae* (non-beta-lactamase–producing strains only)

V. **Dosage**

Age	Type of Infection	Dose Frequency	Total Daily Dose	Duration
5 mo–12 yrs				
	Acute OM	10/mg/kg 24 h Max 400 mg qd or	10/mg/kg/ Max 400 mg qd 5/mg/kg Max 200 mg	10 days 10 days
	Pharyngitis/ tonsillitis	5 mg/kg/12h Max 100 mg qd	10 mg/kg/ divided q12h Max 200 mg	10 days
13 years– older				
	Acute community- acquired pneumonia	200 mg q12h	400 mg	14 days
	Acute bacterial exacerbation of chronic bronchitis	200 mg q12h	400 mg	10 days
	Uncomplicated gonorrhea	single dose	200 mg	
	Skin and skin structure infections	400 mg q12h	800 mg	7–14 days
	Uncomplicated urinary tract infections	100 mg q12h	200 mg	7 days
	Pharyngitis/ tonsillitis	100 mg q12h	200 mg	10 days

VI. **Side effects.** Diarrhea, vomiting, diaper rash, rash, headache, abdominal pain, fever

VII. Contraindications

A. Allergy to the cephalosporin group of antibiotics

B. Pregnancy and lactation

C. During labor and delivery

D. Safety of use in children under 6 months is unknown.

E. Not recommended for treatment of scarlet fever

F. Not recommended for treatment of male rectal infections or gonococcal pharyngeal infections in men or women

VIII. Precautions. Culture and sensitivity testing should be obtained before beginning therapy for urinary tract infections.

IX. Education

A. Keep all medication out of children's reach.

B. Cephalosporin may cause a positive Coombs' test.

C. Store suspension at 36°–46°F.

D. Replace cap tightly.

E. Keep tablets from excessive moisture.

F. Follow directions carefully for mixing the oral suspension.

G. Keep suspension refrigerated.

H. Shake suspension well before administration.

I. Discard unused medication after 14 days.

J. Discontinue use and call office immediately if side effects occur.

VENTOLIN INHALER (AEROSOL BRONCHODILATOR)

I. **Generic name.** Albuterol

II. **Manufacturer/How supplied.** Glaxo-Wellcome; metered-dose aerosol unit with 17-g canister

III. **Route.** Inhalation aerosol

IV. **Uses**

A. Relief of bronchospasm in children age 4 years and older with reversible obstructive airway disease

B. Prevention of exercise-induced bronchospasm

V. **Dosage.** Two inhalations taken about 15–20 minutes before exercise; may be repeated once every 4–6 hours. Some patients find one inhalation sufficient to control bronchospasm.

VI. **Side effects.** Heart palpitations, tachycardia, increased blood pressure, tremor, nausea, vomiting, vertigo, insomnia, unusual drying of the mouth; occasionally, rash, urticaria, bronchospasm, or oropharyngeal edema

VII. **Contraindications**

A. Hypersensitivity to ingredients

B. Pregnancy, labor, delivery, or lactation

C. Safe use in children under age 4 years is not established.

VIII. **Precautions**

A. Use in pregnancy may affect development of the fetus.

B. Use with caution in patients with a history of diabetes mellitus, hyperthyroidism, cardiovascular disorder, or hypertension.

IX. Education

A. Keep all medication out of children's reach.

B. Use of adrenergic aerosols is sometimes associated with paradoxical bronchospasm; if this occurs, discontinue use immediately.

C. Death may result from overuse; strict adherence to dosage and frequency must be followed to ensure safety. Do not take more frequent doses or larger number of inhalations.

D. Do not use other aerosol bronchodilators or epinephrine concomitantly.

E. Can be useful for the treatment of recurrent bouts of bronchospasm; when used judiciously, it is safe over a period of years.

F. If recommended dosage is ineffective, discontinue use and call office immediately.

G. Contents are under pressure. Do not puncture canister. Do not use or store near open fire or heat. Never throw container in an incinerator or an open fire.

H. Overdose is indicated by intense anginal pain and hypertension.

I. Store at 59°–86°F. Exposure to 120°F may cause container to burst.

J. Therapeutic effect may increase when canister is cold.

K. Shake well before using.

VERMOX CHEWABLE TABLETS (ANTHELMINTIC)

I. **Generic name.** Mebendazole

II. **Manufacturer/How supplied.** Janssen; 100-mg tablets in boxes of 12

III. **Route.** Oral

IV. **Action.** Blocks glucose uptake by susceptible helminths, thereby depleting the energy level until it is inadequate for survival

V. **Uses**

A. Treatment of *Trichuris trichiura* (whipworm), *Enterobius vermicularis* (pinworm), *Ascaris lumbricoides* (roundworm), *Necator americanus* (American hookworm), or *Ancylostoma duodenale* (common hookworm)

B. In single or mixed infections, efficacy varies.

VI. **Dosage.** Adults, and children over 2 years: Pinworm, one tablet once; roundworm, whipworm, or hookworm, one tablet twice a day for 3 consecutive days

VII. **Side effects.** Transient symptoms of abdominal pain and diarrhea in cases of massive infection

VIII. **Contraindications**

A. Lactation

B. Pregnancy (may cause fetal damage)

C. Hypersensitivity to the drug

IX. Precautions. Consider the benefits and risks of administering to a child less than 2 years of age. Do not treat children under age 2 without physician's consent.

X. Education

  A. Keep all medication out of children's reach.

  B. Tablets may be chewed, swallowed, or crushed and mixed with food.

  C. If patient is not cured 3 weeks after treatment, a second course of treatment is advised.

  D. Discuss contagiousness, hygiene, transmission of disease, and reinfection.

  E. In case of overdose, call Poison Control Center immediately.

  F. Often all family members are treated at the same time (same dosage for adults and children).

  G. Store medication at 59°–86°F.

ZITHROMAX (MACROLIDE ANTIBIOTIC)

I.   Generic name. Azithromycin

II. Route. Oral

III. Manufacturer/How supplied. Pfizer; capsules: 250 mg; oral suspension: 300, 600, or 900 mg

IV. Uses. Macrolide antibiotic derived from erythromycin and used for the treatment of:

  A. Children: Acute otitis media caused by *Haemophilus influenzae, Moraxella catarrhalis,* or *Streptococcus pneumoniae;* Pharyngitis or tonsillitis caused by *Streptococcus pyogenes*

  B. Adults: Mild to moderate infections of acute bacterial exacerbations of chronic obstructive pulmonary disease due to *H influenzae, M catarrhalis,* or *S pneumoniae;* community-acquired pneumonia due to *S pneumoniae* or *H influenzae* and treatable on an outpatient basis; pharyngitis/tonsillitis caused by *S pyogenes;* uncomplicated skin and skin structure infections due to *Staphylococcus aureus;* nongonococcal urethritis and cervicitis due to *Chlamydia trachomatis.*

V.   Dosage

  A. For acute otitis media in ages 2 years and above:

Body Weight		100 mg/5 ml		200 mg/5 ml		Total ml per treatment
(kg)	(lbs)	Day 1	Day 2–5	Day 1	Day 2–5	course
10	22	5 ml (1 tsp)	2.5 ml (½ tsp)			15 ml
20	44			5 ml (1 tsp)	2.5 ml (½ tsp)	15 ml
30	66			7.5 (1½ tsp)	3.75 (¾ tsp)	22.5 ml
40	88			10 ml (2 tsp)	5 ml (1 tsp)	30 ml

B. For pharyngitis or tonsillitis in ages 2 years and above:

Body Weight (kg)	(lbs)	200 mg/5 ml Suspension Day 1–5	Total ml per Treatment Course
8	18	2.5 ml (½ tsp)	12.5 ml
17	37	5 ml (1 tsp)	25 ml
25	55	7.5 ml (1½ tsp)	37.5 ml
33	73	10 ml (2 tsp)	50 ml
40	88	12.5 ml (2½ tsp)	62.5 ml

C. Age 16 years and older

   1. For treatment of mild to moderate acute bacterial exacerbations of chronic obstructive pulmonary disease, community-acquired pneumonia, pharyngitis or tonsillitis, and uncomplicated skin and skin structure infections: 500 mg on day 1, then 250 mg once daily on days 2–5

   2. For treatment of nongonococcal urethritis and cervicitis: 1 g single dose

VI. Contraindications

A. Allergy to azithromycin, erythromycin, or any macrolide antibiotic

B. Not recommended for treatment of otitis media in children under 6 months

C. Not recommended for treatment of pharyngitis or tonsillitis in children under 2 years

D. Not recommended for use during pregnancy or lactation

VII. Side effects. Nausea, vomiting, diarrhea, abdominal pain, dizziness, headache

VIII. Education

A. Keep all medication out of children's reach.

B. Do not take with food. Take 1 hour before or 2 hours after meals. Do not mix with food or formula.

C. Obtain appropriate culture and sensitivity tests before treatment is instituted.

D. May increase theophylline level of patients taking theophylline

E. Avoid taking aluminum- and magnesium-containing antacids when on Zithromax.

F. Discontinue medication if side effects occur and call the office immediately.

G. Carefully follow directions for reconstituting the oral suspension.

H. Shake bottle before each use.

I. Keep bottle tightly capped.

J. Store at 41°–86°F.

K. Use medication within 10 days. Discard remaining medication after treatment is completed.

REFERENCES

Karch AM. *1998 Lippincott's Nursing Drug Guide.* Philadelphia: JB Lippincott, 1998.

Physicians Desk Reference, 50th ed. Oradell, NJ: Medical Economics, 1997.

Physicians Desk Reference for Nonprescription Drugs, 17th ed. Oradell, NJ: Medical Economics.

Appendices

APPENDIX A: CONVERSION TABLES

TEMPERATURE

°Fahrenheit	°Centigrade
0	-17.8
32.0	0
97.0	36.1
98.0	36.7
98.6	37.0
99.0	37.2
99.5	37.5
100.0	37.7
100.4	38.0
101.0	38.3
102.0	38.8
103.0	39.4
104.0	40.0
105.0	40.5

Conversion for above 0°C
°F to °C: subtract 32, multiply by 5, divide by 9 or 5/9 (°F - 32).
°C to °F: multiply by 9, divide by 5, add 32 or (% x °C) + 32.

LENGTH

Inches	Centimeters	Centimeters	Inches
1	2.5	1	0.4
2	5.1	2	0.8
4	10.2	3	1.2
6	15.2	4	1.6
8	20.3	5	2.0
10	25.0	6	2.4
12	30.5	8	3.1
18	46.0	10	3.9
24	61.0	15	5.9
30	76.0	20	7.9
36	91.0	30	11.8
42	107.0	40	15.7
48	122.0	50	19.7
54	137.0	60	23.6
60	152.0	70	27.6
66	168.0	80	31.5
72	183.0	90	35.4
78	198.0	100	39.4

1 inch = 2.54 cm
1 cm = 0.3937 inch

WEIGHT

Pounds	Kilograms	Kilograms	Pounds
4	1.8	1	2.2
6	2.7	2	4.4
8	3.6	3	6.6
10	4.5	4	8.8
15	6.8	5	11.0
20	9.1	6	13.2
25	11.4	8	17.6
30	13.6	10	22
35	15.9	15	33
40	18.2	20	44
45	20.4	25	55
50	22.7	30	66
55	25.0	35	77
60	27.3	40	88
65	29.5	45	99
70	31.8	50	110
80	36.3	55	121
90	40.9	60	132
100	45.4	65	143
125	56.7	70	154
150	68.2	80	176
175	79.4	90	198
200	90.8	100	220

1 lb = 0.454 kg.
1 kg = 2.204 lb.

APPENDIX B: GROWTH CHARTS

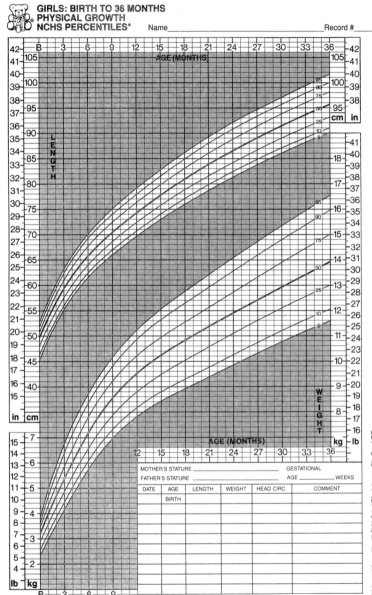

GIRLS: BIRTH TO 36 MONTHS
PHYSICAL GROWTH
NCHS PERCENTILES*   Name_____   Record #_____

*Adapted from: Hamill PVV, Drizd TA, Johnson CL, Reed RB, Roche AF, Moore WM: Physical growth: National Center for Health Statistics percentiles. AM J CLIN NUTR 32:607-629, 1979. Data from the Fels Longitudinal Study, Wright State University School of Medicine, Yellow Springs, Ohio.

© 1982 Ross Products Division, Abbott Laboratories

GIRLS: BIRTH TO 36 MONTHS
PHYSICAL GROWTH
NCHS PERCENTILES*

Name_____ Record #_____

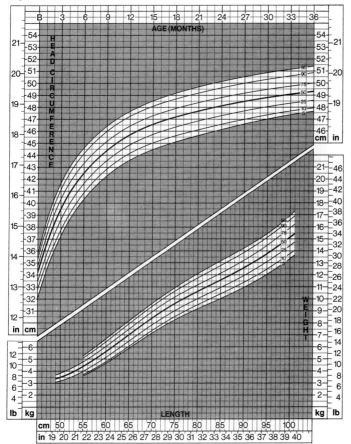

DATE	AGE	LENGTH	WEIGHT	HEAD CIRC.	COMMENT

**GIRLS: 2 TO 18 YEARS
PHYSICAL GROWTH
NCHS PERCENTILES***

Name_____ Record #_____

*Adapted from: Hamill PVV, Drizd TA, Johnson CL, Reed RB, Roche AF, Moore WM: Physical growth: National Center for Health Statistics percentiles. AM J CLIN NUTR 32:607-629, 1979. Data from the National Center for Health Statistics (NCHS), Hyattsville, Maryland.

© 1982 Ross Products Division, Abbott Laboratories

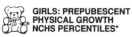

**GIRLS: PREPUBESCENT
PHYSICAL GROWTH
NCHS PERCENTILES***

Name_____Record #_____

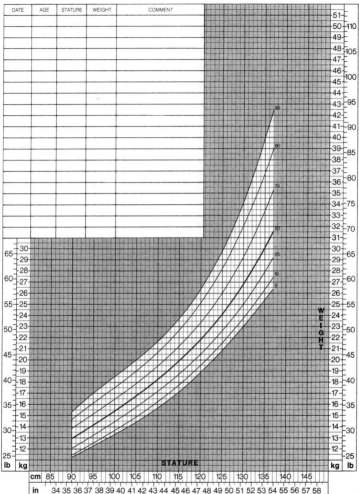

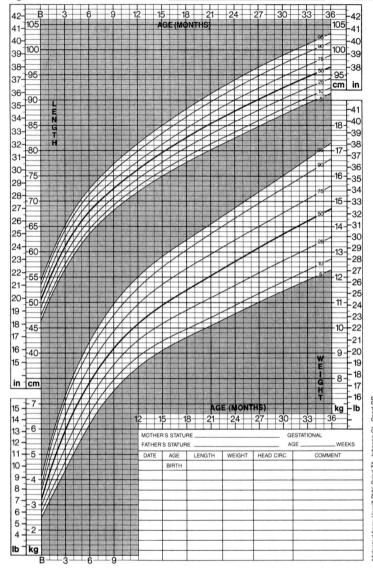

BOYS: BIRTH TO 36 MONTHS
PHYSICAL GROWTH
NCHS PERCENTILES*

Name_____ Record #_____

*Adapted from: Hamill PVV, Drizd TA, Johnson CL, Reed RB, Roche AF, Moore WM: Physical growth: National Center for Health Statistics percentiles. AM J CLIN NUTR 32:607-629, 1979. Data from the Fels Longitudinal Study, Wright State University School of Medicine, Yellow Springs, Ohio.

© 1982 Ross Products Division, Abbott Laboratories

MOTHER'S STATURE _____ GESTATIONAL

FATHER'S STATURE _____ AGE _____ WEEKS

DATE	AGE	LENGTH	WEIGHT	HEAD CIRC.	COMMENT
	BIRTH				

BOYS: BIRTH TO 36 MONTHS
PHYSICAL GROWTH
NCHS PERCENTILES*

Name_____ Record #_____

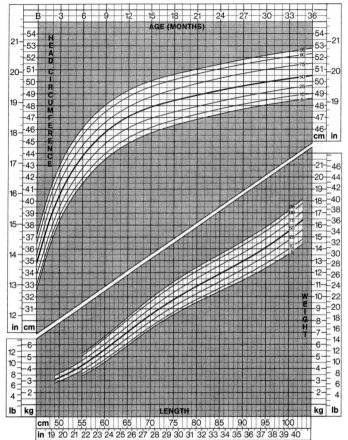

DATE	AGE	LENGTH	WEIGHT	HEAD CIRC.	COMMENT

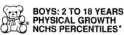

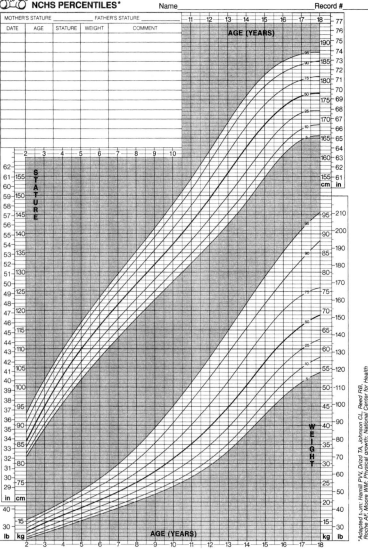

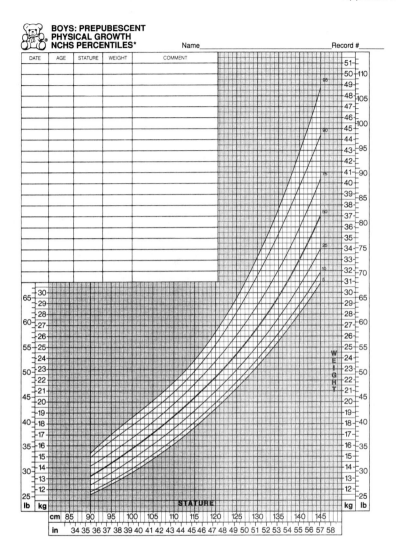

**BOYS: PREPUBESCENT
PHYSICAL GROWTH
NCHS PERCENTILES***

APPENDIX C: IMMUNIZATION SCHEDULES

IMMUNIZATION SCHEDULES

RECOMMENDED CHILDHOOD IMMUNIZATION SCHEDULE
UNITED STATES, JANUARY–DECEMBER 1997

Vaccines are listed under the routinely recommended ages. Bars indicate range of acceptable ages for vaccination. Shaded bars indicate catch-up vaccination: at 11-12 years of age, hepatitis B vaccine should be administered to children not previously vaccinated, and Varicella vaccin should be administered to children not previously vaccinated who lack a reliable history of chickenpox.

Age ▶ / Vaccine ▼	Birth	1 mo	2 mos	4 mos	6 mos	12 mos	15 mos	18 mos	4-6 yrs	11-12 yrs	14-16 yrs
Hepatitis B	Hep B-1	Hep B-2			Hep B-3					Hep B	
Diphtheria, Tetanus, Pertussis			DTaP or DTP	DTaP or DTP	DTaP or DTP		DTaP or DTP		DTaP or DTP	Td	
H. influenzae type b			Hib	Hib	Hib	Hib					
Polio			Polio	Polio		Polio			Polio		
Measles, Mumps, Rubella						MMR			MMR or	MMR	
Varicella						Var				Var	

Please refer to Immunization Guidelines on page 537.

1997 Immunization Guidelines: What's New and Noteworthy

The immunization schedule has been updated, as recommended by the Advisory Committee on Immunization Practices (ACIP) and the American Academy of Pediatrics (AAP).

REQUIREMENTS

Day Care: Effective August 1, 1998. 1 dose of varicella vaccine will be required for children 12 months of age or older without a history of chickenpox, who were born on or after January 1, 1997.

Kindergarten: Since September 1995, 2 doses of measles-containing vaccine for all children, and, since September 1996, 3 doses of hepatitis B vaccine for children born since January 1992.

College: 2 doses of measles-containing vaccine, *regardless* of birth date.

Note: MMR is the vaccine formulation always recommended for the 2nd dose of measles-containing vaccine.

RECOMMENDATIONS

DTaP (diphtheria/tetanus/acellular pertussis) Vaccine
- DTaP is now recommended for all doses of the routine series.
- Whenever feasible, the same brand of DTaP should be used for all doses of the vaccine series. If the provider does not know, or does not have available, the type of DTaP vaccine previously given, any of the licensed DTaP vaccines may be used to complete the series.
- Any licensed DTaP vaccine may be used to complete the vaccination series of children who have had one, two, three, or four doses of whole-cell DTP.
- Contraindications to DTaP are the same as those for DTP.

IPV/Polio Vaccine
- A sequential schedule of 2 doses of inactivated poliovirus vaccine (IVP) and 2 doses of OPV is recommended to reduce the risk of vaccine-associated paralytic polio (VAPP).
- The following schedules are all acceptable by the ACIP and the AAP, and parents and providers may choose among them:
  1. IPV at 2 and 4 mos. OPV at 12–18 mos and 4–6 yrs; or
  2. IPV at 2, 4, 12–18 mos. and 4–6 yrs; or
  3. OPV at 2, 4, 6–18 mos. and 4–6 yrs.
- *Four* doses are needed to complete the primary series if any combination of IPV and OPV is used.
- IPV is the only polio vaccine recommended for immunocompromised persons and their household contacts.

Varicella Vaccine
- 1 dose for children 12–18 months of age without a reliable history of chickenpox.
- 1 dose for susceptible 11–12 year olds without a reliable history of chickenpox or vaccination.

Adolescent Immunization
An adolescent visit at 11–12 years of age, prior to 7th grade, is an opportunity to assess, and immunize if necessary, with:
- Td (tetanus and diphtheria toxoids, adult use), if at least 5 years have elapsed since last does of DTP, DTaP, or DT. Subsequent routine Td boosters are recommended every 10 years.
- 2nd dose of MMR.
- 3 doses of hepatitis B vaccine.
- 1 dose of varicella vaccine for those without a *reliable* history of chickenpox or vaccination.
- Pneumococcal and annual influenza vaccination, if risk factors are present.

IMMUNIZATION GUIDELINES
Massachusetts Department of Public Health
June 1996

As required by state regulations (102 CMR 7.07 and 105 CMR 220.00), the Department of Public Health has established the following requirements for children to attend day care, kindergarten, school and college. These requirements are the minimally acceptable number of immunizations for attendance at day care centers and schools.

Minimal Immunization Requirements

	Day care/Preschool[1]	Kindergarten	Grades 1–6	Grades 7–12	College
Hepatitis B[2]	3 doses	(see footnote 2)			
DTP/DT/Td	≥4 doses DTP	5 doses DTP	≥4 doses DTP OR ≥3 doses Td	≥4 doses DTP or ≥3 doses Td plus 1 Td booster (grade 10, 11 or 12)	1 Td booster within last 10 years
Polio	≥3 doses	4 doses	≥3 doses	≥3 doses	
Hib	3 or 4 doses				
MMR	1 dose	2 doses measles & 1 mumps, 1 rubella	1 dose	2 doses measles & 1 dose mumps & rubella	2 doses measles & 1 dose mumps & rubella

Vaccine Administration Notes

[1] Day care/Preschool: Minimal requirements by 24 months; younger children should be age-appropriately immunized according to schedule.

[2] Hepatitis B: Required for day care/preschool attendance for children born on or after 1/1/92. As of September 1996, 3 doses are required for kindergarten entry for those born in 1992 or later. Infant schedule may vary depending on the hepatitis B status of the mother.

CATCH-UP SCHEDULE FOR CHILDREN NOT YET 7 YEARS OLD
who start late or are >1 month behind schedule

	First visit	Second visit	Third visit	Fourth visit	Fifth visit	Preschool
Age at start of vaccination	Vaccines administered	1 mo. after first visit	1 mo. after second visit	6 wks. after third visit	≥6 mos. after fourth visit	4–6 years old
4-6 months	DTP	DTP	DTP		DTP	DTP¹
	Polio		Polio	Polio		Polio¹
	Hib²	Hib²	Hib²		Hib booster at age ≥ 15 mos.²	
	Hep B³	Hep B³			Hep B³	
					MMR at age 12–15 mos.⁴	
					Varicella at age 12–18 mos.	
7–11 months	DTP	DTP	DTP		DTP	DTP¹
	Polio		Polio	Polio		Polio¹
	Hib²	Hib²			Hib booster at age ≥ 15 mos.²	
	Hep B³	Hep B³			Hep B³	
				MMR at age 12–15 mos.⁴		
				Varicella at age 12–18 mos.		
12–14 months	DTP	DTP	DTP		DTP	DTP¹
	Polio		Polio	Polio		Polio¹
	Hib²	Hib booster at age ≥ 15 mos.²				
	Hep B³	Hep B³			Hep B³	
	MMR at age 12–15 mos.⁴					
	Varicella at age 12–18 mos.					
15–59 months	DTP	DTP	DTP		DTP	DTP¹
	Polio		Polio	Polio		Polio¹
	Hib²					
	Hep B³	Hep B³			Hep B³	
	MMR⁴					
	Varicella at age 12–18 mos.					
5–6 years	DTP	DTP	DTP		DTP	DTP¹
	Polio		Polio	Polio		Polio¹
	Hib vaccine is not routinely recommended for children 5 years (60 months) or older					
	Hep B³	Hep B³			Hep B³	Hep B³ series
	MMR⁴	MMR second dose due at entry to kindergarten or 7th grade				
					Varicella at age 11–12 years if susceptible	

CATCH-UP SCHEDULE FOR INDIVIDUALS 7 YEARS OLD OR OLDER
who were not vaccinated at the recommended time

Vaccine	First Visit	6–8 wks after first visit	6 months after second visit	Every 10 years
Td	1st dose	2nd dose	3rd dose	Booster doses
Polio[5]	1st dose	2nd dose	3rd dose	
MMR[4]	1st dose	2nd dose		
Hepatitis B	1st dose	2nd dose	3rd dose	

Vaccine Administration Notes

[1] Fifth dose of DTP and fourth dose of polio are not needed if most recent doses were given after the fourth birthday.

[2] Hib schedule varies by manufacturer and age child starts vaccination. Give booster at least 2 months after previous dose.

[3] Hepatitis B vaccine is recommended for children born on or after January 1, 1992; sixth graders; and certain high-risk groups.

[4] A second dose of measles, given at least 30 days after the first, is required for kindergarten, 7th grade, and college entry. MMR vaccine is recommended.

[5] Polio is not recommended for those 18 years and older unless there is a potential for exposure.

IMPORTANT FACTS ABOUT DTaP VACCINE

- *Tripedia* is now recommended for the first 3 doses of the diphtheria, tetanus and pertussis vaccine series; and *Tripedia* is approved for the first 4 doses of the 5 dose series.

- *Tripedia* is not yet approved for the fifth dose of the series in children who have received their first four doses as DTaP. However, acellular pertussis vaccine is approved for the fourth and fifth doses of the series in those children who have received whole-cell DTP vaccine for the first three doses.

- Unlike DTP vaccine, which is approved for the 4th dose at $\geq$12 months of age, DTaP vaccines are NOT approved for the 4th dose until $\geq$15 months of age. (Remember the interval between the 3rd and 4th doses must be $\geq$6 months.)

- Lederle's DTaP (*ACEL-IMMUNE*) and Connaught's DTaP (*Tripedia*) are interchangeable for the fourth or fifth dose.

- *Tripedia* may be used to complete the primary series in infants who have received 1 or 2 doses of whole-cell DTP vaccine.

- While Lederle's DTaP (*ACEL-IMMUNE*) is not yet approved for the first three doses of the series, if an infant receives *ACEL-IMMUNE* by mistake for doses 1, 2 or 3, these doses should NOT be repeated.

- Children <7 years of age who have received DT vaccine can receive DTaP. However, children should not receive >6 doses of diphtheria and tetanus-containing vaccines before their 7th birthday.

- DTaP vaccines are not yet approved for use in those $\geq$7 years of age.

- Any contraindication to whole-cell pertussis vaccine is also a contraindication to acellular pertussis vaccine. Any adverse event following whole-cell pertussis vaccine that is considered a precaution is also considered a precaution with future doses of acellular pertussis vaccine.

- All childhood vaccines can be given simultaneously with *Tripedia* and other acellular pertussis vaccines including OPV, IPV, Hib, hepatitis B, MMR, varicella, hepatitis A vaccines.

Ordering DTaP
To order DTaP vaccine, you must use the most recent version of the *Vaccine Order Form,* which is available from your vaccine distributor or your regional immunization office (list enclosed).

Recording Usage of DTaP
Until revised usage forms are available, please record usage of both DTaP and DTP vaccines under the column for DTP on our *Vaccine Usage Report.*

If you have any questions about the availability or use of *Tripedia,* please contact your regional immunization office (list enclosed) or the Massachusetts Immunization Program at 617-983-6800.

ADMINISTRATION OF VACCINES

Simultaneous Administration

In general, vaccines (live or killed/inactivated) can be given at the same time or in combination with immune globulin (10), at separate sites, with the following exceptions:

1. *IG and MMR.* In general IG can be administered with all vaccines, EXCEPT MMRI. If simultaneous administration of IG and MMR becomes necessary due to imminent exposure to disease, it is likely that there will be a decreased immune response to MMR, and the vaccine should be repeated unless serologic testing indicates antibodies have been produced.
2. *Yellow Fever and Cholera.* Decreased immunity may occur when these two vaccines are administered simultaneously. They should therefore be separated by at least 3 weeks. If this is not possible due to lack of time before departure, they can be given at the same time with the understanding that the immune response to both vaccines may be impaired.
3. *Cholera, Typhoid and Plague.* These vaccines are commonly associated with increased local and systemic side effects. Therefore simultaneous administration of any combination of these three vaccines should be avoided if possible.

Non-Simultaneous Administration

When vaccines are *not* given at the same time, the nature (live or inactivated/killed) of the vaccines will determine the interval between the 1st and the 2nd vaccine. Please refer to the following tables.

Time Intervals Between Vaccines When *NOT* Given Simultaneously

Type of Vaccine		Recommended Time Interval
Date 1	Date 2	
live	live	1 month; *1
live	killed	can be given at any time
killed	live	can be given at any time
killed	killed	can be given at any time
IG	live	preferably 3 months; 6 weeks at minimum; *2
live	IG	2 weeks; *2
IG	killed	can be given at any time
killed	IG	can be given at any time

* 1 - If time interval was less, then the 2nd vaccine should be repeated.
* 2 - If time interval was less, then the *vaccine* should be repeated.

Vaccine	Type	Vaccine	Type
Cholera	killed	Plague	killed
DTP, Td or DT	killed	Rabies	killed
Hib	killed	Typhoid	killed
Hepatitis-B	killed	BCG	live
Influenza	killed	MMR	live
IPV	killed	OPV	live
Meningococcal	killed	Yellow Fever	live
Pneumococcal	killed		

APPENDIX D: CLINICAL SIGNS OF DEHYDRATION

Sign	Mild	Moderate	Severe
Weight loss (% of body weight)	3%–5%	6%–9%	10%–15%
Fontanelle	Flat		Sunken
Fever (in absence of infection)	Variable	Present	Present
Skin			
Turgor	Normal	↓	Tenting
Color	Normal	Pallor	Pallor
Mucous membranes	Slightly moist	Dry	Parched
Tears	Present	Variable	Absent
Thirst	Slight	Moderate to marked	Marked
Pulse	May be normal	↑	↑
Intake	↓ – < output	↓ – < output	↓ – < output
Urinary output	↓	↓	↓ to oliguria
Urine specific gravity	Slightly changed	Increased	Markedly increased up to 1.03
Neurologic status	Normal	Irritable	Hyperirritable or lethargic

APPENDIX E: NORMAL RED BLOOD CELL VALUES

Age	Hgb (gm/100 ml)	Hemato-crit (%)	Reticulo-cytes (%)	Mean Corpuscular Volume (μ^3)	Mean Corpuscular Hgb ($\mu\mu g$)	Mean Corpuscular Hgb Conc. (%)
Newborn	16–24	47–60	4.1–6.3	106	38	36
3 mos	10–15	31–41	0.5–1.0	82	27	34
6 mos–6 yrs	11–14	33–42	0.5-1.0	82	27	34
7–12 yrs	11–16	34–40	0.5–1.0	82	27	34
Adolescent						
Female	14	37–47	0.5–1.8	80–94	27–32	33–38
Male	16	42–52	0.5–1.8	80–94	27–32	33–38

APPENDIX F: PEAK EXPIRATORY FLOW RATE

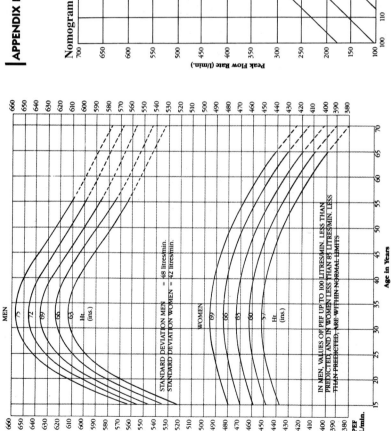

Nomogram

Peak Flow Rate (l/min.)

Height (cm)

+95%

MEAN

-95%

Data from: Godfrey S. et al., *Brit. J. Dis. Chest*, 1970; 64:15-24.

MEN

Ht. (ins.)

75
72
69
66
63

STANDARD DEVIATION MEN = 48 litres/min.
STANDARD DEVIATION WOMEN = 42 litres/min.

WOMEN

Ht. (ins.)

69
66
63
60
57

IN MEN, VALUES OF PEF UP TO 100 LITRES/MIN. LESS THAN PREDICTED, AND IN WOMEN LESS THAN 85 LITRES/MIN. LESS THAN PREDICTED, ARE WITHIN NORMAL LIMITS

Age in Years

PEF L/min.

Data from: Nunn, AJ, Gregg, I, *Brit. Med. J.* 1989; 298:1068-70

Predicted Averages

Table 1
Predicted Average Peak Expiratory Flow for Normal Males

(liters per minute)

Age	Height 60"	65"	70"	75"	80"
20	554	602	649	693	740
25	543	590	636	679	725
30	532	577	622	664	710
35	521	565	609	651	695
40	509	552	596	636	680
45	498	540	583	622	665
50	486	527	569	607	649
55	475	515	556	593	634
60	463	502	542	578	618
65	452	490	529	564	603
70	440	477	515	550	587

Data from: Leiner GC, et al.: Expiratory peak flow rate. Standard values for normal subjects. Use as a clinical test of ventilatory function. *Am Rev Resp Dis* 88:644, 1963.

Table 2
Predicted Average Peak Expiratory Flow for Normal Females

(liters per minute)

Age	Height 55"	60"	65"	70"	75"
20	390	423	460	496	529
25	385	418	454	490	523
30	380	413	448	483	516
35	375	408	442	476	509
40	370	402	436	470	502
45	365	397	430	464	495
50	360	391	424	457	488
55	355	386	418	451	482
60	350	380	412	445	475
65	345	375	406	439	468
70	340	369	400	432	461

Data from: Leiner GC, et al.: Expiratory peak flow rate. Standard values for normal subjects. Use as a clinical test of ventilatory function. *Am Rev Resp Dis* 88:644, 1963.

Table 3
Predicted Average Peak Expiratory Flow for Normal Children and Adolescents

(liters per minute)

Height (inches)	Males & Females	Height (inches)	Males & Females
43	147	56	320
44	160	57	334
45	173	58	347
46	187	59	360
47	200	60	373
48	214	61	387
49	227	62	400
50	240	63	413
51	254	64	427
52	267	65	440
53	280	66	454
54	293	67	467
55	307		

Data from: Polger, G, Promedhat V: *Pulmonary function testing in children: Techniques and standards.* Philadelphia, W.B. Saunders, 1971.

Note: These tables are averages and are based on tests with a large number of people. An individual's PEFR may vary widely. Further, many individuals' PEFR values are consistently higher or lower than the average values. It is recommended that PEFR objectives for therapy be based upon each individual's "personal best," which is established after a period of PEFR monitoring while the individual is under effective treatment.

Reproduced with permission from Guidelines and Management of Asthma—Publication # 91-3042, Objective measures of lung function, p. 23. Bethesda: U.S. Department of Health and Human Services, 1991.

APPENDIX G: NAEP STEP-CARE APPROACH TO ASTHMA

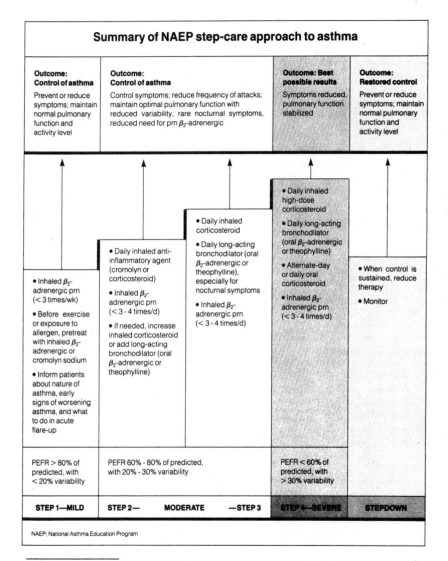

Summary of NAEP step-care approach to asthma

Outcome: Control of asthma	Outcome: Control of asthma	Outcome: Best possible results	Outcome: Restored control
Prevent or reduce symptoms; maintain normal pulmonary function and activity level	Control symptoms; reduce frequency of attacks; maintain optimal pulmonary function with reduced variability, rare nocturnal symptoms, reduced need for prn β_2-adrenergic	Symptoms reduced, pulmonary function stabilized	Prevent or reduce symptoms; maintain normal pulmonary function and activity level
• Inhaled β_2-adrenergic prn (< 3 times/wk) • Before exercise or exposure to allergen, pretreat with inhaled β_2-adrenergic or cromolyn sodium • Inform patients about nature of asthma, early signs of worsening asthma, and what to do in acute flare-up	• Daily inhaled anti-inflammatory agent (cromolyn or corticosteroid) • Inhaled β_2-adrenergic prn (< 3 - 4 times/d) • If needed, increase inhaled corticosteroid or add long-acting bronchodilator (oral β_2-adrenergic or theophylline)	• Daily inhaled corticosteroid • Daily long-acting bronchodilator (oral β_2-adrenergic or theophylline), especially for nocturnal symptoms • Inhaled β_2-adrenergic prn (< 3 - 4 times/d)	• Daily inhaled high-dose corticosteroid • Daily long-acting bronchodilator (oral β_2-adrenergic or theophylline) • Alternate-day or daily oral corticosteroid • Inhaled β_2-adrenergic prn (< 3 - 4 times/d)	• When control is sustained, reduce therapy • Monitor
PEFR > 80% of predicted, with < 20% variability	PEFR 60% - 80% of predicted, with 20% - 30% variability	PEFR < 60% of predicted, with > 30% variability	
STEP 1—MILD	**STEP 2— MODERATE —STEP 3**	**STEP 4—SEVERE**	**STEPDOWN**

NAEP; National Asthma Education Program

Reproduced with permission from Sheffer, A. L. (1992). Where β_2-adrenergics fit into step-care for asthma. *J Respir Dis* 13:10 (Suppl); S51.

APPENDIX H: ABSTRACT OF NEW HAMPSHIRE REPORTING LAW

I. Reporting is mandatory. New Hampshire Law (RSA 169-C-29:30) requires that any person who has reason to suspect that a child under the age of 18 has been abused or neglected must report the case to the Local District Office New Hampshire Division of Welfare.

II. An abused child is one who has

   A. Been sexually molested.

   or

   B. Been sexually exploited.

   or

   C. Been intentionally physically injured.

   or

   D. Been psychologically injured such that he exhibits symptoms of emotional problems generally recognized to result from consistent mistreatment or neglect.

III. A neglected child is one

   A. Who has been abandoned by his parents, guardian, or custodian.

   or

   B. Who is without proper parental care or control, subsistence, education as required by law, or other care or control necessary for his physical, mental, or emotional health, when it is established that his health has suffered or is very likely to suffer serious impairment; and the deprivation is not due primarily to the lack of financial means of the parents, guardian, or custodian.

   or

   C. Whose parents, guardian, or custodian is unable to discharge his responsibilities to and for the child because of incarceration, hospitalization, or other physical or mental incapacity.

NOTE: A child who is under treatment solely by spiritual means through prayer, in accordance with the tenets of a recognized religion by a duly accredited practitioner thereof, shall not for that reason alone be considered to be neglected.

IV. Nature and content of report

   A. Oral. Immediately by telephone or otherwise.

   B. Written. Within 48 hours if requested.

   C. Content (if known):

     1. Name and address of the child suspected of being neglected or abused.

     2. Names of parents or person caring for child.

     3. Specific information indicating neglect or nature of abuse (including any evidence of previous injuries).

     4. Identity of parents or persons suspected in being responsible for neglect or abuse.

     5. Any other information that might be helpful or is required by the bureau.

V. Immunity from liability. Anyone who makes a report in good faith is immune from any liability, civil or criminal. The same immunity applies to participation in any investigation by the bureau or judicial proceedings resulting from such a report.

APPENDIX I: YOUR CHILD AND ORGANIZED SPORTS

A. Be sure your child is ready for an organized sports program.
B. Weigh the time spent on sports against that for other important activities.
C. Consider what your child's participation will mean for your family's mealtime, vacation time, weekends.
D. Know how many hours and months your child will be involved in practices, games, tournaments.
E. Find out about the goals and qualifications of adults in the program.
F. Know the health and safety policies of the program.
G. Know that children are appropriately matched for maturity, size, and skill.
H. Know that each player on the team gets to play.
 I. Plan on how you will behave when your child is a loser, a "bench warmer," or wants to quit.
J. Ask if parents are expected at practices or games.
K. Be ready for the expenses of uniforms, fees, transportation.
L. Observe how parents, coaches, spectators behave in front of children.

Source: From "Your Child and Organized Sports." © 1981 Ross Laboratories. Reprinted with permission of Ross Laboratories, Columbus, OH 43216.

APPENDIX J: ARE YOU DYING TO BE THIN?

The following questionnaire will give you an indication of whether or not you are living a lifestyle that indicates anorexic and/or bulimic tendencies. Anorexia nervosa (key symptom: extreme weight loss due to self-starvation) and bulimia (key symptom: binging followed by purging) are becoming more and more openly acknowledged as publicity increases public awareness and understanding.

Answer the following questions honestly. Write the number of your answer in the space at the left.

_____ 1. I have eating habits that are different from those of my family and friends.
    1. Often   2. Sometimes   3. Rarely   4. Never

_____ 2. I find myself panicking if I cannot exercise as I planned for fear of gaining weight.
    1. Almost always   2. Sometimes   3. Rarely   4. Never

_____ 3. My friends tell me I am thin but I don't believe them because I feel fat.
    1. Often   2. Sometimes   3. Rarely   4. Never

_____ 4. (Females only) My menstrual period has ceased or become irregular due to no known medical reasons.
    1. True   2. False

_____ 5. I have become obsessed with food to the point that I cannot go through a day without worrying about what I will or will not eat.
    1. Almost always   2. Sometimes   3. Rarely   4. Never

_____ 6. I have lost more than 25% of the normal weight for my height (e.g., 30 lbs from 120 lbs).
    1. True   2. False

_____ 7. I would panic if I got on the scale tomorrow and found out I had gained two pounds.
    1. Almost always   2. Sometimes   3. Rarely   4. Never

_____ 8. I find that I prefer to eat alone or when I am sure no one will see me thus am making excuses so I can eat less and less with friends and family.
    1. Often   2. Sometimes   3. Rarely   4. Never

_____ 9. I find myself going on uncontrollable eating binges during which I consume large amounts of food to the point that I feel sick and make myself vomit.
    1. 20 or more times/day   2. 1–2 times/week   3. Rarely   4. Never

_____ 10. I use laxatives as a means of weight control.
    1. On a regular basis   2. Sometimes   3. Rarely   4. Never

_____ 11. I find myself playing games with food (e.g., cutting it up into tiny pieces; hiding food so people will think I ate it; chewing it and spitting it out without swallowing), telling myself certain foods are bad.
    1. Often   2. Sometimes   3. Rarely   4. Never

_____ 12. People around me have become very interested in what I eat and I find myself getting angry at them for pushing food on me.
    1. Often   2. Sometimes   3. Rarely   4. Never

_____ 13. I have felt more depressed and irritable recently than I used to and/or have been spending an increasing amount of time alone.
    1. True   2. False

_____ 14. I keep a lot of my fears about food and eating to myself because I am afraid no one would understand.

    1. Often   2. Sometimes   3. Rarely   4. Never

_____ 15. I enjoy making gourmet, high-calorie meals or treats for others as long as I don't have to eat any myself.

    1. Often   2. Sometimes   3. Rarely   4. Never

_____ 16. The most powerful fear in my life is the fear of gaining weight or becoming fat.

    1. Often   2. Sometime   3. Rarely   4. Never

_____ 17. I find myself totally absorbed when reading books about dieting, exercising and calorie counting to the point that I spend hours studying them.

    1. Often   2. Sometimes   3. Rarely   4. Never

_____ 18. I tend to be a perfectionist and am not satisfied with myself unless I do things perfectly.

    1. Often   2. Sometimes   3. Rarely   4. Never

_____ 19. I go through long periods of time without eating anything (fasting) as a means of weight control.

    1. Often   2. Sometimes   3. Rarely   4. Never

_____ 20. It is important to me to try to be thinner than all of my friends.

    1. Often   2. Sometimes   3. Rarely   4. Never

Scoring

Add scores together and compare with the table below: Also, if #6 is True (1), subtract 8 points from total. Or if #6 is False (2), use total as it is.

Under 30—Strong tendencies toward anorexia nervosa

30–45—Strong tendencies toward bulimia

45–55—Weight conscious, not necessarily with anorexia and bulimic tendencies

Over 55—No need for concern

If you scored below 45, it would be wise for you to (1) seek more information about anorexia nervosa and bulimia and (2) contact a counselor, pastor, or physician, to determine what kind of assistance would be most helpful for you. Anorexia nervosa and bulimia are potentially life-threatening disorders which can be overcome with the proper support and counsel. The earlier you seek help the better, although it is never too late to start on the road to recovery.

For more information contact:
K. Kim Lampson Reiff, Ph.D.,
Sherwood Forest Office Park #104
2661 Bel-Red Road
Bellevue, WA 98008.

APPENDIX K: DSM-IV DIAGNOSTIC CRITERIA FOR EATING DISORDERS

Anorexia Nervosa (307.1)

A. Refusal to maintain body weight at or above a minimally normal weight for age and height (eg, weight loss leading to maintenance of body weight less than 85% of that expected; or failure to make expected weight gain during period of growth, leading to body weight less than 85% of that expected).

B. Intense fear of gaining weight or becoming fat, even though underweight.

C. Disturbance in the way in which one's body weight or shape is experienced, undue influence of body weight or shape on self-evaluation, or denial of the seriousness of the current low body weight.

D. In postmenarcheal females, amenorrhea, (ie, the absence of at least three consecutive menstrual cycles). A woman is considered to have amenorrhea if her periods occur only following hormone (eg, estrogen administration.)

Bulimia Nervosa (307.51)

A. Recurrent episodes of binge eating. An episode of binge eating is characterized by both of the following:
   (1) eating, in a discrete period of time (eg, within any 2-hour period), an amount of food that definitely is larger than most people would eat during a similar period of time and under similar circumstances
   (2) a sense of lack of control over eating during the episode (eg, a feeling that one cannot stop eating or control what or how much one is eating)

B. Recurrent inappropriate compensatory behavior in order to prevent weight gain, such as self-induced vomiting; misuse of laxatives, diuretics, enemas, or other medications; fasting; or excessive exercise.

C. The binge eating and inappropriate compensatory behaviors both occur, on average, at least twice a week for 3 months.

D. Self-evaluation is unduly influenced by body shape and weight.

E. The disturbance does not occur exclusively during episodes of anorexia nervosa.

American Psychiatric Association: *Diagnostic and Statistical Manual of Mental Disorders.* 4th ed. Washington, DC: American Psychiatric Association; 1994

APPENDIX L: FLUORIDE DOSAGE SCHEDULE

	Water F Content		
Ages	0–0.3 ppm	0.3 ppm–0.6 ppm	>0.6 ppm
6 mo.–2 yrs.	0.25 mg F (0.5 ml Luride)*	0	0
2–3 yrs.	0.5 mg F (1 ml Luride)	0.25 mg F (0.5 ml Luride)	0
3–14 yrs	1.0 mg F (2 ml Luride)	0.5 mg F (1 ml Luride)	0

* Luride Drops dosage now expressed in milliliters. Prescriptions should be written/dispensed accordingly.

APPENDIX M: RANKING OF TOPICAL STEROIDS

Group I *Do not use: 1000 times as potent as hydrocortisone.*
Diprolene cr, ung, 0.05%   Temovate cr, ung, 0.05% (clobetasol)
(betamethasone)   Ultravate, 0.05% (halobetasol)
Psorcon ung, 0.05% (diflorasone)

Group II *Use only for advanced disease on small areas, for specific time (eg, 5–7 days).*
Never use on face or groin.
Cyclocort ung, 0.1% (amcinonide)   Lidex cr, gel, ung, 0.05%
Diprosone ung, 0.05%   (fluocinonide)
(betamethasone)   Maxiflor ung, 0.05% (diflorasone)
Florone ung, 0.05% (diflorasone)   Maxivate ung, 0.05%
Halog cr, 0.1% (halcinonide)   (betamethasone)
                                     Topicort cr, ung 0.25%
                                     (desoximetasone)

Group III
Aristocort cr (HP) 0.5%   Maxiflor cr 0.05% (diflorasone)
(triamcinolone)   Maxivate cr 0.05% (betamethasone)
Diprosone cr 0.05% (betamethasone)   Valisone ung 0.1% (betamethasone)
Florone cr 0.05% (diflorasone)

Group IV
Aristocort ung 0.1% (triamcinolone) Kenalog ung 0.05% (triamcinolone)
Benisone ung 0.025%   Synalar cr (HP), ung 0.2%
(betamethasone)   (fluocinolone)
Cordran ung 0.05%   Topicort LP cr 0.05%
(flurandrenolide)   (desoximetasone)

Group V *Fairly safe for long-term use on small body surface. Try to limit to 2–3 wk.*
Never use on face or groin.
Locoid cr, ung 0.1%   Maxivate lot 0.05% (betamethasone)
(hydrocortisone)   Synalar cr 0.025% (fluocinolone)
Benisone cr 0.025% (betamethasone)   Valisone cr, lot 0.01%
Cordran cr 0.05% (flurandrenolide)   (betamethasone)
Diprosone lot 0.05%   Westcort cr 0.2% (hydrocortisone)
(betamethasone)   Elocon cr, lot, ung 0.1%
Kenalog cr, lot 0.1% (triamcinolone) (mometasone)

Group VI
DesOwen cr 0.05% (desonide)   Synalar solution 0.01%
Aclovate cr, ung 0.05%   (fluocinolone)
(alclometasone)   Tridesilon cr 0.05% (desonide)

Group VII *Safe for long-term use but too weak for lichenified dermatitis. Best for*
maintenance and modest disease.
Nutracort cr, lot 1% (Hydrocortisone; other topical corticosteroids with
dexamethasone, flumethasone, prednisolone, and methyl prednisolone)

APPENDIX N: QUICK CONVERSION GUIDE FOR PEDIATRIC DOSAGES

Pounds	Kilograms	2mg/kg	5mg/kg	7.5mg/kg	20mg/kg	30mg/kg	40mg/kg
15	6.8	13.5mg	34mg	51mg	136mg	204mg	272mg
20	9	18	45	68	180	270	360
25	11.4	23	57	86	228	342	456
30	13.6	27	68	102	273	408	544
35	15.9	32	80	119	318	477	636
40	18.1	36	91	136	363	543	724
50	22.7	45	114	170	455	681	908
60	27.3	55	137	205	546	816	1088
70	31.8	64	159	239	636	954	1272
80	36.3	73	182	272	726	1090	1452
90	40.9	82	205	307	820	1230	1640

INDEX

NOTE: A *t* following a page number indicates tabular material.

A

Abdomen
assessment of
at initial visit, 11–12
at 2 week visit, 28
at 2 month visit, 41
at 3 year visit, 134
at 6 year visit, 150
traumatic injury to, abuse and, 18
Abstract thinking. *See* Formal (abstract)
thinking
Accidents. *See* Injuries
Acetaminophen
for acute cervical adenitis, 256, 257
for fever, 302
for hand/foot/mouth disease, 308
for herpangina, 310
for herpes zoster, 321
for herpetic gingivostomatitis, 324
for mycoplasmal pneumonia, 357
for otitis media, 361
for roseola, 384
for scarlet fever, 392
for streptococcal pharyngitis, 404
for urinary tract infection, 428
for varicella, 433
Aclovate, 463
for diaper rash, 272
Acne, 209–213
Acquired immune deficiency syndrome. *See*
AIDS
Actifed, 464
for allergic rhinitis and conjunctivitis, 229
for otitis media, 361
Acular, for allergic conjunctivitis, 229, 264
Acyclovir
for herpes simplex infection, 314, 317, 318
for herpes zoster, 321
side effects of, 318
for varicella, 433, 434
Adenitis
acute cervical, 255–257
chronic, acute cervical adenitis differentiated
from, 256
Adenopathy, in mononucleosis, 332
Adolescence, definition of, 165
Adolescents
HIV infection/AIDS and, 222
suicide risk and, 176, 181, 407
Adrenalin, 464–465. *See also* Epinephrine
Advil (Children's). *See also* Ibuprofen
for fever, 302

Aerosol-holding chambers (Aerochamber), for
asthma, 247
Affection
at 24 to 36 months, 124
at 3 to 6 years, 140
at 6 to 9 years, 156
Agammaglobulinemia, X-linked, AIDS differentiated from, 219
Aggression
at 14 to 18 months, 98–99
at 24 to 36 months, 124
at 3 to 6 years, 140
AIDS (acquired immune deficiency syndrome), 215–222
blood tests for, 219
congenital/pediatric, 216, 217, 218, 221–222
treatment of, 220
Albuterol, 246, 508–509, 519–520
for asthma, 243, 245, 246
side effects of, 246
Alclometasone, 463
for diaper rash, 272
Allergies/allergic reactions
asthma and, 240
conjunctivitis, 227–231, 262, 263, 264
contact dermatitis
diaper rash caused by, 271
miliaria rubra differentiated from, 351
tinea cruris differentiated from, 414
tinea pedis differentiated from, 419
diaper dermatitis caused by, 271
environmental control for child with,
290–292
to hymenoptera, 223–225
rhinitis, 227–231
sinusitis and, 228, 400, 401
Aluminum sulfate and calcium acetate. *See* Domeboro solution
Alupent. *See also* Metaproterenol
for asthma, 245
Ambivalence, at 24 to 36 months, 124
Amenorrhea, in anorexia nervosa, 232
Amoxicillin, 465–466
with clavulanic acid, 471
for external otitis, 297
for otitis media, 360
for sinusitis, 401
for Lyme disease, 344
for otitis media, 360
for serous otitis media, 397
for sinusitis, 401
for urinary tract infection, 428

Amoxil, 465–466. *See also* Amoxicillin
Ampicillin, 466–467
  for pneumonia, 440*t*
Anal fissure, 269
Anal intercourse, HIV infection/AIDS transmission and, 215, 220
Anaphylaxis
  differential diagnosis of, 224
  hymenoptera sting causing, 223, 224, 225
Anaprox, 467–468. *See also* Naproxen
Anemia, iron-deficiency, 338–341
Anorexia nervosa, 232–236
Ant (fire) stings, allergic response to, 223–225
Antibiotics. *See specific agent and/or specific disorder*
Anticipatory guidance
  for period of 2 to 8 weeks, 20–34
  for period of 2 to 4 months, 42–49
  for period of 4 to 6 months, 54–59
  for period of 6 to 8 months, 66–74
  for period of 8 to 14 months, 81–89
  for period of 14 to 18 months, 95–100
  for period of 18 to 24 months, 106–113
  for period of 24 to 36 months, 119–128
  for period of 3 to 6 years, 136–144
  for period of 6 to 9 years, 152–161
  for period of 9 to 11 years, 169
  for period of 12 to 17 years, 184–188
  sibling rivalry and, 197
Anticonvulsants, for bulimia, 251
Antidepressants, for bulimia, 251
Antihistamines
  for allergic rhinitis and conjunctivitis, 228
  with decongestant, 464
    for allergic rhinitis and conjunctivitis, 229
    for otitis media, 361
  for otitis media, 361
  for pediculosis, 367
  side effects of, 230
  for varicella, 432
Antimicrobial chemoprophylaxis, for otitis media, 361
Antimicrobials. *See specific agent and/or specific disorder*
Antiprostaglandins, for dysmenorrhea, 281–282
Antipyretics, 302
Antiretroviral drugs, for HIV infection/AIDS, 220
Antisocial behavior
  in 9 to 11 year old, 167
  in 12 to 17 year old, 181
Anus, assessment of, at initial visit, 12
Anxieties. *See* Fears and anxieties
Aphthous stomatitis, 237–238
Appearance and behavior
  at 2 week visit, 28
  at 2 month visit, 41
  at 4 month visit, 52
  at 6 month visit, 64
  at 8 month visit, 80
  at 14 month visit, 94
  at 24 month visit, 117

  at 3 year visit, 134
  at 6 year visit, 150
  at 9 to 11 year visit, 167–168
  at 12 to 17 year visit, 181–182
Aristocort, 468–469. *See also* Triamcinolone
Arms. *See* Extremities
Aspirin, 469–470
  for dysmenorrhea, 281
Assertiveness
  at 24 to 36 months, 124
  at 3 to 6 years, 140
  at 6 to 9 years, 156
Astemizole, for allergic rhinitis and conjunctivitis, 229
Asthma, 240–248
  exercise-induced, 244–245
Atabrine, for giardiasis, 278
Atarax, 470
  for varicella, 432
Ataxia–telangiectasia, AIDS differentiated from, 219
Athlete's foot (tinea pedis), 412, 417–419
Atopic child. *See also* Allergies/allergic reactions
  environmental control for, 290–292
Atopic dermatitis, diaper rash caused by, 271
Attapulgite, 482–483
Audiography, in serous otitis media, 397
Augmentin, 471
  for external otitis, 297
  for otitis media, 360
  for sinusitis, 401
Auralgan Otic Solution, 471–472
  for otitis media, 361
Autonomy, Erikson's stage of
  for 8 to 14 month old, 78, 86
  for 14 to 18 month old, 93, 98
  for 18 to 24 month old, 104, 112
Aveeno
  for pityriasis rosea, 378
  for poison ivy/poison oak, 381
  for varicella, 432
Axillary temperature
  normal, 301
  taking, 301
Azithromycin, 521–522
Azmacort, 472–473. *See also* Triamcinolone
AZT, for HIV infection/AIDS, 220

B
B19 parvovirus, erythema infectiosum caused by, 293
Baby food, homemade, 69. *See also* Feeding/feeding problems
Babysitter, 87
  selection of, 58
Bacitracin
  for herpes simplex infection, 314
  for herpes zoster, 321
  for poison ivy/poison oak, 381
  for scabies, 388
  for varicella, 433

Back, assessment of, at initial visit, 12
Bacterial conjunctivitis, 262, 263, 264
Bacterial croup (epiglottitis), viral croup differentiated from, 435
Bactiuria, asymptomatic, 427
Bactrim, 473–474. *See also* Trimethoprim–sulfamethoxazole
for otitis media, 360
for urinary tract infection, 428
Bactroban, 474–475
for impetigo, 329
for intertrigo, 336
for poison ivy/poison oak, 381
Baking soda baths, for varicella, 432
Bathing, for fever reduction, 301
Beclomethasone, for asthma, 245
Beclovent, for asthma, 245
Bed-wetting (nocturnal enuresis), 284–289
Bee sting
allergic response to, 223–225
stinger removal and, 224, 225
Behavior. *See* Appearance and behavior
Behavioral traits, parental perception of, 6
Behavioral treatment, for enuresis, 286–287
Benadryl. *See also* Diphenhydramine
for hymenoptera sting, 224
for pediculosis, 367
for pityriasis rosea, 378
for poison ivy/poison oak, 381
for scabies, 388
for varicella, 432
Benzagel. *See also* Benzoyl peroxide
for acne, 210
Benzocaine, for herpes simplex infection, 317, 318
Benzoyl peroxide, for acne, 210, 211
Beta agonists, for asthma, 244, 245
Betadine, for herpes simplex infection, 317
Biaxin, 475–476
for external otitis, 297
for mycoplasmal pneumonia, 357
for sinusitis, 401
Binge eating, in bulimia, 249
Birth control pills. *See* Oral contraceptives
Birth history, 4–5
Bisexuality, HIV/AIDS exposure and, 215
Bladder control. *See also* Enuresis; Toilet training; Urine
daytime, 193
nighttime, 193
Bladder-stretching exercises, for enuresis, 286, 287–288
Blepharitis
herpes simplex, conjunctivitis differentiated from, 263
hordeolum differentiated from, 326
marginal, 347–348
seborrhea and, 347, 394
Blistex, for herpes simplex infection, 314
Blood dyscrasias, mononucleosis differentiated from, 332
Blood transfusion, HIV/AIDS exposure and, 215

Body habitus, assessment of, 9
Body louse, 364. *See also* Pediculosis
Body temperature
determination of, 301
elevated. *See* Fever
normal, 301
Bordetella pertussis, 371
Borrelia burgdorferi, Lyme disease caused by, 342
Bottle-feeding
colic and, 259
diarrhea and, 276–277
supplementary, 21–22
Bowel control, 192. *See also* Stools; Toilet training
Bowel movements. *See* Stools
B pertussis, 371
Breast-feeding, 19–23
baby's feeding schedule and, 21
colic and, 259
diarrhea and, 276
guidelines for mother and, 19–21
introduction of solid foods and, 68
signs of adequate nutrition and, 21
supplementary feeding and, 22
weaning and, 22–23
Breast milk, expression of, for supplementary feeding, 21–22
Breasts
assessment of
at 9 to 11 year visit, 168
at 12 to 17 year visit, 182
sore, breast-feeding and, 20
Bromfed DM, 476–477
Bromfed PD, 477
Brompheniramine
with pseudoephedrine, 477
with pseudoephedrine and dextromethorphan, 476–477
Bronchial hyperreactivity, in asthma, 240
Bronchiolitis, differential diagnosis of, 437–440t
asthma in, 243
Bronchitis, differential diagnosis of, 437–440t
asthma in, 243
Bronchodilators, for asthma, 244
Bronchopneumonia, asthma differentiated from, 243
Budenoside, for sinusitis, 401
Bulimia, 249–252
Burns
abuse and, 18, 201
prevention of, 15
in 8 to 14 month old, 76
Burow's solution (Domeboro solution), 482
for diaper rash, 272
for herpes simplex infection, 314
for herpes zoster, 321
for intertrigo, 335
otic, for external otitis, 297
for poison ivy/poison oak, 381
for tinea cruris, 415
for tinea pedis, 418

C

Calamine lotion
for hymenoptera sting, 224
for intertrigo, 335
for miliaria rubra, 352
for pityriasis rosea, 378
for poison ivy/poison oak, 381
for varicella, 432
Caldesene Medicated Powder
for diaper rash, 272
for intertrigo, 335
in tinea cruris prevention, 415
Candida albicans (candidiasis)
diaper rash caused by, 253–254, 271, 411
intertrigo and, 335, 336
miliaria rubra differentiated from, 351
oral (thrush), 410–411
identification of
at 2 week visit, 28
at 2 month visit, 41
tinea corporis differentiated from, 412
tinea cruris differentiated from, 414
tinea pedis differentiated from, 417
vulvovaginitis in prepubertal child and, 451
Canker sores (aphthous stomatitis), 237–238
Carbinoxamine, with pseudoephedrine and dextromethorphan (Rondec), 510–511
Cardiovascular system. *See* Heart/cardiovascu-
lar system
Caregiver arrangements
assessment/anticipatory guidance and, at 8 to
14 months, 87
selecting babysitter/day care center and, 58
Caregiver-child interaction. *See* Parent (caregiver)-child interaction
Carrier state, after streptococcal pharyngitis,
405
Cat. *See also* Pets
ringworm transmitted by, 413
Cat-scratch fever, acute cervical adenitis differ-
entiated from, 256
Causality, development of, in 8 to 14 month
old, 86
CD4+ T lymphocytes, in AIDS, 215
Cefaclor, 477–478
Cefadroxil, 485–486
Cefixime, 512–513
for urinary tract infection, 428
Cefpodoxime, 517–519
Cefprozil, 479–480
for otitis media, 361
for sinusitis, 401
Ceftin, 478–479
for otitis media, 360
Cefuroxime, 478–479
for otitis media, 360
Cefzil, 479–480
for otitis media, 361
for sinusitis, 401
Central nervous system, assessment of develop-
ment of. *See* Neurologic assessment
Cephalexin, 491–492
for acute cervical adenitis, 256

Cephalosporins. *See also specific agent*
for otitis media, 361
for scarlet fever, 392
for streptococcal pharyngitis, 404
Cervical adenitis, acute, 255–257
Cetirizine (Zyrtec), for allergic rhinitis and
conjunctivitis, 229
Chalasia, vomiting and, 447
Chalazion, hordeolum differentiated from,
326
Chemical conjunctivitis, 262, 263, 264
Chemoprophylaxis, for otitis media, 361
Chest. *See* Respiratory system
Chickenpox (varicella), 320, 431–434
herpetic gingivostomatitis differentiated
from, 324
Child abuse, 17–18, 201–204
assessment of indications/risk factors for,
201–203
at initial visit, 7
at 2 week visit, 25
at 2 month visit, 27, 40, 44
at 4 month visit, 49, 51
at 6 month visit, 61, 64
at 8 month visit, 76
at 14 month visit, 90–91
at 18 month visit, 102
at 24 month visit, 114–115
at 3 year visit, 130
at 6 year visit, 147
at 9 to 11 year visit, 163
at 12 to 17 year visit, 177
management of, 204
predisposing factors to, 203
role of health care provider and, 203
vulvovaginitis in prepubertal child and, 451
Childrearing practices
assessment/anticipatory guidance and
at 2 to 4 months, 46
at 4 to 6 months, 58
at 6 to 8 months, 72–73
at 8 to 14 months, 87
at 14 to 18 months
emotional development and, 98–99,
110–111
intellectual development and, 111–112
social development and, 112
at 24 to 36 months
emotional development and, 124–125
social development and, 127
at 3 to 6 years, 139
emotional development and, 140–141
intellectual development and, 142
language development and, 142
social development and, 144
at 6 to 9 years
emotional development and, 157
intellectual development and, 158
language development and, 158–159
physical development and, 156
social development and, 160
at 9 to 11 years, 174
child abuse and, 201–204

common concerns of, 189–205
limit setting, 194–196
sibling rivalry and, 197–200
temper tantrums and, 189–191
toilet training and, 192–193
Chlamydia trachomatis (chlamydial infection), conjunctivitis caused by, 262
Chloraseptic
for aphthous stomatitis, 237
for herpangina, 310
for herpetic gingivostomatitis, 324
Chlorpheniramine
for poison ivy/poison oak, 381
with pseudoephedrine (PediaCare 2), 503–504
with pseudoephedrine and dextromethorphan (PediaCare 3), 503–504
Chlor-Trimeton, for poison ivy/poison oak, 381
Chronic granulomatous disease (Wiskott-Aldrich syndrome), AIDS differentiated from, 219
CIBA Eye Scrub
for hordeolum, 326
for marginal blepharitis, 347
Clarithromycin, 475–476
for external otitis, 297
for mycoplasmal pneumonia, 357
for sinusitis, 401
Claritin, 480–481
Clemastine, 513–514
for allergic rhinitis and conjunctivitis, 229
with phenylpropanolamine, for allergic rhinitis and conjunctivitis, 229
Cleocin T lotion, for acne, 210
Clindamycin, for eradication of carrier state after streptococcal pharyngitis, 405
Clothing, for child with fever, 301–302
Clotrimazole, 495, 499–500
for candidal diaper rash, 253
for tinea corporis, 412
for tinea cruris, 415
for tinea pedis, 418
Cloxacillin, for acute cervical adenitis, 256
Colace (docusate sodium), 481–482
for constipation, 268
with encopresis, 268
Cold agglutinins, in mycoplasmal pneumonia, 357
Cold injury, frostbite, 304–306
"Cold sore", 313–315. *See also* Herpes simplex infection
Colic, 33, 258–261
Coly-Mycin S Otic, for external otitis, 297
Comedones, 209, 210
Compresses, hot, for hordeolum, 326
Concrete thinking
in 6 to 9 year old, 149, 157
in 9 to 11 year old, 166, 172
in 12 to 17 year old, 180, 187
Condoms, for HIV/AIDS prevention, 220

Conduction hearing loss, serous otitis media causing, 396
Condyloma acuminatum, 457
Conjunctivitis, 262–265
allergic, 227–231, 262, 263, 264
bacterial, 262, 263, 264
chemical, 262, 263, 264
hordeolum differentiated from, 326
Consolidation, as Piaget stage of development, 79
Constipation, 267–270
in 8 to 14 month old, 85
in 6 to 9 year old, 155
with encopresis, 268–269, 270
Contact dermatitis
diaper rash caused by, 271
miliaria rubra differentiated from, 351
poison ivy/poison oak, 380–381
tinea cruris differentiated from, 414
tinea pedis differentiated from, 418
Contagious diseases. *See* Infection/contagious diseases
Cool-mist vaporizer, for croup, 436, 440t
Cooperation
at 24 to 36 months, 124
at 3 to 6 years, 140
Cord care, 422
Corneal abrasion, conjunctivitis differentiated from, 264
Corneal ulcer, conjunctivitis differentiated from, 264
Corporal punishment, abuse and, 17
Corticosteroids. *See also specific agent*
for asthma, 244, 245–246
for diaper rash, 272
fluorinated
for herpes simplex infection, 315
for wart removal, 455
for mononucleosis, 333
for seborrhea, 395
Cortisporin Otic, for external otitis, 297
Cough, in croup, 435, 437t, 438t
Coxsackie virus A
hand/foot/mouth disease caused by, 308
herpangina caused by, 310
"Crab" louse, 364. *See also* Pediculosis
Cradle cap (seborrhea of scalp), 394–395
Cramps, menstrual (dysmenorrhea), 280–283
Crib, injury prevention and, 16
Crib toys, for 2 to 8 week old, 33–34
Crixivan, for HIV infection/AIDS, 220
Cromolyn, 490–491
action of, 246
for asthma, 244, 245, 246, 490–491
nasal
action of, 230
for allergic rhinitis and conjunctivitis, 228, 229, 230
side effects of, 246, 490
Crotamiton, 488–489
for scabies, 387, 388

Croup
  bacterial (epiglottitis), viral croup differenti-
    ated from, 435
  viral (laryngotracheobronchitis), 435–441
  differential diagnosis of, 437–440*t*
  asthma in, 243
Crying
  colic causing, 258
  interpretation of, 32–33
Cryosurgery
  for molluscum contagiosum, 354
  for wart removal, 455, 456
Cyproheptadine, for pityriasis rosea, 378
Cystic fibrosis, asthma differentiated from,
    243
Cystitis, enuresis and, 285
Cystogram, radionuclide, in urinary tract infec-
    tion, 428
Cystourethrogram, voiding, indications for,
    428
Cysts, acne, 209, 210

D
Dacryostenosis, conjunctivitis differentiated
    from, 264
Day care center, 87
  selection of, 58, 87
DDAVP, 288
  for enuresis, 286, 288
  side effects of, 288
ddI, for HIV infection/AIDS, 220
Decongestants
  for allergic rhinitis and conjunctivitis, 228
  with antihistamine, 464
    for allergic rhinitis and conjunctivitis, 229
  for otitis media, 361
  for otitis media, 361
Deer ticks, Lyme disease transmitted by, 342,
    344–345
DEET, for Lyme disease prevention, 344
Dehydration, prevention of. *See* Hydration
Dental care, assessment of. *See also* Teeth
  at 8 month visit, 78
  at 18 month visit, 104, 110
  at 6 year visit, 155
Depression, suicide risk and, 408
Dermatitis
  allergic contact
    diaper rash caused by, 271
    miliaria rubra differentiated from, 351
    tinea cruris differentiated from, 414
    tinea pedis differentiated from, 418
  atopic, diaper rash caused by, 271
  candidal, diaper rash caused by, 253–254,
    271, 411
  poison ivy/poison oak, 380–381
  primary irritant, diaper rash caused by,
    271–273
  seborrheic
    blepharitis and, 377
    pityriasis rosea differentiated from, 377
    of scalp (cradle cap), 394–395
    tinea cruris differentiated from, 414

Desensitization, for allergic rhinitis and con-
    junctivitis, 229
Desitin
  for diaper rash, 272
  for irritation caused by pinworms, 374
Desquam-X. *See also* Benzoyl peroxide
  for acne, 210
Developmental process, assessment of. *See also*
    Growth and development
  at 2 week visit, 26
  at 2 month visit, 38
  at 4 month visit, 50
  at 6 month visit, 62
  at 8 month visit, 78
  at 14 month visit, 92
  at 18 month visit, 103
  at 24 month visit, 116
  at 6 year visit, 146
  at 9 to 11 year visit, 165
  at 12 to 17 year visit, 178
Dextromethorphan, 503–504
  with carbinoxamine and pseudoephedrine
    (Rondec), 510–511
  with guaifenesin, (Tussi-Organidin DM),
    517
  with pseudoephedrine and brompheniramine
    (Bromfed DM), 476–477
  with pseudoephedrine and chlorpheniramine
    (PediaCare 3), 503–504
  with pseudoephedrine and guaifenesin
    (Dorcol/Novahistine), 484–485,
    502–503
Diabetes insipidus, enuresis and, 285
Diabetes mellitus, enuresis and, 285
Diaper rash
  candidal, 253–254, 271, 411
  primary irritant, 271–273
Diarrhea, 274–279
  infectious, 275–276
  parenteral, 276
  starvation, 276, 445
  in viral gastroenteritis, 442
Dicloxacillin
  for acute cervical adenitis, 256
  for impetigo, 329
Didanosine, for HIV infection/AIDS, 220
Diet history. *See also* Nutrition
  at initial visit, 5
  at 6 month visit, 62
  at 8 month visit, 78
  at 14 month visit, 92
  at 18 month visit, 103
  at 6 year visit, 148
Diflucan, for nail infection, 418
DiGeorge anomolad, AIDS differentiated
    from, 219
Digestion/digestive system. *See* Gastrointesti-
    nal system
Dimetapp
  for allergic rhinitis and conjunctivitis, 229
  for otitis media, 361
Diphenhydramine
  for allergic rhinitis and conjunctivitis, 229

for hymenoptera sting, 224
for pediculosis, 367
for pityriasis rosea, 378
for poison ivy/poison oak, 381
for scabies, 388
for varicella, 432
Diprosone cream, for wart removal, 456
Discipline
  for 24 to 36 month old, 127
  for 3 to 6 year old, 144
  limit setting and, 194–196
Disequilibrium, as Piaget stage of development, 79
Diurnal enuresis, 284–289
Divorce. *See also* Single parent; Step-parents
  adolescent affected by, 185
Docusate sodium, 481–482
  for constipation, 268
  with encopresis, 268
Dog. *See also* Pets
  ringworm transmitted by, 413
Domeboro solution (Burow's solution), 482
  for diaper rash, 272
  for herpes simplex infection, 314
  for herpes zoster, 321
  for intertrigo, 335
  otic, for external otitis, 297
  for poison ivy/poison oak, 381
  for tinea cruris, 415
  for tinea pedis, 418
Donnagel, 482–483
Donnatal, 483–484
Dorcol, 484–485
Doxycycline, for Lyme disease, 344
Drooling, at 4 to 6 months, 57
Drowning, prevention of, 16
Drugs/medications
  abuse of. *See* Substance abuse
  breast-feeding and, 19
DTP vaccine, 370, 371
Duofilm, for wart removal, 455, 456
Duricef, 485–486
Dyprotex, for diaper rash, 272
Dysmenorrhea, primary, 280–283

E
Earache
  in external otitis, 296
  in otitis media, 359
Ear canal, abscess in, external otitis differentiated from, 297
Ear drops
  for external otitis, 297
  instillation of, 297–298, 361
  for otitis media, 361
Ears, assessment of. *See also* Hearing
  at initial visit, 7, 10
  at 8 month visit, 80
  at 14 month visit, 94
  at 3 year visit, 134
  at 6 year visit, 150

Eating disorders. *See* Anorexia nervosa; Bulimia
Eating habits. *See also* Feeding/feeding problems
  in 6 month old, 70
  in 8 to 14 month old, 78
  in 14 to 18 month old, 92, 97
  in 18 to 24 month old, 103, 109
  in 24 to 36 year old, 122
EBV. *See* Epstein-Barr virus
ECM. *See* Erythema chronicum migrans
E coli, diarrhea caused by, 276, 278
  viral gastroenteritis differentiated from, 442
Eczema, intertrigo differentiated from, 335
Egocentricity
  of 3 to 6 year old, 140
  of 6 to 9 year old, 156
Electrodesiccation, for wart removal, 457
Elimination patterns
  at 2 to 8 weeks, 27, 32
  at 2 to 4 months, 39, 45
  at 4 to 6 months, 50, 57
  at 6 to 8 months, 62, 71
  at 8 to 14 months, 78, 85
  at 14 to 18 months, 92–93, 97
  at 18 to 24 months, 103–104, 110
  at 24 to 36 months, 116–117, 122–123
  at 3 to 6 years, 131, 139
  at 6 to 9 years, 148–149, 154–155
  at 12 to 17 years, 179
Elimite. *See also* Permethrin
  for scabies, 387–388
ELISA, in Lyme disease, 343
Emotional abuse, 201. *See also* Child abuse
Emotional development
  at 2 weeks, 27–28
  at 2 to 4 months, 39–40, 45–46
  at 4 to 6 months, 51, 57
  at 6 to 8 months, 63, 72
  at 8 to 14 months, 79, 86
  at 14 to 18 months, 93, 98
  at 18 to 24 months, 104, 110
  at 24 to 36 months, 117, 123–125
  at 3 to 6 years, 133–134, 139–141
  at 6 to 9 years, 149, 156–157
  at 9 to 11 years, 166, 172
  at 12 to 17 years, 180, 187
Emotional neglect, 201, 202. *See also* Child abuse
Encopresis, 267, 268, 268–269, 270
Endocrine system, assessment of
  at initial visit, 8
  at 3 year visit, 133
Enema, for constipation, 268
Enterobius vermicularis, 374
Enterovirus infections, scarlet fever differentiated from, 392
Enuresis, 284–289. *See also* Toilet training; Urine
  urinary tract infection and, 285, 426
Environment, safe, in injury prevention, 15
Environmental control, for atopic child, 290–292

Epidermophyton floccosum, tinea cruris caused by, 414
Epiglottis, assessment of, at initial visit, 11
Epiglottitis (bacterial croup), viral croup differentiated from, 435
Epinephrine, 464–465
  for asthma, 244, 246
  for hymenoptera sting, 224–225
  side effects of, 246, 464
EpiPen. *See also* Epinephrine
  for hymenoptera sting, 225
Epistaxis, in allergic rhinitis, 230
Epstein-Barr virus, mononucleosis caused by, 331
Equilibrium, as Piaget stage of development, 79
Equinovarus prewalkers, for metatarsus adductus, 349, 349–350
Erikson's stages of growth and development. *See also specific stage* and Emotional development
  for 2 week old, 27–28
  for 2 to 4 month old, 40, 45
  for 4 to 6 month old, 51, 57
  for 6 to 8 month old, 63, 72
  for 8 to 14 month old, 79, 86
  for 14 to 18 month old, 93, 98
  for 18 to 24 month old, 104, 110
  for 24 to 36 month old, 117, 123–125
  for 3 to 6 year old, 139–141
  for 6 to 9 year old, 149
  for 9 to 11 year old, 166, 172
  for 12 to 17 year old, 180, 187
Erycette, 486–487. *See also* Erythromycin
Erythema chronicum migrans, in Lyme disease, 342, 343, 345
Erythema infectiosum (fifth disease), 293–294
  scarlet fever differentiated from, 392
Erythromycin, 487–488
  for acute cervical adenitis, 256
  for blepharitis, 347
  for impetigo, 329
  for Lyme disease, 344
  for mycoplasmal pneumonia, 357, 440t
  ophthalmic, 347, 489–490
  for pertussis, 371
  for pneumonia, 440t
  for scarlet fever, 392
  for streptococcal pharyngitis, 404
  topical, 486–487
  for vulvovaginitis in prepubertal child, 451
Escherichia coli, diarrhea caused by, 276, 278
  viral gastroenteritis differentiated from, 442
Eurax, 488–489. *See also* Crotamiton
  for scabies, 387
Eustachian tube
  autoinflation of, for serous otitis media, 397
  obstruction of, otitis media differentiated from, 360
  in serous otitis media, 396
Exanthems
  in scarlet fever, 391
  viral

erythema infectiosum and, 293
  miliaria rubra differentiated from, 351
  mononucleosis differentiated from, 332
Exanthem subitum (roseola), 383–384
  scarlet fever differentiated from, 392
Excretory system. *See* Elimination patterns; Genitourinary system
Exelderm cream, for tinea versicolor, 420
Exercise
  for 6 to 9 year old, 155
  for 9 to 11 year old, 172
  for 12 to 17 year old, 186
  asthma and, 244–245
Exsel shampoo, for seborrhea, 394
External otitis, 296–298
  acute otitis media differentiated from, 297, 360
Extremities, assessment/anticipatory guidance and
  at initial visit, 12
  at 2 weeks, 28
  at 2 to 4 months, 41, 45
  at 6 to 8 months, 64
Eye medications, instillation of, 265, 326
Eyes, assessment of. *See also* Vision
  at initial visit, 7, 10
  at 2 week visit, 28
  at 2 month visit, 41
  at 6 month visit, 64
  at 8 month visit, 80
  at 18 month visit, 105
  at 24 month visit, 118
  at 3 year visit, 134
  at 6 year visit, 150, 155

F

Face, assessment of, at initial visit, 7, 9–10
Failure to thrive, abuse and, 18
Falls
  abuse and, 18
  prevention of injury from, 15–16
  in 8 to 14 month old, 76
Family history, 3
Family status, assessment/anticipatory guidance and. *See also* Parents
  at 2 to 8 weeks, 26, 32
  at 2 to 4 months, 38, 44
  at 4 to 6 months, 50, 56
  at 6 to 8 months, 62, 68
  at 8 to 14 months, 78, 83–84
  at 14 to 18 months, 92, 96
  at 18 to 24 months, 103, 108–109
  at 24 to 36 months, 116, 121–122
  at 3 to 6 years, 138
  at 6 to 9 years, 148, 154
  at 9 to 11 years, 165, 171
  at 12 to 17 years, 178, 185–186
Father. *See also* Family status; Parent (caregiver)-child interaction
  of 14 to 18 month old, 96–97
  abusive, characteristics of, 17

Fears and anxieties
  at 24 to 36 months, 124
  at 3 to 6 years, 140
Feeding/feeding problems. *See also* Anorexia
    nervosa; Bulimia; Nutrition
  assessment/anticipatory guidance and
    at initial visit, 5
    at 4 to 6 months, 56–57
    at 6 to 8 months, 68–71
    at 8 to 14 months, 78
  colic and, 258–261
  establishing good eating habits and, 70
  homemade baby foods and, 69
  introduction of new foods and, 68–69
  vomiting and, 447
Feeding schedule. *See also* Nutrition
  at 4 to 6 months, 56
  for breast-fed baby, 21
Feet, assessment of, at initial visit, 12
Feosol Elixir, for iron-deficiency anemia, 340,
    489
Fer-In-Sol, for iron-deficiency anemia, 340
Ferrous sulfate, for iron-deficiency anemia,
    340, 489
Fever, 300
  control of, 300–302
Fiber, dietary, for constipation, 268, 269
Fifth disease (erythema infectiosum), 293–294
  scarlet fever differentiated from, 392
Fine motor skills
  at initial visit, 5–6
  at 4-6 months, 57
  at 8 to 14 months, 85
  at 14 to 18 months, 93, 97
  at 18 to 24 months, 104
  at 24 to 36 months, 117, 123
  at 3 to 6 years, 139
Fire, prevention of injury from, 15
  in 8 to 14 month old, 76
Fire ant stings, allergic response to, 223–225
Flagyl, for giardiasis, 278
Fluids, forcing. *See* Hydration
Fluocinolone, for diaper rash, 272
Fluorescent antibody tests, in Lyme disease,
    343
Fluoride (sodium), 495–496
Flurazepam, for nail infection, 418
Foods. *See* Feeding/feeding problems
Foreign body
  in ear, external otitis differentiated from, 297
  nasal, sinusitis and, 401
  in trachea/bronchi
    asthma differentiated from, 243
    viral croup differentiated from, 435
  in vagina, 451
Formal (abstract) thinking
  in 9 to 11 year old, 166, 172
  in 12 to 17 year old, 180, 187
Formula feeding
  colic and, 259
  diarrhea and, 276–277
  supplementary, 21–22
Frostbite, 304–306

Frustration. *See also* Temper tantrums
  manifestations of, 189–190
Furniture, prevention of injury from, 16
Furunculosis, external otitis differentiated
    from, 297

G
Gamma-benzene hexachloride (Kwell), 368,
    492–493, 493
  for pediculosis capitis, 366
  for pediculosis corporis, 366
  for pediculosis pubis, 366–367
  for scabies, 388
Garamycin, for diaper rash, 272
Gastrocolic reflex, 269
Gastroenteritis. *See also* Diarrhea; Vomiting
  viral, 442–445
Gastrointestinal system, assessment of. *See also*
    Nutrition
  at 2 month visit, 39
  at 3 year visit, 133
Genital herpes, 316–318
  HSV-1 causing, 313, 316
Genitalia, assessment of
  at initial visit, 12
  at 8 month visit, 80
  at 3 year visit, 134
  at 6 year visit, 150
  at 9 to 11 year visit, 168
  at 12 to 17 year visit, 182
Genitourinary system, assessment of. *See also*
    Elimination patterns
  at initial visit, 7
  at 2 month visit, 39
  at 3 year visit, 133
Gentamicin, for diaper rash, 272
Giardiasis, diarrhea in, 276, 278
Gingiva (gums), assessment of, at initial visit,
    10
Gingivostomatitis, herpetic, 313, 323–325
  hand/foot/mouth disease differentiated from,
    308, 324
  herpangina differentiated from, 310, 324
Glomerulonephritis, enuresis and, 285
Gly-Oxide, for herpetic gingivostomatitis, 324
Gonorrhea/gonococcal infection
  conjunctivitis and, 262
  urethritis and, urinary tract infection differen-
    tiated from, 428
  vulvovaginitis in prepubertal child and, 451
Granuloma, umbilical, 424
Granulomatous disease, chronic (Wiskott-Ald-
    rich syndrome), AIDS differentiated
    from, 219
Grifulvin
  for tinea corporis, 412
  for tinea pedis, 418
Griseofulvin
  for tinea corporis, 412
  for tinea pedis, 418
Gross motor skills
  at initial visit, 5
  at 4-6 months, 57

Gross motor skills *(continued)*
  at 8 to 14 months, 85
  at 14 to 18 months, 93
  at 18 to 24 months, 104
  at 24 to 36 months, 117, 123
  at 3 to 6 years, 139
Group A beta-hemolytic streptococci
  acute cervical adenitis caused by, 255
  pharyngitis caused by, 403–405
  scarlet fever caused by, 391
  sinusitis and, 401
  vulvovaginitis caused by, 451
Growth and development. *See also specific*
    aspect
  assessment/anticipatory guidance and
    at initial visit, 5–6, 8
    at 2 weeks, 27–28
    at 2 to 4 months, 39–40
    at 4 to 6 months, 51, 57–59
    at 6 to 8 months, 63–64, 71–74
    at 8 to 14 months, 79, 85–89
    at 14 to 18 months, 93–94, 97–100
    at 18 to 24 months, 104, 110–113
    at 24 to 36 months, 117, 123–128
    at 3 to 6 years, 133–134, 139–145
    at 6 to 9 years, 149–150, 155–161
    at 9 to 11 years, 165–167, 172–174
    at 12 to 17 years, 180–181, 186–188
  parental reaction/perception of child's accom-
    plishment and, 6
Growth/growth measurements, 9. *See also*
    Physical growth and development
  at 2 month visit, 40–41
  at 4 month visit, 52
  at 6 month visit, 64
  at 8 month visit, 80
  at 14 month visit, 94
  at 18 month visit, 104–105
  at 24 month visit, 117
  at 3 year visit, 131–132, 134
  at 6 year visit, 150
  at 9 to 11 year visit, 167
  at 12 to 17 year visit, 181
Growth spurt
  at 6 to 9 years, 156
  at 9 to 11 years, 165–166
Guaifenesin
  with dextromethorphan (Tussi-Organidin
    DM), 517
  with dextromethorphan and pseudoephed-
    rine (Dorcol/Novahistine), 484–485,
    502–503
Gums
  assessment of, at initial visit, 10
  inflammation of. *See* Gingivostomatitis
Guttate psoriasis, pityriasis rosea differentiated
    from, 377

H

Haemophilus influenzae
  conjunctivitis caused by, 262
  otitis media caused by, 359
  pneumonia caused by, 439*t*

sinusitis caused by, 400
  vulvovaginitis caused by, 451
Hair, assessment of
  at 14 month visit, 94
  at 9 to 11 year visit, 168
  at 12 to 17 year visit, 182
Haloprogin, for tinea pedis, 418
Halotex, for tinea pedis, 418
Hand. *See* Extremities
Hand/foot/mouth disease, 308–309
  herpangina differentiated from, 308, 310
  herpetic gingivostomatitis differentiated
    from, 308, 324
Handicapped child, sibling rivalry issues and,
    199–200
Head, assessment of
  at initial visit, 7, 9–10
  at 2 week visit, 28
  at 2 month visit, 41, 45
  at 4 month visit, 52
  at 6 month visit, 64
  at 18 month visit, 105
Head injury, abuse and, 18
Head louse, 364. *See also* Pediculosis
Health care workers, AIDS/HIV risk and, 217,
    221
Health habits/patterns. *See also specific type*
  at 2 to 8 weeks, 26–27, 32
  at 2 to 4 months, 38–39, 44–45
  at 4 to 6 months, 50–51, 56–57
  at 6 to 8 months, 62, 68–71
  at 8 to 14 months, 78, 84–85
  at 14 to 18 months, 92–93, 97
  at 18 to 24 months, 103–104, 109–110
  at 24 to 36 months, 116–117, 122–123
  at 3 to 6 years, 131, 138–139
  at 6 to 9 years, 148–149, 154–155
  at 9 to 11 years, 165, 171–172
  at 12 to 17 years, 178–180, 186
Hearing, assessment of. *See also* Ears
  at 2 to 4 months, 45
  at 4 months, 51
  at 8 months, 79
  at 14 to 18 months, 93
  at 3 to 6 years, 132
Hearing loss, serous otitis media causing, 396
Heart/cardiovascular system, assessment of
  at initial visit, 7, 11
  at 2 week visit, 27, 28
  at 2 month visit, 41
  at 6 month visit, 64
  at 18 month visit, 105
  at 3 year visit, 133, 134
  at 6 year visit, 150
  at 9 to 11 year visit, 168
  at 12 to 17 year visit, 182
Heat rash (miliaria rubra), 351–352
HEENT. *See* Ears; Eyes; Head; Nose; Throat
Hematopoietic system, assessment of, at 8
    month visit, 79
Hemoccult stool test, in diarrhea, 275

HEPA filters, for environmental control for atopic child, 290
Hepatitis, mononucleosis differentiated from, 332
Herpangina, 310–311
aphthous stomatitis differentiated from, 237
hand/foot/mouth disease differentiated from, 308, 310
herpetic gingivostomatitis differentiated from, 310, 324
Herpes simplex infections. *See also* Gingivostomatitis, herpetic
aphthous stomatitis differentiated from, 237
blepharitis, conjunctivitis differentiated from, 263
hand/foot/mouth disease differentiated from, 308
herpangina differentiated from, 310
keratitis, conjunctivitis differentiated from, 264
type 1, 313–315
type 2, 316–318
vulvovaginitis in prepubertal child and, 451
Herpes simplex virus. *See also* Herpes simplex infections
type 1, 313, 316, 323
type 2, 316
Herpes zoster, 320–321, 432
Herpetic whitlow, 313
Herplex, for herpes simplex infection, 314
Heterophil antibody test, in mononucleosis, 332
High risk sexual behavior
herpes simplex infections and, 318
HIV/AIDS exposure and, 215, 220
Hips. *See* Extremities
Hirschsprung's disease, constipation differentiated from, 268
Hismanal, for allergic rhinitis and conjunctivitis, 229
Histofreezer, for wart removal, 455, 456
History, initial, in well child care, 3–8
HIV-1, 215. *See also* AIDS
blood tests for, 219
transmission of, 215
Hivid, for HIV infection/AIDS, 220
Home environment, control of allergens in, 290–292
Homosexuality, HIV/AIDS exposure and, 215
Hordeolum (stye), 326–327
Hornet sting, allergic response to, 223–225
Hospitalizations, history of, 7
Hot compresses, for hordeolum, 326
HSV-1. *See* Herpes simplex virus, type 1
HSV-2. *See* Herpes simplex virus, type 2
Human herpes virus 6, roseola and, 383
Human immunodeficiency virus, type 1, 215.
See also AIDS
blood tests for, 219
transmission of, 215
Human papilloma virus, warts caused by, 454
Human parvovirus B19, erythema infectiosum caused by, 293

Hydration
for croup, 436
for diarrhea, 276, 277
fever affecting, 301
for hand/foot/mouth disease, 309
for herpangina, 311
for herpetic gingivostomatitis, 324
for streptococcal pharyngitis, 404
for viral gastroenteritis, 443–444
Hydrocephalus, vomiting and, 447
Hydrocortisone
for diaper rash, 272
for intertrigo, 335
for miliaria rubra, 352
for poison ivy/poison oak, 381
for scabies, 388
for seborrhea, 395
Hydroxyzine, 470
for varicella, 432
Hygiene
acne and, 212
assessment/anticipatory guidance and, at 9 to 11 years, 165
Hyperhidrosis, tinea pedis differentiated from, 417
Hyperthermia
cold sponging for, 301
for wart removal, 455
Hypopigmentation, postinflammatory/posttraumatic, tinea versicolor differentiated from, 420

I

Ibuprofen, 498–499
for acute cervical adenitis, 256, 257
for children, 302, 498
for dysmenorrhea, 282
for fever, 302
for herpetic gingivostomatitis, 324
for roseola, 384
for streptococcal pharyngitis, 404
Identity versus role confusion, Erikson's stage of
for 9 to 11 year old, 172
for 12 to 17 year old, 180, 187
Idoxuridine, for herpes simplex infection, 314
"Id" reaction, 417
Illnesses
history of, 7
reaction to, at 8 to 14 months, 86
Ilotycin, 489–490. *See also* Erythromycin
for blepharitis, 347
Imipramine, 288, 516–517
for bulimia, 251
for enuresis, 286, 288
side effects of, 288
Immune system, assessment of
at 2 week visit, 27
at 2 month visit, 39
at 6 month visit, 63
at 8 month visit, 79
at 3 year visit, 133
Immunization history, 6

Immunodeficiency
acquired, 215–222. *See also* AIDS
congenital, AIDS differentiated from,
218–219
Impetigo, 328–330
herpes simplex infection differentiated from,
314
scabies differentiated from, 387
varicella differentiated from, 432
Industry versus inferiority, Erikson's stage of,
for 6 to 9 year old, 156
Infection/contagious diseases
chronic, iron-deficiency anemia differentiated
from, 339
diarrhea caused by, 275–276
history of, 7
prevention of, in 12 to 17 year old, 179
vomiting caused by, 448
Infectious mononucleosis, 331–334
acute cervical adenitis differentiated from,
256
streptococcal pharyngitis differentiated from,
332, 404
Initiative versus guilt, Erikson's stage of
for 3 to 6 year old, 139–141
for 6 to 9 year old, 149
Injuries. *See also* Child abuse
history of, 7
prevention of/safety strategies, 15–16
for 2 to 8 week old, 24–25, 34
for 2 to 4 month old, 36–37, 47
for 4 to 6 month old, 48–49, 59
for 6 to 8 month old, 60–61, 73–74
for 8 to 14 month old, 75–76, 88–89
for 14 to 18 month old, 90, 100
for 18 to 24 month old, 101–102, 112–113
for 24 to 36 month old, 114, 127–128
for 3 to 6 year old, 129–130, 144–145
for 6 to 9 year old, 146–147, 155, 161
for 9 to 11 year old, 163, 174
for 12 to 17 year old, 177, 178–179, 186
Insect bites
allergic response to, 223–225
varicella differentiated from, 432
Intal, for asthma, 245, 490–491. *See also* Cromolyn
Intellectual development
for 2 week old, 28
for 2 to 4 month old, 40, 46
for 4 to 6 month old, 51, 57–58
for 6 to 8 month old, 63, 72
for 8 to 14 month old, 79, 86
for 14 to 18 month old, 93, 99
for 18 to 24 month old, 104, 111
for 24 to 36 month old, 117
for 3 to 6 year old, 134, 141–143
for 6 to 9 year old, 149, 157–159
for 9 to 11 year old, 166, 172–173
for 12 to 17 year old, 180, 187
Intertrigo, 335–336
tinea cruris differentiated from, 414
Intuitive learning, in 18 to 24 month old, 104
Intussusception, vomiting and, 447

Invirase, for HIV infection/AIDS, 220
Iritis, conjunctivitis differentiated from, 264
Iron, dietary/supplemental, in iron-deficiency
anemia, 340, 489
Iron-deficiency anemia, 338–341
Isolation, as punishment, 196
Isomil formula, for child with diarrhea, 277
Ixodes dammini tick, Lyme disease transmitted
by, 342, 344–345

J
Jealousy, of siblings, 197–200. *See also* Sibling
rivalry; Siblings
"Jock itch," 414–415
Johnson's Baby Shampoo, for hordeolum, 347

K
Kawasaki syndrome, scarlet fever differentiated from, 392
Keflex, 491–492
for acute cervical adenitis, 256
Kenalog. *See also* Triamcinolone
for aphthous stomatitis, 237, 238
Keratitis, herpes simplex, conjunctivitis differentiated from, 264
Ketoconazole
for tinea corporis, 412
for tinea cruris, 414
for tinea versicolor, 420, 421
Ketoprofen, for dysmenorrhea, 282
Ketorolac, for allergic conjunctivitis, 229, 264
KOH test (potassium hydroxide test)
in candidal diaper rash, 253
in tinea pedis, 417
in tinea versicolor, 420
Koplik's spots, in rubeola (measles), 332, 384,
392
Kwell, 369, 492–493, 493
for pediculosis capitis, 366
for pediculosis corporis, 366
for pediculosis pubis, 366–367
for scabies, 388

L
Lactose-free formula, for diarrhea, 277
Lactulose, for constipation with encopresis,
268
Language skills/development
at initial visit, 6
at 4 to 6 months, 51, 57
at 6 to 8 months, 63, 72
at 8 to 14 months, 79, 86
at 14 to 18 months, 93, 99
at 18 to 24 months, 104, 111
at 24 to 36 months, 123
at 3 to 6 years, 131, 139, 142
at 6 to 9 years, 149, 155–156, 158–159
at 9 to 11 years, 172, 173
at 12 to 17 years, 180
Laryngotracheobronchitis (viral croup),
435–441
differential diagnosis of, 437–440t
asthma in, 243

Laser surgery, for wart removal, 457
Lead poisoning, iron-deficiency anemia differentiated from, 339
Learning. *See also* Intellectual development
 in 6 to 9 year old, 149
Legs. *See* Extremities
Leukemia
 acute cervical adenitis differentiated from, 256
 mononucleosis differentiated from, 332
Lice, 364–368
Lidocaine, for herpes simplex infection, 317
Limit setting, 194–196. *See also* Discipline
 for 24 to 36 month old, 127
Lindane (Kwell), 369, 492–493, 493
 for pediculosis capitis, 366
 for pediculosis corporis, 366
 for pediculosis pubis, 366–367
 for scabies, 388
Lips. *See also* Mouth
 assessment of at initial visit, 10
Lorabid, 493–495
 for otitis media, 361
 for sinusitis, 401
Loracarbef, 493–495
 for otitis media, 361
 for sinusitis, 401
Loratadine, 480–481
Lotrimin, 495. *See also* Clotrimazole
 for candidal diaper rash, 253
 for tinea corporis, 412
 for tinea cruris, 415
 for tinea pedis, 418
Lungs. *See* Respiratory system/chest
Luride, 495–496
Lyme disease, 342–345
Lymph nodes
 assessment of
  at initial visit, 11
  at 9 to 11 year visit, 168
  at 12 to 17 year visit, 182
 enlargement/inflammation of. *See* Adenitis; Adenopathy
Lytren. *See also* Oral rehydration
 for diarrhea, 277
 for viral gastroenteritis, 443

M
Macewen's sign, 10
Malassezia furfur, tinea versicolor caused by, 420
Maltsupex, for constipation, 268
Marginal blepharitis, 347–348
Masturbation
 in 24 to 36 month old, 127
 in 12 to 17 year old, 180
Maxivate cream, for wart removal, 456
Measles (rubeola)
 mononucleosis differentiated from, 332
 roseola differentiated from, 384
 scarlet fever differentiated from, 392
Mebendazole, 375, 520–521
 for pinworms, 374, 375

side effects of, 375
Medic Alert bracelets, for hymenoptera allergy, 225
Mefenamic acid, 507–508
 for dysmenorrhea, 282
Memory
 in 4 to 6 month old, 57
 in 6 to 8 month old, 63, 72
 in 8 to 14 month old, 86
Meningococcemia, roseola differentiated from, 384
Menstrual cramps (dysmenorrhea), 280–283
Menstruation
 onset of, in 12 to 17 year old, 179–180
 resumption of, breast-feeding and, 19
Metaproterenol, for asthma, 245
Metatarsus adductus, 349–350
Metered-dose inhalers, for asthma, 245, 246–247
Metronidazole, for giardiasis, 278
Micatin. *See also* Clotrimazole
 for tinea cruris, 415
Miconazole, 496–497, 497
 for candidal diaper rash, 253
Microsporum, tinea corporis caused by, 412, 413
Middle ear infection. *See* Otitis media
Miliaria rubra (heat rash/prickly heat), 351–352
Milk of magnesia, for constipation with encopresis, 268
Mineral oil, for constipation with encopresis, 268
Mites, scabies caused by, 386
Molluscum contagiosum, 353–354
Moniliasis, vulvovaginitis in prepubertal child and, 451
Monistat, 496–497, 497. *See also* Miconazole
 for candidal diaper rash, 253
Mononucleosis, 331–334
 acute cervical adenitis differentiated from, 256
 streptococcal pharyngitis differentiated from, 332, 404
Monospot test, in mononucleosis, 332
Moraxella catarrhalis
 conjunctivitis caused by, 262
 otitis media caused by, 359
 sinusitis caused by, 400
Mother. *See also* Family status; Parent (caregiver)-child interaction
 abusive, characteristics of, 17
 working
  of 8 to 14 month old, 84
  of 14 to 18 month old, 96
  of 24 to 36 month old, 121
  return to work and, 38
Motor skills. *See also* Fine motor skills; Gross motor skills
 at initial visit, 5–6
 at 8 to 14 months, 85

Motrin, 498–499. *See also* Ibuprofen
for children, 498
Mouth, assessment of
at initial visit, 7, 10
at 2 week visit, 28
at 2 month visit, 41
Mumps, acute cervical adenitis differentiated
from, 256
Mupirocin, 474–475
for impetigo, 329
for intertrigo, 336
for poison ivy/poison oak, 381
Musculoskeletal system, assessment of
at initial visit, 12
at 8 month visit, 80
at 14 month visit, 94
at 18 month visit, 105
at 24 month visit, 118
at 3 year visit, 132, 135
at 6 year visit, 150
at 9 to 11 year visit, 168
at 12 to 17 year visit, 182
Mycelex, 499–500. *See also* Clotrimazole
Mycoplasma pneumoniae pneumonia, 356–
358, 439*t*
Mycostatin, 500–501. *See also* Nystatin
for candidal diaper rash, 253
for thrush, 410
Myringotomy, for serous otitis media, 398

N
Nails, fungal infection of, 418
Naproxen, 467–468
for dysmenorrhea, 281
Nasacort, 230, 501
action of, 230
for allergic rhinitis and conjunctivitis, 229,
230
Nasalcrom (cromolyn sodium nasal solution)
action of, 230
for allergic rhinitis and conjunctivitis, 228,
229, 230
Nasal foreign body, sinusitis and, 401
Nasopharyngeal culture, in pertussis, 371
Neck, assessment of
at initial visit, 11
at 3 year visit, 134
Negativism, in 14 to 18 month old, 99
*Neisseria gonorrhoeae. See also under Gono-
coccal*
conjunctivitis caused by, 262
vulvovaginitis caused by, 451
Neonatal health history, 4–5
Neosporin
in cord care, 422
for diaper rash, 272
for herpes simplex infection, 314
for herpes zoster, 321
for molluscum contagiosum, 354
for scabies, 388
for varicella, 433
Neuralgia, postherpetic, 321

Neurologic assessment
at initial visit, 8
at 2 week visit, 27
at 2 month visit, 39, 41, 45
at 4 month visit, 51, 57
at 6 month visit, 63
at 8 month visit, 79
at 3 year visit, 132–133, 135
at 6 year visit, 150
Nipples, sore, breast-feeding and, 20–21
Nix, 502. *See also* Permethrin
for pediculosis capitis, 365–366
Nizoral
for tinea corporis, 412
for tinea cruris, 414
for tinea versicolor, 420
Nizoral shampoo, for seborrhea, 394
Nocturnal emissions, in 12 to 17 year old, 180
Nocturnal enuresis, 284–289. *See also* Enuresis
Norvir, for HIV infection/AIDS, 220
Nose, assessment of, at initial visit, 7, 10
Nosebleeds. *See* Epistaxis
Novahistine, 502–503
Nucleoside analogs, for HIV infection/AIDS,
220
Nutrition. *See also* Feeding/feeding problems;
Feeding schedule
assessment/anticipatory guidance and
at initial visit, 5
at 2 to 8 weeks, 26–27, 32
at 2 to 4 months, 38–39, 44–45
at 4 to 6 months, 50, 56
at 6 to 8 months, 62, 68–70
at 8 to 14 months, 78, 84–85
at 14 to 18 months, 92, 99
at 18 to 24 months, 103, 109
at 24 to 36 months, 116, 122
at 3 to 6 years, 131, 138
at 6 to 9 years, 148, 154
at 9 to 11 years, 165, 171
at 12 to 17 years, 179, 186
breast feeding and, 21
establishing good eating habits and, 70
homemade baby foods and, 69–70
introducing new foods and, 68–69
Nutrition history. *See* Diet history
Nystatin, 500–501
for candidal diaper rash, 253
for candidal intertrigo, 336
for thrush, 410

O
Object permanence, development of. *See also*
Memory
at 4 to 6 months, 57
at 6 to 8 months, 63, 72
Occlusal-HP, for molluscum contagiosum,
354
Ophthalmia neonatorum, 264
Oral candidiasis (thrush), 410–411
identification of
at 2 week visit, 28
at 2 month visit, 41

Oral contraceptives
acne and, 211, 213
for dysmenorrhea, 282
Oral rehydration. *See also* Hydration
for diarrhea, 276, 277
Lytren for, 277, 443
Pedialyte for, 277, 443, 505
Ricelyte for, 277, 443
for viral gastroenteritis, 443–444
Oral temperature
normal, 301
taking, 301
Oral ulcers (aphthous stomatitis), 237–238
Ortho-Novum. *See also* Oral contraceptives
for dysmenorrhea, 282
Ortho Tri-Cyclen. *See also* Oral contraceptives
acne and, 211
Otitis
external, 296–298
acute otitis media differentiated from, 297, 360
media
acute, 359–363
external otitis differentiated from, 297, 360
serous, 396–398
acute otitis media differentiated from, 360
Otoscopy, pneumatic, in serous otitis media, 397
Over-the-counter medications, for acne, 213
Oxacillin, 508
Oxiconazole
for tinea corporis, 412
for tinea pedis, 418
Oxistat
for tinea corporis, 412
for tinea pedis, 418

P

Pad and bell technique, for enuresis, 286–287, 288
Pain
in ear. *See* Earache
reaction to, at 8 to 14 months, 85
Palate, assessment of, at initial visit, 11
PanOxyl. *See also* Benzoyl peroxide
for acne, 210
Papilloma virus, warts caused by, 454
Paranasal sinuses, bacterial infection of, 400–402
Parent (caregiver)-child interaction, assessment of
at 2 week visit, 28
at 4 month visit, 52
at 6 month visit, 64
at 8 month visit, 80
at 14 month visit, 94
at 18 month visit, 105
at 24 month visit, 118
at 3 year visit, 135
at 6 year visit, 151
at 9 to 11 year visit, 168
at 12 to 17 year visit, 182

Parents. *See also* Family status; Parent (caregiver)-child interaction
abusive, characteristics of, 17
developmental changes in. *See* Developmental process
single
of 6 month old, 62
of 8 to 14 month old, 84
of 14 to 18 month old, 96
of 18 to 24 month old, 108
of 24 to 36 month old, 121
of 12 to 17 year old, 185
Parvovirus B19, erythema infectiosum caused by, 293
Passivity, at 3 to 6 years, 140
Pastia's lines, in scarlet fever, 391
P carinii pneumonia prophylaxis, in HIV infection/AIDS, 220
Peak expiratory flow rate (PEFR), in asthma, 247
Peak flow meter, in asthma, 247
PediaCare, 503–504
Pedialyte, 505. *See also* Oral rehydration
for diarrhea, 277
for viral gastroenteritis, 443
Pedialyte freezer pops, 444. *See also* Oral rehydration
Pediapred. *See also* Prednisone
for asthma, 245
PediaProfen. *See also* Ibuprofen
for fever, 302
Pediculosis (capitis/corporis/pubis), 364–368
Pediculus humanus capitis, 364
Pediculus humanus corporis, 364
Peer group, in social development of 9 to 11 old, 173–174
PEFT. *See* Peak expiratory flow rate
Penicillin, 505–506
for Lyme disease, 344
for pneumonia, 440t
for scabies, 388
for scarlet fever, 392
for streptococcal pharyngitis, 404
for vulvovaginitis in prepubertal child, 451
Pen-V, 505–506
for Lyme disease, 344
Periactin, for pityriasis rosea, 378
Periungual warts, 455
Permethrin, 502
for pediculosis capitis, 365–366
for scabies, 387–388
Persa-Gel. *See also* Benzoyl peroxide
for acne, 210
Personality traits
of 24 to 36 month old, 123–124
parent's perception of, 6
Pertussis, 370–372
asthma differentiated from, 243
Petroleum jelly, for herpes simplex infection, 314
Pets
environmental control for atopic child and, 290–291

Pets *(continued)*
  ringworm transmitted by, 413
PFTs. *See* Pulmonary function tests
Pharyngitis
  herpetic, 324
  in mononucleosis, 331, 332
  streptococcal, 403–405
    mononucleosis differentiated from, 332, 404
    viral, streptococcal pharyngitis differentiated from, 404
Phenazopyridine, 509–510
Phenergan, with codeine, 506–507
Phenoxymethyl penicillin. *See also* Penicillin
  for Lyme disease, 344
Phenytoin, for bulimia, 251
Phthirus pubis, 364. *See also* Pediculosis
Physical abuse, 201, 201–202. *See also* Child abuse
Physical examination
  at initial visit, 9–12
  at 2 week visit, 28–29
  at 2 month visit, 40–41
  at 4 month visit, 52
  at 6 month visit, 64
  at 8 month visit, 80
  at 14 month visit, 94
  at 18 month visit, 104–105
  at 24 month visit, 117–118
  at 3 year visit, 134–135
  at 6 year visit, 150–151
  at 9 to 11 year visit, 167–168
  at 12 to 17 year visit, 181–182
Physical growth and development. *See also* Growth/growth measurements
assessment/anticipatory guidance and
  at initial visit, 5
  at 2 weeks, 27, 28
  at 2 to 4 months, 39, 40–41, 45
  at 4 to 6 months, 51, 52, 57, 64
  at 6 to 8 months, 63, 64, 71
  at 8 to 14 months, 79, 80, 85–86
  at 14 to 18 months, 93–94, 94, 97–98
  at 18 to 24 months, 104, 104–105, 110
  at 24 to 36 months, 117, 123
  at 3 to 6 years, 131–132, 134, 139
  at 6 to 9 years, 149–150, 150, 155–156
  at 9 to 11 years, 165–166, 167, 172
  at 12 to 17 years, 180, 181, 186–187
measurements recording, 9
Physical neglect, 201, 202. *See also* Child abuse
Piaget's stages of growth and development. *See also specific stage and* Intellectual development
  for 2 week old, 28
  for 2 month old, 40
  for 4 to 6 month old, 51, 57–58
  for 6 to 8 month old, 63, 72
  for 8 to 14 month old, 79, 86
  for 14 to 18 month old, 93, 99
  for 18 to 24 month old, 104, 111
  for 24 to 36 month old, 117
  for 3 to 6 year old, 141–142

Piaget's stages of growth and development. *(cont'd.)*
  for 9 to 11 year old, 166, 172–173
  for 12 to 17 year old, 180, 187
Pilosebaceous follicles, in acne, 209
Pinna, in external otitis, 296
Pinworms, 374–375
  vulvovaginitis in prepubertal child and, 450, 451
Pityriasis rosea, 377–378
  tinea corporis differentiated from, 377, 412
  tinea versicolor differentiated from, 420
Plantar warts, 454–457
Pneumatic otoscopy, in serous otitis media, 397
Pneumocystis carinii pneumonia prophylaxis, in HIV infection/AIDS, 220
Pneumonia
  differential diagnosis of, 437–440*t*
  mycoplasmal (walking), 356–358, 439*t*
  P carinii, prophylaxis for in HIV infection/ AIDS, 220
Poisoning, prevention of, 16
  in 8 to 14 month old, 76
Poison ivy/poison oak dermatitis, 380–381
Polytrim, for conjunctivitis, 264
Ponstel, 507–508. *See also* Mefenamic acid
Postherpetic neuralgia, 321
Potassium hydroxide test
  in candidal diaper rash, 253
  in tinea pedis, 417
  in tinea versicolor, 420
Preadolescence, definition of, 165
Precipitated sulfur, for scabies, 388
Prednisone
  for asthma, 243, 245
  for emergency clearing of acne, 212
  for hymenoptera sting, 224
  for mononucleosis, 333
  for pityriasis rosea, 378
  for poison ivy/poison oak, 381
Pregnancy, HIV infection/AIDS and, 221
Pregnancy history, 4
Preoperative learning, in 18 to 24 month old, 104
Prepuberty, Erikson's stage of, 166
Prickly heat (miliaria rubra), 351–352
Primary enuresis, 284, 286–287, 288–289
Privileges, restriction of, as punishment, 196
Prochlorperazine, for vomiting associated with dysmenorrhea, 282
Projectile vomiting, 447
Promethazine, with codeine, 506–507
"Prom" pills, for emergency clearing of acne, 212
ProSobee formula, for child with diarrhea, 277
Prostaglandins, in dysmenorrhea, 280
Prostaphilin, 508
Protease inhibitors, for HIV infection/AIDS, 220
Proventil, 508–509. *See also* Albuterol
  for asthma, 245

Pseudoephedrine, 504, 511–512
  for allergic rhinitis and conjunctivitis, 229
  with brompheniramine (Bromfed PD), 477
  with brompheniramine and dextromethor-
      phan (Bromfed DM), 476–477
  with carbinoxamine and dextromethorphan
      (Rondec), 510–511
  with chlorpheniramine (PediaCare 2),
      503–504
  with chlorpheniramine and dextromethor-
      phan (PediaCare 3), 503–504
  with guaifenesin and dextromethorphan,
      (Dorcol/Novahistine), 484–485,
      502–503
  for otitis media, 361
  in PediaCare Drops, 504
Psoriasis
  pityriasis rosea differentiated from, 377
  primary irritant diaper rash differentiated
      from, 271
  seborrhea differentiated from, 394
  tinea corporis differentiated from, 412
  tinea cruris differentiated from, 414
Pubic louse, 364. *See also* Pediculosis
Pulmonary function tests, in asthma, 242
Pulse rate, fever and, 301
Purging, in bulimia, 249
Pustules, acne, 209, 210
Pyelonephritis, enuresis and, 285
Pyloric stenosis, vomiting and, 447
Pyridium, 509–510

Q

Quinacrine, for giardiasis, 278

R

Radionuclide cystogram, in urinary tract infec-
      tion, 428
Rales, in asthma, 241
Rapid strep test, in streptococcal pharyngitis,
      403–404
Rash. *See* Exanthems
Rectal intercourse, HIV infection/AIDS trans-
      mission and, 215, 220
Rectal temperature
  normal, 301
  taking, 301
Rectum, assessment of, at initial visit, 12
Reflexes
  at 8 months, 80
  at 14 months, 94
  at 6 months, 64
Reflux (regurgitation), 26
Rehydration. *See also* Hydration
  for diarrhea, 276, 277
  in viral gastroenteritis, 443–444
Respiratory rate, fever and, 301
Respiratory system/chest
  assessment of
    at initial visit, 7, 11
    at 2 week visit, 27, 28
    at 2 month visit, 41

  at 3 year visit, 133, 134
  at 12 to 17 year visit, 182
  in mycoplasmal pneumonia, 356
Retin-A
  for acne, 210, 211
  for molluscum contagiosum, 354
  for wart removal, 455
Reverse-last shoes, for metatarsus adductus,
      349, 349–350
Review of systems, at 3 year visit, 131
Rewarming, after frostbite, 305
Rhinitis
  allergic, 227–231
    seasonal versus perennial, 227, 228
    sinusitis and, 228, 400, 401
  medicamentosus, 228
  vasomotor, 228
Rhinocort, for sinusitis, 401
Rhonchi, in asthma, 241
Rhus toxins, poison ivy/poison oak caused by,
      380
Ricelyte. *See also* Oral rehydration
  for diarrhea, 277
  for viral gastroenteritis, 443
RID, for pediculosis corporis, 366
Rifampin, for eradication of carrier state after
      streptococcal pharyngitis, 405
Ringworm
  of body (tinea corporis), 412–413
    pityriasis rosea differentiated from, 377, 412
    seborrhea differentiated from, 394
  of foot (tinea pedis), 412, 417–419
  of groin (tinea cruris), 414–415
  of scalp (tinea capitis), 412
    seborrhea differentiated from, 394
Rinne test, in serous otitis media, 396
Risk factors
  at 2 weeks, 28
  at 2 to 4 months, 40, 42, 46
  at 4 to 6 months, 48, 51, 54, 58
  at 6 to 8 months, 60, 63–64, 66, 72
  at 8 to 14 months, 75, 79, 81, 87
  at 14 to 18 months, 90, 93–94, 95, 99
  at 18 to 24 months, 101, 104, 106, 109, 110,
      111, 112
  at 24 to 36 months, 114, 117, 119, 123, 126,
      127
  at 3 to 6 years, 129, 134, 137, 139, 140, 142,
      144
  at 6 to 9 years, 146, 150, 152, 157, 158, 160
  at 9 to 11 years, 163, 167, 172, 173, 174
  at 12 to 17 years, 176, 181
Rondec-DM, 510–511
Roseola (exanthem subitum), 383–384
  scarlet fever differentiated from, 392
Rubella
  roseola differentiated from, 383
  scarlet fever differentiated from, 392
Rubeola (measles)
  mononucleosis differentiated from, 332
  roseola differentiated from, 384
  scarlet fever differentiated from, 392

S

Safety strategies, 15–16
  for 2 to 8 week old, 24–25, 34
  for 2 to 4 month old, 36–37, 47
  for 4 to 6 month old, 48–49, 59
  for 6 to 8 month old, 60–61, 73–74
  for 8 to 14 month old, 75–76, 88–89
  for 14 to 18 month old, 90, 100
  for 18 to 24 month old, 101–102, 112–113
  for 24 to 36 month old, 114, 127–128
  for 3 to 6 year old, 129–130, 144–145
  for 6 to 9 year old, 146–147, 155, 161
  for 9 to 11 year old, 163, 174
  for 12 to 17 year old, 177, 178–179, 186
Salicylic acid
  for molluscum contagiosum, 354
  for wart removal, 455
Salmonella (salmonellosis), diarrhea caused
  by, 276, 277
  viral gastroenteritis differentiated from, 442
Sarcoptes scabiei, 386
Scabicides, 387, 388, 389
Scabies, 386–389
  varicella differentiated from, 432
Scalp, seborrhea of (cradle cap), 394–395
Scarlet fever, 391–393
School, environmental control for atopic child
  and, 292
School performance/adjustment, assessment
  of at initial visit, 6
School readiness, assessment of at 6 years,
  142–143
Screening tests, history of, 7
Seborrhea
  blepharitis and, 347, 394
  pityriasis rosea differentiated from, 377
  of scalp (cradle cap), 394–395
  tinea cruris differentiated from, 414
Secondary enuresis, 284, 287, 289
Secondary sex characteristics. *See* Sexual maturation
Selenium sulfide (Selsun), 421
  for seborrhea, 394
  for tinea versicolor, 420–421, 421
Self-concept, in 6 to 9 year old, 156
Self-control
  in 8 to 14 month old, 86
  in 14 to 18 month old, 98
  in 18 to 24 month old, 112
  stages in development of, 189
Self-esteem
  in 14 to 18 month old, 98
  in 18 to 24 month old, 104, 110
  in 6 to 9 year old, 156
Self-identity, in 6 to 9 year old, 156
Self-identity versus role confusion, Erikson's
  stage of
  for 9 to 11 year old, 172
  for 12 to 17 year old, 180, 187
Selsun, 421
  for seborrhea, 394
  for tinea versicolor, 420–421, 421

Sensorimotor stage of development (Piaget),
  28, 40
Separation anxiety, in 4 to 6 month old, 56
Septra, 473–474. *See also* Trimethoprim–
  sulfamethoxazole
  for otitis media, 360
  for urinary tract infection, 428
Serous otitis media, 396–398
  acute otitis media differentiated from, 360
Sertraline, for bulimia, 251
Severe combined immunodeficiency, AIDS differentiated from, 219
Sexual abuse, 18, 201, 202–203. *See also* Child
  abuse
  vulvovaginitis in prepubertal child and, 451
Sexual contact
  herpes simplex infections and, 318
  HIV/AIDS transmission by, 215, 220
Sexual experimentation, in 9 to 11 year old,
  167
Sexual identity
  in 24 to 36 month old, 126–127
  in 3 to 6 year old, 144
  in 6 to 9 year old, 156, 160–161
  in 9 to 11 year old, 173
Sexually active adolescents, information provided to, 179
Sexual maturation, assessment of
  at initial visit, 8
  in 6 to 9 year old, 156
  in 9 to 11 year old, 166, 166–167
  in 12 to 17 year old, 180
Shaken baby syndrome, 18
Shigellosis, diarrhea in, 276, 278
Shyness, at 3 to 6 years, 140
Sibling rivalry, 197–200
  in step-families, 199
Siblings. *See also* Family status
  of 2 month old, 38
  of 4 month old, 50
  of 8 to 14 month old, 84
  of 14 to 18 month old, 97
  of 18 to 24 month old, 109
  of 24 to 36 month old, 121–122
  of 12 to 17 year old, 186
  birth of, 197–198
  handicapped children and, 199–200
  interactions among, 198–199. *See also* Sibling
    rivalry
  in step-families, 185–186, 199
Silver nitrate, for umbilical granuloma, 424
Simethicone, for colic, 260
Single parent
  of 6 month old, 62
  of 8 to 14 month old, 84
  of 14 to 18 month old, 96
  of 18 to 24 month old, 108
  of 24 to 36 month old, 121
  of 12 to 17 year old, 185
Sinusitis
  allergic rhinitis and, 228, 400, 401
  bacterial, 400–402

Skeletal system, assessment of. *See also* Muscu-
    loskeletal system
  at initial visit, 8
  at 3 year visit, 132
Skin, assessment of
  at initial visit, 7, 9
  at 2 week visit, 28
  at 2 month visit, 41
  at 6 month visit, 64
  at 8 month visit, 80
  at 14 month visit, 94
  at 18 month visit, 105
  at 24 month visit, 118
  at 3 year visit, 132, 134
  at 6 year visit, 150
  at 9 to 11 year visit, 168
  at 12 to 17 year visit, 182
Slapped-check rash, in erythema infectiosum,
    293, 294, 392
Sleep Dry program, for enuresis, 287, 288
Sleep patterns
  at 2 weeks, 27
  at 2 to 4 months, 39, 45
  at 4 to 6 months, 50, 57
  at 6 to 8 months, 62, 70–71
  at 8 to 14 months, 78, 85
  at 14 to 18 months, 92, 97
  at 18 to 24 months, 103, 109
  at 24 to 36 months, 116, 122
  at 3 to 6 years, 131, 139
  at 6 to 9 years, 148, 155
  at 9 to 11 years, 165
  at 12 to 17 years, 179
Smallpox, varicella differentiated from, 432
SMZ (sulfamethoxazole), with trimethoprim.
    See Trimethoprim–sulfamethoxazole
Social development
  for 18 to 24 month old, 112
  for 24 to 36 month old, 126–127
  for 3 to 6 year old, 134, 143–144
  for 6 to 9 year old, 150, 159–161
  for 9 to 11 year old, 166–167, 173–174
  for 12 to 17 year old, 180–181, 187–188
Social health problems, for 6 to 9 year old,
    147
Social history, 3–4
Sodium fluoride, 495–496
Sodium Sulamyd
  for blepharitis, 347
  for conjunctivitis, 264
  for hordeolum, 326
Sore throat. *See* Pharyngitis
Spanking, 195
Speech. *See* Language skills/development
Spirometry, in asthma, 242
Sponge bath, for fever reduction, 301
Staphylococcus (staphylococcal infection)
  acute cervical adenitis caused by, 255
  aureus
    blepharitis caused by, 347
    conjunctivitis caused by, 262
    hordeolum (stye) caused by, 326
    impetigo caused by, 328

sinusitis caused by, 400
food poisoning caused by, viral gastroenteri-
    tis differentiated from, 442
pneumonia caused by, 439*t*
Starvation diarrhea, 276, 445
Step-parents, 185
Step-siblings, 185–186, 199. *See also* Siblings
Stimulation, assessment/anticipatory guidance
    and
  at 2 to 8 weeks, 33–34
  at 2 to 4 months, 46
  at 4 to 6 months, 58
  at 6 to 8 months, 73
  at 8 to 14 months, 88
  at 14 to 18 months, 100
  at 18 to 24 months, 112
Stomatitis
  aphthous, 237–238
  herpetic. *See* Gingivostomatitis, herpetic
Stools. *See also* Constipation; Diarrhea; Toilet
    training
  assessment/anticipatory guidance and
    at 2 weeks, 27
    at 2 to 4 months, 45
    at 4 to 6 months, 50, 57
    at 6 to 8 months, 62, 71
    at 8 to 14 months, 78, 85
  culture of, in diarrhea, 275
  starvation, 276, 445
Stool softeners, for constipation, 268
Straight-last shoes, for metatarsus adductus,
    349
Stranger anxiety, 68
"Strawberry tongue," in scarlet fever, 391
Strep throat. *See Streptococcus* (streptococcal
    infection), pharyngitis caused by
Streptococcus (streptococcal infection)
  acute cervical adenitis caused by, 255
  impetigo caused by, 328
  pharyngitis caused by, 403–405
    mononucleosis differentiated from, 332,
      404
  pneumoniae
    conjunctivitis caused by, 262
    otitis media caused by, 359
    sinusitis caused by, 400
  pyogenes, sinusitis caused by, 400
  scarlet fever caused by, 391
  sinusitis caused by, 401
  vulvovaginitis caused by, 451
Stridor
  congenital, 436
  in viral croup, 436, 437*t*, 438*t*
Stubbornness, at 24 to 36 months, 124
Stye (hordeolum), 326–327
Substance abuse
  in 9 to 11 year old, 167
  in 12 to 17 year old, 176
  HIV infection/AIDS transmission and, 220,
    221
Subungual warts, 455

Sudafed, 511–512
  for allergic rhinitis and conjunctivitis, 229
  for otitis media, 361
Sudden infant death syndrome, abuse and, 18
Suffocation, prevention of, 16
Suicide
  aspirin used for, 470
  prevention of, 407–408
  risk of, in adolescent, 176, 181, 407
Sulamyd
  for blepharitis, 347
  for conjunctivitis, 264
  for hordeolum, 326
Sulfacetamide (Sulamyd)
  for blepharitis, 347
  for conjunctivitis, 264
  for hordeolum, 326
Sulfamethoxazole, with trimethoprim. See Tri-
    methoprim–sulfamethoxazole
Sulfur, precipitated, for scabies, 388
Sun exposure, acne and, 210, 212
Suprax, 512–513
  for urinary tract infection, 428
Swimmer's ear (external otitis), 296–298
Synalar, for diaper rash, 272
Syncope, vasopressor, hymenoptera sting dif-
    ferentiated from, 224
Syphilis, secondary, pityriasis rosea differenti-
    ated from, 377
Systems review, at initial visit, 7–8

T
Talipes equinovarus, metatarsus adductus dif-
    ferentiated from, 349
Tavist, 513–514
  for allergic rhinitis and conjunctivitis, 229
Tavist-D, for allergic rhinitis and conjunctivi-
    tis, 229
Teeth. See also Dental care
  assessment of
    at initial visit, 10
    at 6 month visit, 63, 64
    at 8 month visit, 78, 80
    at 14 month visit, 94
    at 18 month visit, 105
    at 24 month visit, 118
    at 3 year visit, 132
    at 6 year visit, 149, 150, 155
    at 9 to 11 year visit, 168, 172
    at 12 to 17 year visit, 182
  schedule of eruption of, 71t
Teething
  at 6 to 8 months, 63, 71
  at 8 to 14 months, 78
Television watching/control
  at 3 to 6 years, 143
  restriction as punishment and, 196
Temovate cream, for wart removal, 456
Temperament
  of 24 to 36 month old, 124
  of 3 to 6 year old, 140
  of 6 to 9 year old, 156–157

Temperature
  determination of, 301
  elevated. See Fever
  normal, 301
Temper tantrums, 189–191
  at 14 to 18 months, 98–99
Tetracycline, 514–515
  for acne, 211, 213
  for aphthous stomatitis, in mouth rinse, 237
  for Lyme disease, 344
  for mycoplasmal pneumonia, 357
Thalassemia trait, iron-deficiency anemia dif-
    ferentiated from, 339
Theophylline
  action of, 246
  for asthma, 244, 245, 246, 248
  monitoring levels of, 248
  side effects of, 246
Thermometers, 302
Throat
  assessment of
    at initial visit, 7, 11
    at 3 year visit, 134
    at 6 year visit, 150
  sore. See Pharyngitis
Throat culture
  in mononucleosis, 332
  in streptococcal pharyngitis, 403, 405
Thrush, 410–411
  identification of
    at 2 week visit, 28
    at 2 month visit, 41
Thyroglossal duct cyst, acute cervical adenitis
    differentiated from, 256
Thyroid gland, assessment of, at initial visit, 11
Ticks
  Lyme disease transmitted by, 342, 344–345
  removal of, 345
Tinactin, 515–516
  for tinea cruris, 415
  for tinea pedis, 418
Tinea
  capitis, 412
    seborrhea differentiated from, 394
  corporis, 412–413
    pityriasis rosea differentiated from, 377, 412
    seborrhea differentiated from, 394
  cruris, 414–415
  pedis, 412, 417–419
  versicolor, 420–421
T lymphocytes, in AIDS, 215
TMP–SMX. See Trimethoprim–
    sulfamethoxazole
Tobramycin, for conjunctivitis, 264
Tobrex, for conjunctivitis, 264
Toddler, definition of, 96
Tofranil, 516–517. See also Imipramine
  for enuresis, 286
Toilet training, 192–193
  assessment/anticipatory guidance and
    at initial visit, 6
    at 8 to 14 months, 78, 85
    at 14 to 18 months, 92–93, 97

at 18 to 24 months, 103–104, 110
at 24 to 36 months, 116–117, 122–123
constipation and, 268–269
Tolnaftate, 515–516
for tinea cruris, 415
for tinea pedis, 418
Tongue, assessment of
at initial visit, 10
at 2 month visit, 41
Tonsils
assessment of, at initial visit, 11
in mononucleosis, 331, 332
Toys (crib), for 2 to 8 week old, 33–34
Trachea, assessment of at initial visit, 11
Trachoma, conjunctivitis differentiated from, 264
Trans-plantar patch, for wart removal, 455, 456
Trans-Ver-Sal patch, for wart removal, 455, 456
Trauma. See Child abuse; Injuries
Traveler's diarrhea, 276
Tretinoin
for acne, 210, 211
for molluscum contagiosum, 354
for wart removal, 455
Triamcinolone, 468–469, 472
for aphthous stomatitis, 237, 238
for asthma, 472
nasal inhaler (Nasacort), 230, 501
action of, 230
for allergic rhinitis and conjunctivitis, 229, 230
Trichloroacetic acid, for molluscum contagiosum, 353
Trichomonas vaginitis, in prepubertal child, 451
Trichophyton
mentagrophytes, tinea pedis caused by, 417
rubrum, tinea pedis caused by, 417
tinea corporis caused by, 412
tinea cruris caused by, 414
Trimethoprim–sulfamethoxazole, 473–474
for E coli diarrhea, 278
for otitis media, 360
for P carinii pneumonia prophylaxis, 220
for pertussis, 371
for serous otitis media, 397
for shigellosis, 278
for urinary tract infection, 428
Tri-Norinyl. See also Oral contraceptives
for dysmenorrhea, 282
Triprolidine, with pseudoephedrine (Actifed), 464
for allergic rhinitis and conjunctivitis, 229
for otitis media, 361
Trust, Erikson's stage of
for 2 week old, 27–28
for 2 to 4 month old, 40, 45
for 4 to 6 month old, 51, 57
for 6 to 8 month old, 63, 72
for 8 to 14 month old, 79
for 14 to 18 month old, 93
T-Stat pads, for acne, 210, 211

Tuberculosis, acute cervical adenitis differentiated from, 256
Tussi-Organidin DM, 517
Tylenol. See also Acetaminophen
for acute cervical adenitis, 256
Tympanic membrane
in acute otitis media, 359–360
in external otitis, 296
hyperemia of, 360
in serous otitis media, 396
Tympanometry, in serous otitis media, 397

U
U-bag urine collection, 429
Ulcers
corneal, conjunctivitis differentiated from, 264
oral (aphthous stomatitis), 237–238
Ultrasound, in urinary tract infection, indications for, 428
Umbilical cord/umbilicus
assessment of, at initial visit, 12
care of, 422
Umbilical granuloma, 424
Umbilical polyp, 424
Urachus, patent, 424
Urethritis
enuresis and, 285
urinary tract infection differentiated from, 428
Urinary retention, in herpes simplex infections, 317
Urinary tract infection, 426–430
enuresis and, 285, 426
roseola differentiated from, 384
Urine, assessment/anticipatory guidance and.
See also Toilet training
at 2 to 4 months, 45
at 2 weeks, 27
at 4 to 6 months, 51, 57
at 6 to 8 months, 62, 71
at 8 to 14 months, 85
Urine culture, in urinary tract infection, 427–428
Urine specimen, collection of, 429
Urticaria, in streptococcal pharyngitis, 403
Urushiol, poison ivy/poison oak caused by, 380
UTI. See Urinary tract infection
Uveitis, conjunctivitis differentiated from, 264
Uvula, assessment of, at initial visit, 11

V
Vaginitis
in prepubertal child, 450–452
urinary tract infection differentiated from, 428
Valisone, for seborrhea, 395
Vanceril, for asthma, 245
Vantin, 517–519
Vaporizer, cool-mist, for croup, 436, 440t
Varicella, 320, 431–434
herpetic gingivostomatitis differentiated from, 324
Varicella zoster immune globulin, 434

Varicella zoster virus
  herpes zoster caused by, 320–321
  varicella caused by, 431
Varicella zoster virus vaccine, 431
Vasomotor rhinitis, 228
Vasopressor syncope, hymenoptera sting differentiated from, 224
VCUG. *See* Voiding cystourethrogram
Venereal warts, 457
Ventolin inhaler, 519–520. *See also* Albuterol
  for asthma, 245
Vermox, 520–521. *See also* Mebendazole
  for pinworms, 374
Verruca
  plantaris (plantar warts), 454–457
  vulgaris (common warts), 454–457
Vesicoureteral reflux, 428
Viral conjunctivitis, 262, 263, 264
Viral croup (laryngotracheobronchitis), 435–441
  differential diagnosis of, 237–240*t*
  asthma in, 243
Viral exanthems
  erythema infectiosum and, 293
  miliaria rubra differentiated from, 351
  mononucleosis differentiated from, 332
Viral gastroenteritis, 442–445
Viral infections. *See also specific disease*
  acute cervical adenitis caused by, 255
  asthma and, 240
  sinusitis and, 401
Viral pneumonia, 439*t*
Vision, assessment/anticipatory guidance and.
  See also Eyes
  at 2 months, 45
  at 4 months, 51
  at 8 months, 79
  at 14 to 18 months, 93
  at 3 to 6 years, 132
Vitamin C, for iron-deficiency anemia, 340
Vitiligo, tinea versicolor differentiated from, 420
Voiding cystourethrogram, indications for, 428
Volvulus, vomiting and, 447
Vomiting, 446–449
  in viral gastroenteritis, 442
V-Sol Otic Solution, for external otitis, 297
Vulvovaginitis
  in prepubertal child, 450–452
  urinary tract infection differentiated from, 428
VZIG (varicella zoster immune globulin), 434
VZV. *See* Varicella zoster virus
VZV vaccine, 431

W

Walking pneumonia, 356–358
Warts
  common and plantar, 454–457
  venereal, 457
Wasp sting, allergic response to, 223–225
Water, prevention of injury from, 16
Weaning, 22, 58, 68

Weight loss, in anorexia nervosa, 232, 233
Well child care. *See also* Anticipatory guidance
  breast-feeding guidelines in, 19–23
  child abuse guidelines in, 17–18
  initial visit in
    history and, 3–8
    physical examination and, 9–13
  injury prevention guidelines in, 15–16
  schedule of visits for, 13–14. *See also* Well child visit
Well child visit. *See also* Anticipatory guidance
  at 2 weeks, 24–29
  at 2 months, 36–41
  at 4 months, 48–52
  at 6 months, 60–65
  at 8 months, 75–80
  at 14 months, 90–94
  at 18 months, 101
  at 24 months, 114–118
  at 3 years, 129–135
  at 6 years, 146–150
  at 9 to 11 years, 162–168
  at 12 to 17 years, 176–183
Wet Stop program, for enuresis, 287, 288
Wheezing
  in asthma, 241
  in croup, 435
White blood cell count, in mononucleosis, 332
Whitlow, herpetic, 313
Whooping cough (pertussis), 370–372
  asthma differentiated from, 243
Wiskott-Aldrich syndrome, AIDS differentiated from, 219
Wood's light, tinea versicolor lesions and, 420
Working mother
  of 8 to 14 month old, 84
  of 14 to 18 month old, 96
  of 18 to 24 month old, 108
  of 24 to 36 month old, 121
  return to work and, 38

X

X-linked agammaglobulinemia, AIDS differentiated from, 219
Xylocaine Viscous Solution
  for aphthous stomatitis, 237
  for herpetic gingivostomatitis, 324

Y

Yellow jacket sting, allergic response to, 223–225

Z

Zalcitabine, for HIV infection/AIDS, 220
Zidovudine, for HIV infection/AIDS, 220
Zithromax, 521–522
Zoloft, for bulimia, 251
Zoster, 320–321, 432
Zovirax. *See also* Acyclovir
  for herpes simplex infection, 314, 317
  for herpes zoster, 321
  for varicella, 433, 434
Zyrtec, for allergic rhinitis and conjunctivitis, 229